Testicular Vascular Lesions

Manuel Nistal
Pilar González-Peramato

Testicular Vascular Lesions

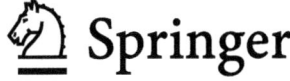 Springer

Manuel Nistal
Department of Anatomy, Histology and
Neuroscience
School of Medicine
Universidad Autónoma de Madrid
Madrid, Madrid, Spain

Pilar González-Peramato
Department of Pathology
University Hospital La Paz
School of Medicine
Universidad Autónoma de Madrid
Madrid, Madrid, Spain

ISBN 978-3-031-57846-5   ISBN 978-3-031-57847-2   (eBook)
https://doi.org/10.1007/978-3-031-57847-2

This Springer imprint is published by the registered company Springer Nature Switzerland AG
The registered company address is: Gewerbestrasse 11, 6330 Cham, Switzerland

If disposing of this product, please recycle the paper.

To my dearest daughter Natalia and the long-awaited grandson Jorge

To Maytechu for the happy reunion

Manuel Nistal

To my husband, Alvaro

To my children Álvaro, Teresa, and Javier

In memoriam, to my parents Antonio and Pilar

Pilar González-Peramato

Preface

Pathology has been fundamental to the advances in diagnostic procedures that have facilitated treatment individualization. The contribution of pathologists in both the tumoural and non-tumoural field of the testis has been very important. While the information provided by histological studies continues to be the basis for classifying neoplasms, in the non-tumoural field, testicular biopsy has been progressively marginalized over the last decades. Genetics, molecular biology, and the application of other techniques have been incorporated into the study of the patient. The most surprising thing in these studies is that their results always relate them with possible testicular lesions, based on the classic descriptions of those lesions, but the existence of which in that specific patient is unknown. The type of testicular lesion cannot be detected by karyotype, whether in the field of congenital anomalies, nor is it alone a determinant in the reproductive capacity of an infertile male. Molecular studies can pinpoint the genetic cause of an anomaly, but the expression of a genetic defect can be variable and therefore cannot be used to predict the functional capacity of the testis. The same can be said in many cases of hormonal determinations. Each contributes value to the diagnosis, but it is only the pathology that allows us to know what is happening inside the testicle, the actual nature of the lesions, their progressiveness, or to suggest a treatment.

The readers will find in this book a different viewpoint of approaching the nature of some testicular lesions: the study of vascular lesions. Most of the references in the scientific literature in this field are reduced to citing testicular torsions and varicocele. Without underestimating the fact that the studies focus on the seriousness of the loss of a testicle due to torsion of the cord or the negative impact of varicocele on fertility, the field of vascular pathology is much broader and the references to the different processes are scarce.

This book contains the testicular pathology produced by lesions associated with arterial, venous, and lymphatic vessel lesions in an orderly fashion. Sometimes, as is logical, the alterations are purely testicular, in others, the majority, the testicle is the target organ of systemic pathologies. The first ten chapters are dedicated to arterial pathology, the following five to venous pathology, and the final four to pathology of the lymphatic vessels.

In the review of testicular specimens in our files, previously undescribed vascular, arterial, venous, and lymphatic vessel lesions have been observed and have been incorporated in the respective chapters. Whether they are mere histologic findings or represent entities with a certain category is left to the readers' consideration.

Madrid, Madrid, Spain   Manuel Nistal
Madrid, Madrid, Spain   Pilar González-Peramato

Acknowledgements

First, our thanks are due to our publishers, the Springer-Verlag team, in particular, our Senior Editor, Sylvana Freyberg, for giving us the opportunity of publishing this book.

The authors would like to heartily thank the University Hospital La Paz, one of the first big hospitals in Spain, where two of the authors have developed/undertaken their professional activity for many years. Special thanks go to all the staff members and residents of the Department of Pathology at University Hospital La Paz for their support and for calling our attention to items and cases of special diagnostic and descriptive interest. We also express our appreciation and gratitude to the technical staff of the Department of Pathology at University Hospital La Paz for their careful preparation of the slides shown in this book. We also thank the Universidad Autónoma de Madrid where we have carried out our teaching and research activity.

Our deepest thanks and appreciation also go to a large number of colleagues, co-workers, and friends who throughout the years have generously contributed cases in consultation, many of them very rare, and so, precious material.

Finally, we wish to acknowledge C.F. Warren for her help to improve the English grammar and syntax of our manuscripts to transform them into readable documents.

Contents

Part I   Arterial Pathology: Introduction

**1   Large- and Medium-Sized Vessel Systemic Vasculitis
with Testicular Involvement**............................... 7
1.1   Giant Cell Arteritis (Temporal Arteritis) 7
1.2   Polyarteritis Nodosa (PAN) 7
1.3   Kawasaki Disease (KD)............................. 10
1.4   Behçet's Disease 11
1.5   Cogan Disease 11
References.. 12

2   Small Vessel Vasculitis with Testicular Involvement 15
2.1   Microscopic Polyangiitis (MPA) 15
2.2   Granulomatosis with Polyangiitis (Wegener's
Granulomatosis) (GPA) 15
2.3   Testicular Eosinophilic Granulomatosis with Polyangiitis
(EGPA) (Churg-Strauss) 18
2.4   Immunoglobulin A (IgA) Vasculitis (Henoch-Schönlein
Purpura) (IgAV)................................... 19
References.. 20

3   Vasculitis with Isolated Testicular Involvement 23
3.1   Isolated Arteritis of the Testis, Epididymis,
and Spermatic Cord 23
3.2   Testicular Vasculitis Associated with Germ Cell Tumour 26
3.2.1   Testicular Granulomatosis Polyangiitis-Like
Granulomatosis Associated with Seminoma 26
3.2.2   PAN-Like Vasculitis and Combined
Nonseminomatous Germ Cell Tumour 27
3.2.3   Vasculitis in the Contralateral Testis 28
References.. 30

**4 Testicular Vasculitis Associated with Sepsis Due
    to Viruses and Bacteria**.................................. 33
   4.1 Cytomegalovirus-Associated Vasculitis of Testis
        and Epididymis 33
   4.2 SARS-Cov-2-Associated Vasculitis of the Testis
        and Epididymis 36
   4.3 Necrotizing Vasculitis in Whipple's Disease 37
   References.. 41

**5 Testicular Vasculitis Associated with Treatment
    with Sex Hormones**...................................... 43
   5.1 Vasculitis Associated with Treatment with Oestrogens
        and Antiandrogens in Patients with Gender
        Identity Dysphoria.................................... 43
   5.2 Bilateral Vasculitis Associated with Testosterone
        Treatment.. 46
   References.. 50

6 Thromboangiitis Obliterans (TAO) or Buerger Disease 53
   6.1 Thromboangiitis Obliterans........................... 53
   References.. 56

7 The Complexity of Testicular Lesions in Arteriosclerosis...... 59
   7.1 Atherosclerosis...................................... 59
   7.2 Arteriolosclerosis.................................... 63
   7.3 Mönckeberg Medial Calcific Sclerosis 65
   7.4 Arteriosclerosis Obliterans (ASO)..................... 68
   7.5 Arteriolar Hyalinosis of the Testis..................... 71
   References.. 74

**8 Testicular and Paratesticular Lesions Associated
    with Arteriosclerosis**.................................... 77
   8.1 Cholesterol Thromboembolism (Atheromatous
        Embolism) 77
   8.2 Intracavitary Nodular Polypoid Calcifying
        Proliferation in the Rete Testis........................ 80
   8.3 Ischemic Epididymitis 84
   8.4 Hematoma of Paratesticular Structures 87
   References.. 90

**9 Vascular Tumours and Pseudotumorous Vascular
    Lesions of the Testicle**................................... 93
   9.1 Testicular Hemangioma............................... 93
   9.2 Testicular Hemangiomatosis 98
   9.3 Testicular Pseudoangioma............................. 104
   9.4 Aneurysm of the Testicular Artery..................... 106
   9.5 Arteriovenous Malformation of the Spermatic Cord........ 106
   References.. 109

10 Testicular Biopsy as the Most Sensitive Diagnostic Method for Amyloidosis 113
   10.1 Amyloidosis 113
   References 117

Part II Venous Pathology: Introduction

11 Impact of Spermatic Cord Torsion on Testicular Structure and Function 125
   11.1 Introduction 125
   11.2 Parenchymal Injuries in Children and Adults 125
   11.3 Injuries to Veins, Arteries, and Nerves of the Cord After Torsion 133
      11.3.1 Intraparenchymal Vein Thrombosis 133
      11.3.2 Obliteration of Spermatic Cord Arteries 133
      11.3.3 Morton-Like Neuroma in the Spermatic Cord 134
   11.4 Management of Vanishing Testis Secondary to Testicular Torsion 138
   11.5 Impact of Spermatic Cord Torsion on Testicular Function 141
   References 142

12 Peculiar Lesions Associated with Spermatic Cord Torsion 145
   12.1 Spermatic Cord Lipomembranous Fat Necrosis 145
   12.2 Pseudosarcomatous Periorchitis Secondary to Testicular Torsion 148
   12.3 Lymphoma-Like Orchitis Secondary to Transient Testicular Torsion 152
   References 156

13 Varicocele, the Most Common Cause of Treatable Infertility 159
   13.1 Clinical Evaluation of Varicocele 159
   13.2 The Diversity of Pathogenetic Mechanisms 161
   13.3 Value of Testicular Biopsy in Fertility Studies 162
   13.4 Peculiarities of Intratesticular Varicocele 164
   References 167

14 Pathology of Intratesticular Veins of Uncertain Significance ... 171
   14.1 Phlebosclerosis of the Intraparenchymal Veins 171
   14.2 Hypertrophic Fibrosis of the Adventicia of the Intratesticular Veins 174
   14.3 Adventitial Smooth Muscle Hyperplasia of Intratesticular Veins 177
   References 180

15 **Venous Thrombosis. Segmental Infarction**
    and Polypoid Granulomatous Endophlebitis 183
    15.1 Venous Thrombosis 183
          15.1.1 Spermatic Vein Thrombosis 183
          15.1.2 Pampiniform Plexus Thrombosis 183
          15.1.3 Intraparenchymal Vein Thrombosis 184
    15.2 Segmental Infarction 188
    15.3 Polypoid Granulomatous Endophlebitis
          of the Spermatic Cord 190
    References 194

Part III Pathology of the Lymphatic Vessels: Introduction

16 **Insufficiency of the Lymph Vascular System**
    of the Testis 203
    16.1 Chronic Hydrocele 203
    16.2 Scrotal Elephantiasis 206
    References 208

17 **Testicular Lymphangiectasias**
    and Pseudolymphangiectasias 211
    17.1 Testicular Lymphangiectasias 211
    17.2 Testicular Pseudolymphangiectasia. Microcystic
          Testicular Oedema 217
    References 221

18 **Tumour Lesions of the Testicular Lymphatic Vessels** 223
    18.1 Lymphangioma of Paratesticular Structures 223
    18.2 Benign Lymphangioendothelioma 224
    18.3 Haemangiolymphangioma 229
    References 230

19 **Pathology Secondary to Metastatic Tumours**
    in the Lymphatic Vessels of the Spermatic Cord 231
    19.1 Anterograde and Retrograde Carcinomatous
          Lymphangitis 231
    19.2 Sarcoid-like Granulomatous Lymphangitis
          of the Spermatic Cord Associated with Testicular
          Germ Cell Tumours (Intravascular Granulomas) 232
    References 235

Part I

Arterial Pathology: Introduction

The high frequency of abdominal cavity surgery has markedly increased the importance of knowing/understanding the anatomy of the testicular artery in order to avoid irreversible testicular lesions [1]. The testicle is irrigated by the testicular artery, which originates from the anterolateral aspect of the abdominal aorta at the level of the second lumbar vertebra, 2.5–5 cm caudal to the origin of the renal artery. It descends retroperitoneally obliquely in front of the psoas muscle. Before crossing the deep inguinal ring, it crosses the genitofemoral nerve, ureter, and the inferior part of the external iliac artery before joining the spermatic cord and reaching the testicle. But, it is not uncommon for it to originate from other arteries, such as the main artery of the kidney or the accessory renal artery, the middle adrenal artery or one of the lumbar arteries, the common or internal iliac artery or even the superior epigastric artery [2–4]. Exceptionally, it can be double and each arm even has a different origin or even be missing, or may be absent, in which case the testicular vascularization will proceed from the vesical or prostatic arteries. Variants in its course are also important, such as running posterior to the inferior vena cava or forming an arch over the renal pedicles on both sides [5, 6]

The testicular artery descends within the spermatic cord surrounded by several venous, lymphatic, and nervous trunks (Fig. 1). Along the spermatic cord, it gives the superior and inferior epididymal arteries, which usually arise from a common trunk, as collaterals. Before reaching the testicle, the testicular artery bifurcates into an anterior/superior and posterior/inferior branch. Although the testicular artery is the main source of blood supply to the testicle, anastomoses with the deferential and cremasteric arteries are frequent (Fig. 2).

Before reaching the lower pole of the testicle, the testicular artery penetrates the tunica albuginea and divides into capsular arteries, which are situated in the tunica vasculosa, leading tortuously from the inferior pole to the superior pole of the testicle, along its anterior aspect. At different levels of this course, they give rise to arteries that follow the interlobular conjunctival septa towards the rete testis. These branches are known as centripetal arteries. Along their course, the centripetal arteries change direction, and, with numerous branches, they head towards the albuginea (recurrent rami); these are the centrifugal arteries from which the arterioles of the testicular intersti-

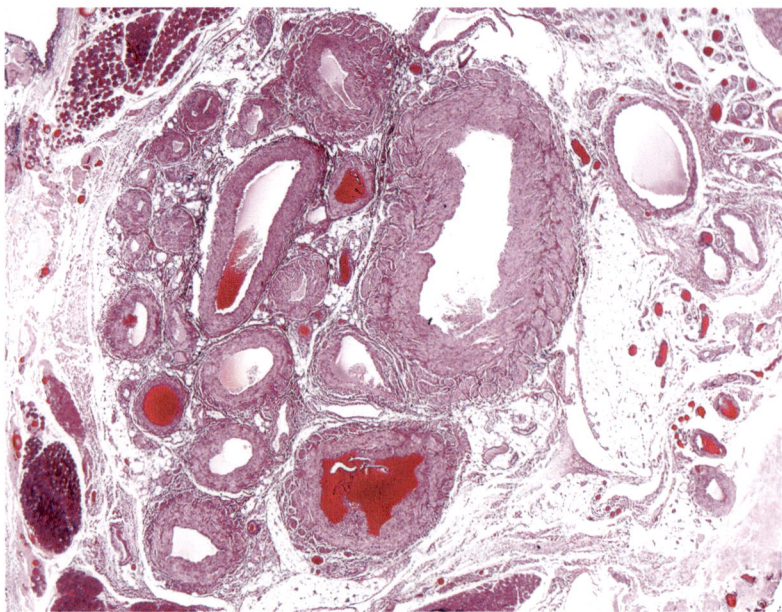

Fig. 1 Cross section of the spermatic cord. The testicular artery is located in the central part and surrounded by several veins. In contrast to the thin wall of the artery and its small branches, the thick wall of the veins with longitudinal smooth muscle bundles in the adventitia stands out

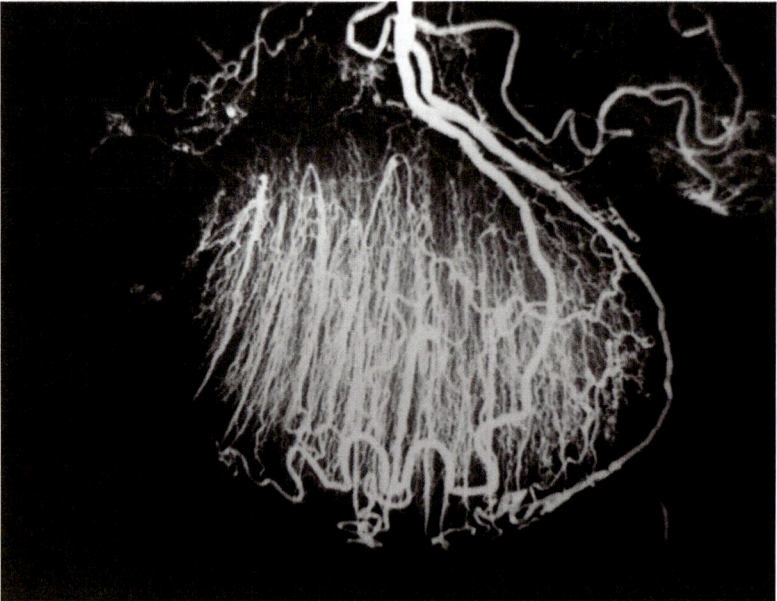

Fig. 2 The two branches of the testicular artery lead to the inferior pole. They pierce the albuginea and, after a sinuous course under the albuginea, give rise to the centripetal arteries

tium arise. Before changing direction again, the centripetal arteries give rise to fine spiral or corkscrew arteries that reach the testicular mediastinum (Figs. 3 and 4).

Arterioles give rise to capillaries that extend through the interstitium between Leydig cell clusters (forming intertubular capillaries) or in the proximity of the tunica propria (forming peritubular capillaries). The former are of a continuous type, their cells show little pinocytosis, strong adherent fascia-like junctions, and have low permeability. The endothelial cells of the peritubular capillaries are partially fenestrated.

The testicular artery or its branches can be affected in the same way as those of other territories in different pathologies. Vasculitis lesions can be observed in autopsy studies and sometimes in surgical specimens. Following the nomenclature adopted for the classification of vasculitis, most vasculitis seen in the testis, epididymis and spermatic cord are small vessel vasculitis, although in some cases medium-sized vessels may be involved. Testicular vasculitis can be secondary or primary (idiopathic) [7]. Among secondary small vessel vasculitis, ANCA (anti-neutrophil cytoplasmic antibody)-associated vasculitis such as microscopic polyangiitis, granulomatosis with polyangiitis, eosinophilic granulomatosis with polyangiitis, Behçet's disease, and Cogan's syndrome stand out. Immune complex-mediated small-vessel vasculitis such as rheumatoid arthritis and systemic lupus erythematosus, IgA (Henoch-Schönlein) can also occur.

Vasculitis associated with bacterial, viral, or paraneoplastic diseases or with drugs is also seen in the testis [8]. Structural lesions like testicular artery aneurysms or arteriovenous fistulas are rare. Other vessel lesions such as arte-

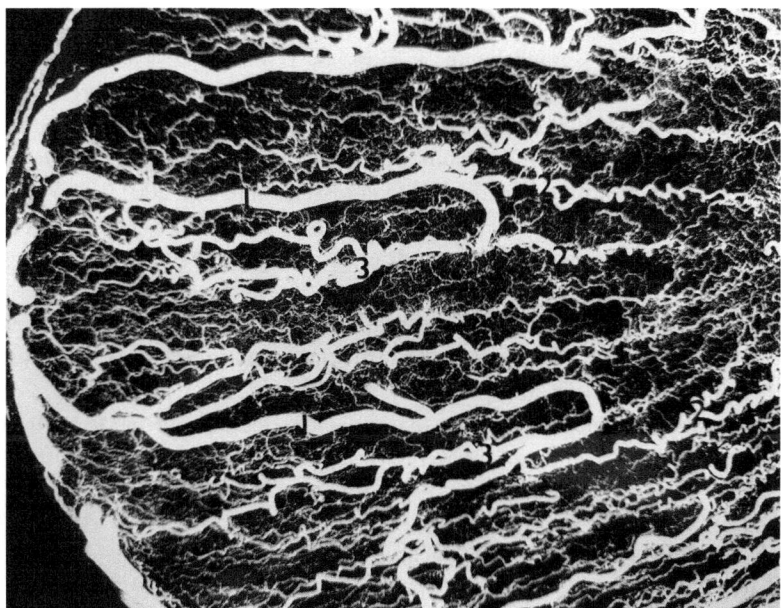

Fig. 3 Centripetal arteries (1) follow the interlobular septum, as they approach the testicular mediastinum they give rise to highly spiralized arteries (2). Along their course, the centripetal arteries give collaterals to the centrifugal arteries, which are directed towards the periphery of the parenchyma they are irrigating

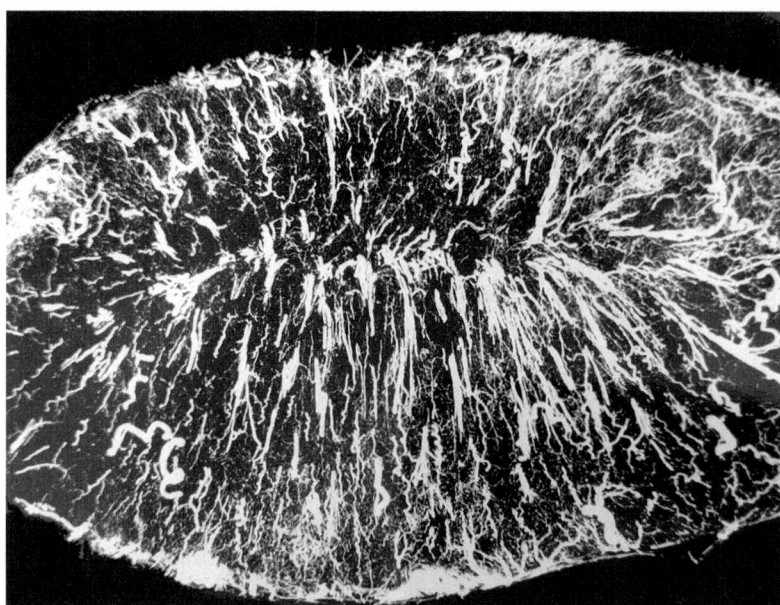

Fig. 4 In this section, close to the testicular mediastinum, note the bending of the centripetal arteries which transforms them into the centrifugal arteries that spread towards the albuginea

riosclerosis, atherosclerosis, arteriolosclerosis, arteriosclerosis obliterans (ASO) Mönckeberg medial calcific sclerosis, thromboembolism, or thromboangiitis obliterans (TAO) appear with age.

References
1. Cussenot O, Desgrandchamps F, Bassi S, Teillac P, Lassau JP, Le Duc A. Anatomic basis of laparoscopic surgery in the male pelvis. Surg Radiol Anat. 1993;15:265–9.
2. Asala S, Chaudhary SC, Masumbuko-Kahamba N, Bidmos M Anatomical variations in the human testicular blood vessels. Ann Anat. 2001:183:545–9.
3. Kotian SR, Pandey AK, Padmashali S, Jaison J, Kalthur SG. A cadaveric study of the testicular artery and its clinical significance. J Vasc Bras. 2016;15:280–6.
4. Balci S, Ardali Duzgun S, Arslan S, Balci H, Karcaaltincaba M, Karaosmanoglu AD. Anatomy of testicular artery: a proposal for a classification with MDCT angiography. Eur J Radiol. 2021;142:109885.
5. Felix W. Mesonephric arteries (aa. mesonephrica). In: Keibel F, Mall FP (eds) Manual of human embryolology, vol. 2. Lippincott, Philadelphia; 1912, p. 820–5.
6. Nallikuzhy TJ, Rajasekhar SSSN, Malik S, Tamgire DW, Johnson P, Aravindhan K. Variations of the testicular artery and vein: a meta-analysis with proposed classification. Clin Anat. 2018;31:854–69.
7. Hernández-Rodríguez J, Tan CD, Koening CL, Khasnis A, Rodríguez ER, Hoffman GS. Testicular vasculitis: findings differentiating isolated disease from systemic disease in 72 patients. Medicine (Baltimore). 2012;91:75–85.

8. Jennette JC, Falk RJ, Bacon PA, Basu N, Cid MC, Ferrario F, Flores-Suarez LF, Gross WL, Guillevin L, Hagen EC, Hoffman GS, Jayne DR, Kallenberg CG, Lamprecht P, Langford CA, Luqmani RA, Mahr AD, Matteson EL, Merkel PA, Ozen S, Pusey CD, Rasmussen N, Rees AJ, Scott DG, Specks U, Stone JH, Takahashi K, Watts RA. 2012 revised International Chapel Hill Consensus Conference Nomenclature of Vasculitides. Arthritis Rheum. 2013;65:1–11.

Large- and Medium-Sized Vessel Systemic Vasculitis with Testicular Involvement

1

1.1 Giant Cell Arteritis (Temporal Arteritis)

Giant cell arteritis, also known as temporal arteritis, is the most common autoinflammatory and autoimmune vasculitis affecting medium and large vessels. The incidence of the disease increases from the age of 50 years and peaks at between 70 and 79 years of age [1]. The highest incidence is observed in individuals of Scandinavian descent, specifically in Norway with an annual incidence of 32.8 per 100,000 in inhabitants over 50 years of age [2]. The aetiology is unknown although it is related to immunological processes triggered by inflammatory or environmental agents [3].

Granulomatous vasculitis like those affecting the temporal artery has been observed in other locations such as the heart, renal arteries, gallbladder artery, and in veins of the lower extremities. The vessels of the spermatic cord and testis may be affected in the context of generalized disease [4]. The clinical presentation is that of a testicular mass simulating an orchitis [5] or a malignant tumour [6]. The lesions are formed by a granulomatous reaction with abundant CD4+ T cells, macrophages, and giant cells preferentially located in the intima of the vessels in relation centred in the internal elastic lamina, which has a fragmented appearance [7].

Another granulomatous vasculitis, with a histological image that is similar to giant cell arteritis, is Takayasu's disease [8], but this disease has clear differences from classical giant cell arteritis in genetics, epidemiology, pathogenic mechanisms, response to treatment and complications of treatment [9]. Testicular involvement developed in the course of the disease in a 7-year-old patient with Takayasu disease [10].

1.2 Polyarteritis Nodosa (PAN)

Polyarteritis nodosa (PAN) is a form of multisystem necrotising vasculitis affecting small- and medium-sized muscular arteries of the kidney, liver, heart, adrenal glands, gastrointestinal tract, joints, spleen, lungs, and central nervous system without accompanying glomerulonephritis that spares arterioles, capillaries, and venules [11]. The annual incidence is estimated at 0.7/100,000, preferentially affecting males between the fourth and sixth decade of age. PAN accounts for 9% of vasculitis in childhood, ranking third behind IgA vasculitis/Henoch-Schönlein purpura (IgAV/HSP) and Kawasaki disease [12].

In PAN, both the testis and epididymis are affected [13]. The estimated frequency in autopsy series is 60% and 86%. Only 2–18% of the cases are symptomatic [14]. In 10% of cases, epididymal and/or testicular involvement is the first manifestation of systemic vasculitis. In these cases, the clinical presentation may be orchitis, epididymitis, torsion or testicular tumour [15, 16].

The definitive diagnosis of the condition is histological. The testicle or epididymis often shows arterial lesions at different evolutive times (fibrinoid necrosis, inflammatory reaction, thrombosis, or aneurysm), even in the same organ. Initially, the parenchyma shows more or less extensive areas of infarction followed by tubular sclerosis with interstitial fibrosis (Figs. 1.1, 1.2, 1.3, 1.4, 1.5, and 1.6).

The aetiology of PAN is unknown, and most cases are idiopathic. There are patients in whom it is associated with autoimmune diseases (rheumatoid arthritis, lupus erythematosus), infectious diseases (hepatitis B and C, HIV), or tumours. Three PAN patients with testicular involvement had an associated neoplasm (prostate adenocarcinoma, acute myelogenous leukaemia, hairy-cell leukaemia, and hepatocellular carcinoma). In

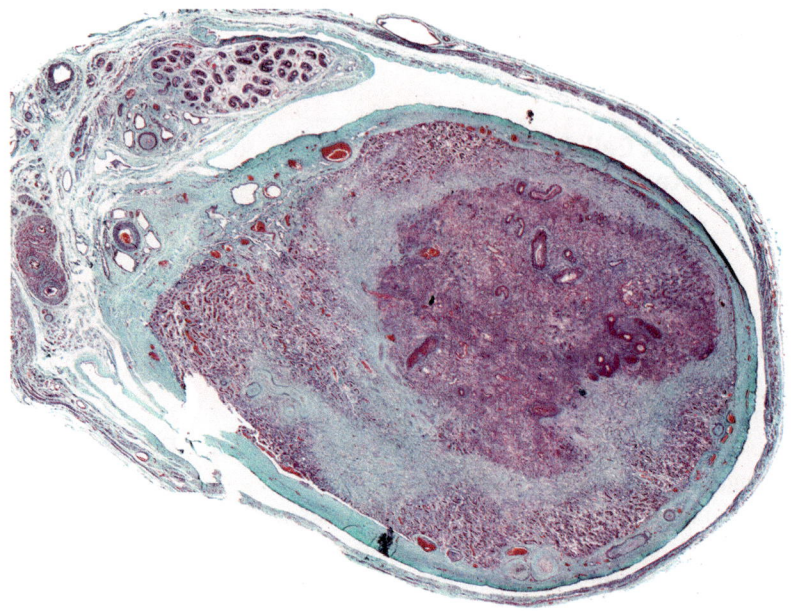

Fig. 1.1 Polyarteritis nodosa. Longitudinal section of testis, epididymis, and tunica vaginalis. The testicle has a central necrotic area surrounded by fibrous tissue. Preserved testicular parenchyma (Masson's trichrome) is visible only in the subalbuginea area

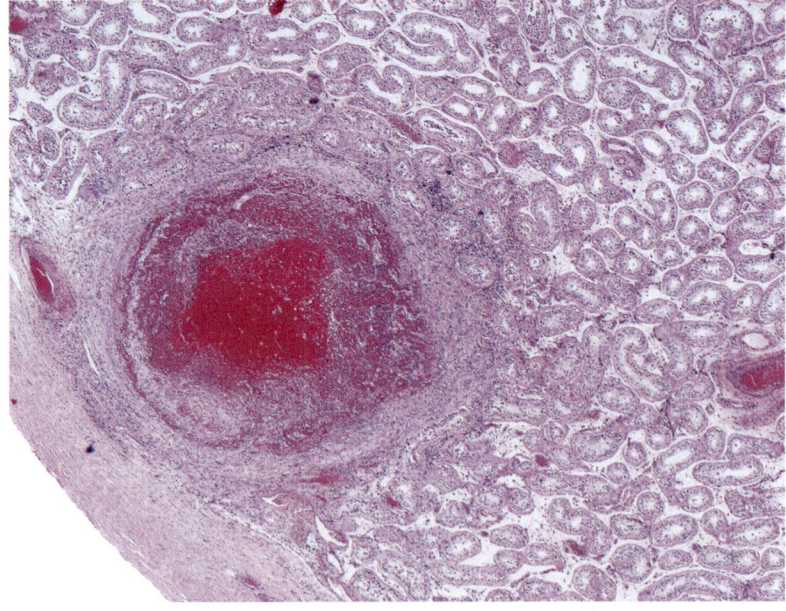

Fig. 1.2 Polyarteritis nodosa. Subalbuginea artery with partial necrosis of the wall and thrombosis. It is surrounded by an inflammatory infiltrate extending to the nearby seminiferous tubules. The remaining parenchyma is better preserved

Fig. 1.3 Polyarteritis nodosa. Along an interlobular artery there are some normal segments and others with fibrinoid necrosis, thrombosis, and lymphoid infiltrates around them

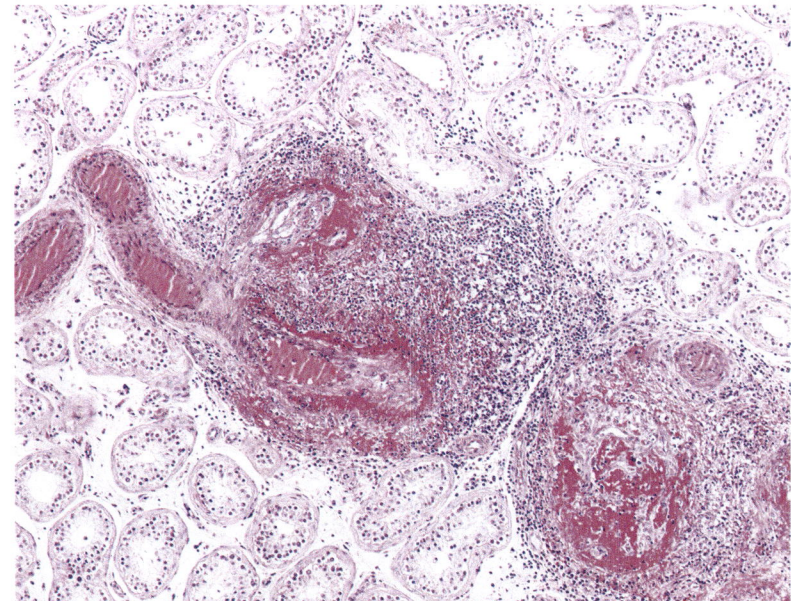

Fig. 1.4 Polyarteritis nodosa. Cross section of an intraparenchymal artery with extensive fibrinoid necrosis of the wall surrounded by lymphoid infiltrates. The seminiferous tubules have decreased calibre and a maturation arrest in spermatogonia

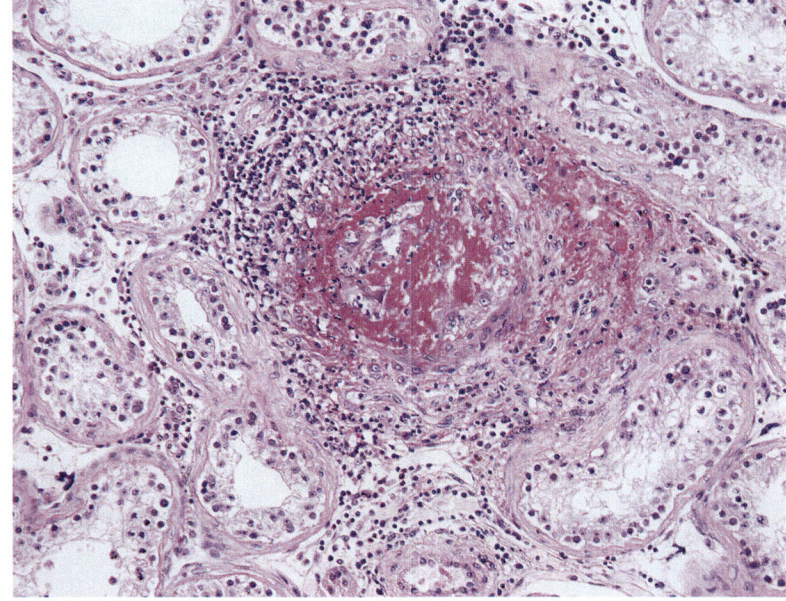

contrast to microscopic polyangiitis, Wegener's disease and Churg-Strauss syndrome, antineutrophil cytoplasmic antibodies (ANCAs) are not present in classic PAN [11].

A vasculitis that may be related to PAN is known as lymphocytic thrombophilic arteritis or macular lymphocytic arteritis [17]. This vasculitis has an indolent course and is accompanied by livedo racemosa or macular hyperpigmentation. It affects the small- and medium-sized arteries of the hypodermis and deep dermis and is characterized by the deposit of a thick fibrin ring in the intima and a dense infiltrate of mononuclear cells, mainly lymphocytes and some histiocytes, around the vessel. The presence of polynuclear neutrophils and eosinophils is residual. In rare cases, other organs can be involved, including the testis, resulting in bilateral testicular infarcts [18].

Fig. 1.5 Polyarteritis nodosa. Intraparenchymal artery with fibrinoid necrosis of all layers and partially recanalized thrombosis

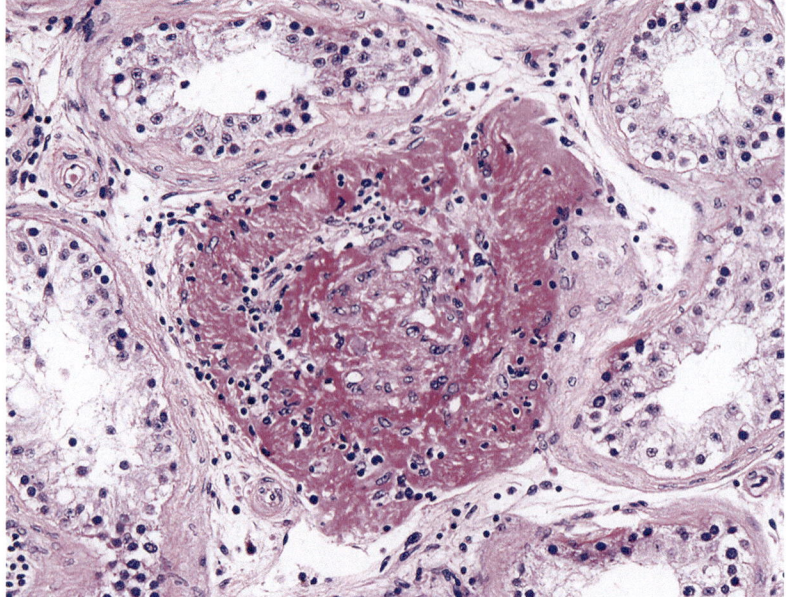

Fig. 1.6 Polyarteritis nodosa. The section of the epididymis shows an artery with luminal stenosis, discontinuous fibrosis of the media and adventitia with minimal lymphoid infiltrates that are interpreted as sequelae of the vasculitis. Next to the artery, an arteriole shows fibrinoid necrosis of the wall

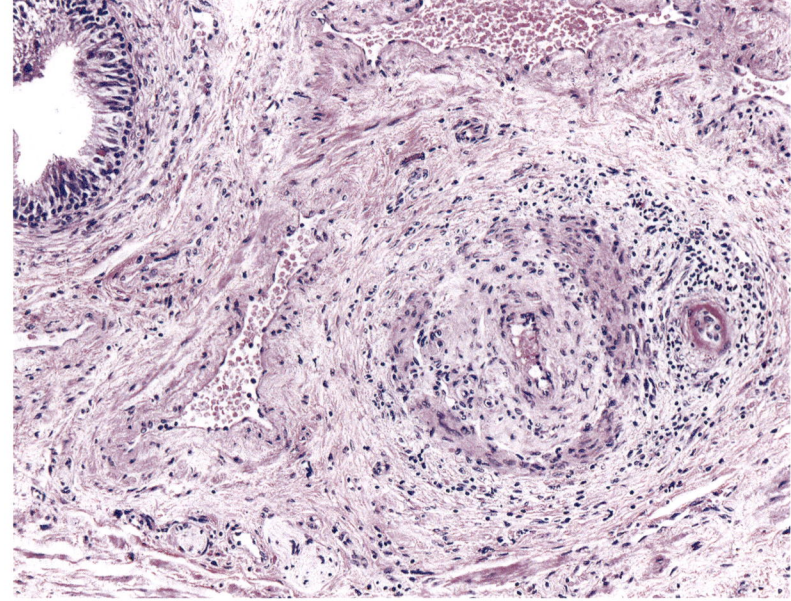

1.3 Kawasaki Disease (KD)

This multisystem vasculitis preferentially affects children under 5 years of age with mucocutaneous lymph node syndrome. After 5 or more days with fever, patients develop most of the following symptoms: bilateral conjunctival injection, oral and upper respiratory tract mucosal changes (oedema, erythema) in the mouth and upper respiratory tract, polymorphous rash, oedema, and erythema of the extremities and cervical adenopathy [19]. Medium and small arteries are preferentially affected. KD is considered the most frequent cause of acquired coronary artery disease in children.

Testicular involvement is a rare complication. In most cases, it manifests simply as a hydrocele, but in others, the clinical presentation is that of an acute scrotum [20, 21], which implies the need for a correct differential diagnosis among possible causes: torsion of the spermatic cord or testicular appendages, incarcerated inguinal hernia, orchio-epididymitis, testicular tumour, and acute idiopathic scrotal oedema. Treatment with immunoglobulin, aspirin, and prednisolone resolves scrotal swelling in most cases [20, 22].

The few histological studies, both on surgical specimens [23] and autopsies, have revealed a testicular arteritis or arteritis of the vessels of the spermatic cord [24, 25] that is morphologically indistinguishable from PAN [26].

1.4   Behçet's Disease

This systemic vasculitis clinically manifests as recurrent aphthous oral and genital ulcers, relapsing uveitis, and skin lesions (folliculitis, erythema nodosum-like lesions) and a positive pathergy test. Other frequently associated pathologies are arthritis, thrombophlebitis, and various neurological syndromes [27, 28]. It has a higher prevalence in countries along the ancient silk route extending from Japan to the Mediterranean and Middle Eastern countries than in northern European and North American countries and this may reflect a genetic predisposition as well as environmental triggering factors [29]. It preferentially affects individuals between 20 and 40 years of age.

There is a strong association between Behçet's disease and human leukocyte antigen (HLA) type B51 and HLA-12. Many patients with Behçet's disease carry the B5101 allele, so this may be a predisposing marker for the disease [30]. Exposure to an infectious agent would produce an autoinflammatory response in genetically predisposed individuals. The inflammatory mechanism, mediated by natural killer cells and heat shock proteins, gives rise to clinical manifestations through inflammatory repair processes in the blood vessels of the affected tissues.

In 40% of cases, the vascular tree is affected [27]. The main arteries affected are the large calibre arteries like the aorta, pulmonary artery, popliteal artery, femoral artery, subclavian artery and, less frequently, the common carotid artery. Arteritis is initially manifested by increased neutrophil emigration followed by occlusive-thrombotic and aneurysmal phenomena. The perivascular infiltrate is dominated by T, CD4+ and CD8+ lymphocytes and HLA-DR cells [31]. This occlusive vasculitis leads to infarcts or haemorrhages in the various affected organs. Both superficial and deep veins develop thrombophlebitis [32]. Inflammation of the vein wall is considered the hallmark of the pathogenesis of Behçet's disease [33]. Venous wall thickening is secondary to a process also initiated by neutrophilic hyperfunction, which produces reactive oxygen species (ROS). ROS cause endothelial dysfunction, necrosis, and platelet activation followed by thrombus formation [34].

Testicular and epididymal involvement simulates orchitis or epididymo-orchitis [35] and usually appears several years after the onset of the disease. It has a variable incidence related to the geographical area and age of the patients: 2% in France, 6% in Turkey, 12% in Greece, 31% in Iraq, and 44% in Russia [36]. The incidence of orchio-epididymitis is higher in adult (11.3%) than in young patients (7.7%). The duration of testicular symptoms is 1–2 weeks and is thought to be secondary to vasculitis. The involvement may be recurrent, and, in these cases, nodules are observed in the affected area. A complication, as with other vasculitis, is testicular infarction [37]. Patients with Behcet's disease very often develop AA-type amyloidosis, which has an unfavourable prognosis [38].

In some cases, the vasculitis resolves spontaneously, without treatment, or with analgesics alone, but most cases require the administration of colchicine and/or non-steroidal anti-inflammatory drugs. In more resistant cases, the additional use of corticosteroids is justified [36].

1.5   Cogan Disease

Cogan disease is a rare, multisystemic autoimmune vasculitis affecting large- and medium-sized vessels that predominantly occurs in children and young adults [39]. Initially described as an association of ophthalmologic (interstitial keratitis) and auditory (sensorineural deafness and vestibular dysfunction) pathology, it can present with other types of ocular pathology [40]. In 70% of patients, the disease is systemic, and vasculitis is considered the underlying pathology [41, 42]. Most cases have been described in Caucasian patients of both sexes. It is exceptional in Arabic and Middle Eastern countries [43].

Unilateral testicular swelling and acute testicular pain, mimicking orchitis, may be observed due to vasculitis of the testicular artery in 5% of patients with Cogan's disease [44, 45]. Histological studies are very rare [46–48]. Foci of fibrinoid necrosis, abundant epithelioid cells, and giant cells in the vessel wall are described. These observations suggest a differential diagnosis with other arteritis such as Wegener's granulomatosis, microscopic polyangiitis, and Takayasu's disease. There is no specific marker for Cogan's syndrome, which is why ophthalmologists, otorhinolaryngologists, and internists need to collaborate when this is suspected [49, 50].

The different types of treatment, including steroids, immunosuppressive drugs (methotrexate, azathi-oprine, and cyclophosphamide), and TNF-αantagonist (infliximab) have recently been reviewed in a large series of patients [50].

References

1. Gonzalez-Gay MA, Vazquez-Rodriguez TR, Lopez-Diaz MJ, Miranda-Filloy JA, Gonzalez-Juanatey C, Martin J, Llorca J. Epidemiology of giant cell arteritis and polymyalgia rheumatica. Arthritis Rheum. 2009;61:1454–61.
2. Barra L, Pope JE, Pequeno P, Saxena FE, Bell M, Haaland D, Widdifield J. Incidence and prevalence of giant cell arteritis in Ontario, Canada. Rheumatology. 2020;59:3250–8.
3. Dinkin M, Johnson E. One giant step for giant cell arteritis: updates in diagnosis and treatment. Curr Treat Options Neurol. 2021;23:6.
4. Arnillas E, de la Fuente J, Núñez M, Domínguez F. Giant cell arteritis with epididymal involvement. Med Clin. 2009;132:485.
5. Patil A, Upadhyaya S, Kashyap V, Kumar R, Mishra N. An unusual case of giant cell arteritis with monoarthritis and orchitis at presentation. Arch Rheumatol. 2017;32:268–70.
6. Sundaram S, Smith DH. Giant cell arteritis mimicking a testicular tumour. Rheumatol Int. 2001;20:215–6.
7. Zerbino DD. Giant-cell vasculitis (arteritis and phlebitis). Arkh Patol. 1981;43:42–7.
8. Mendiola Ramírez K, Portillo Rivera AC, Galicia Reyes A, García Montes JA, Maldonado Velázquez Mdel R, Faugier FE. Type III Takayasu's arteritis in a pediatric patient. Case report and review of the literature. Reumatol Clin. 2012;8:216–9.
9. Watanabe R, Berry GJ, Liang DH, Goronzy JJ, Weyand CM. Pathogenesis of giant cell arteritis and takayasu arteritis-similarities and differences. Curr Rheumatol Rep. 2020;22:68.
10. Brunette MG, Bonny Y, Spigelblatt L, Barrette G. Long-term immunosuppressive treatment of a child with Takayasu's arteritis and high IgE immunoglobulins. Pediatr Nephrol. 1996;10:67–9.
11. Jennette JC, Falk RJ, Bacon PA, Basu N, Cid MC, Ferrario F, Flores-Suarez LF, Gross WL, Guillevin L, Hagen EC, Hoffman GS, Jayne DR, Kallenberg CG, Lamprecht P, Langford CA, Luqmani RA, Mahr AD, Matteson EL, Merkel PA, Ozen S, Pusey CD, Rasmussen N, Rees AJ, Scott DG, Specks U, Stone JH, Takahashi K, Watts RA. 2012 revised international Chapel Hill consensus conference nomenclature of vasculitides. Arthritis Rheum. 2013;65:1–11.
12. Kasap Cuceoglu M, Sener S, Batu ED, Kaya Akca U, Demir S, Sag E, Atalay E, Balık Z, Basaran O, Bilginer Y, Ozen S. Systematic review of childhood-onset polyarteritis nodosa and DADA2. Semin Arthritis Rheum. 2021;51:559–64.
13. Azar N, Guillevin L, Huong Du LT, Herreman G, Meyrier A, Godeau P. Symptomatic urogenital manifestations of polyarteritis nodosa and Churg-Strauss angiitis: analysis of 8 of 165 patients. J Urol. 1989;142:136–8.
14. Shurbaji MS, Epstein JI. Testicular vasculitis: implications for systemic disease. Hum Pathol. 1988;19:186–9.
15. Teichman JM, Mattrey RF, Demby AM, Schmidt JD. Polyarteritis nodosa presenting as acute orchitis: a case report and review of the literature. J Urol. 1993;149:1139–40.
16. Eilber KS, Freedland SJ, Rajfer J. Polyarteritis nodosa presenting as hematuria and a testicular mass. J Urol. 2001;166:624.
17. Lee JS, Kossard S, McGrath MA. Lymphocytic thrombophilic arteritis: a newly described medium-sized vessel arteritis of the skin. Arch Dermatol. 2008;144:1175–82.
18. Wee E, Nikpour M, Balta S, Williams RA, Kelly RI. Lymphocytic thrombophilic arteritis complicated by systemic involvement. Australas J Dermatol. 2018;59:223–5.
19. Newburger JW, Fulton DR. Kawasaki disease. Curr Opin Pediatr. 2004;16:508–14.
20. Jibiki T, Sakai T, Saitou T, Kanazawa M, Ide T, Fujita M, Iida Y, Yamazaki S, Ishiwada F, Sato J. Acute scrotum in Kawasaki disease: two case reports and a literature review. Pediatr Int. 2013;55:771–5.
21. Roy S, Chakrabartty S. Kawasaki disease presenting as acute scrotum. Indian J Pediatr. 2018;85:796.

22. Connolly KD, Timmons D. Epididymo-orchitis in Kawasaki disease. Arch Dis Child. 1979;54:728.

23. Katayama O, Murakami M. A case of Kawasaki disease with scrotum hydrops. Jpn J Pediatr. 1981;34:578–81.

24. Tanaka N, Sekimoto K, Naoe S, Kawasaki disease. Relationship with infantile periarteritis nodosa. Arch Pathol Lab Med. 1976;100:81–6.

25. Landing BH, Larson EJ. Are infantile periarteritis nodosa with coronary artery involvement and fatal mucocutaneous lymph node syndrome the same? Comparison of 20 patients from North America with patients from Hawaii and Japan. Pediatrics. 1977;59:651–62.

26. Roberts FB, Fetterman GH. Polyarteritis nodosa in infancy. J Pediatr. 1963;63:519–29.

27. Yazici H, Seyahi E, Hatemi G, Yazici Y. Behçet syndrome: a contemporary view. Nat Rev Rheumatol. 2018;14:107–19.

28. Hatemi G, Uçar D, Uygunoğlu U, Yazici H, Yazici Y. Behçet syndrome. Rheum Dis Clin N Am. 2023;49(3):585–602.

29. Verity DH, Marr JE, Ohno S, Wallace GR, Stanford MR. Behçet's disease, the silk road and HLA-B51: historical and geographical perspectives. Tissue Antigens. 1999;54:213–20.

30. Koumantaki Y, Stavropoulos C, Spyropoulou M, Messini H, Papademetropoulos M, Giziaki E, Marcomichelakis N, Palimeris G, Kaklamanis P, Kaklamani E. HLA-B*5101 in Greek patients with Behçet's disease. Hum Immunol. 1998;59:250–5.

31. Mahammad A, Mandl T, Stufeet C, Segel MM. Incidence, prevalence and clinical characteristics of Behçet's disease in southern Sweden. Rheumatology. 2013;52:304–10.

32. Rodríguez-Carballeira M, Solans R, Larrañaga JR, García-Hernández FJ, Rios-Fernández R, Nieto J, Solanich X, Martínez-Valle F, Fonseca E, Muñoz FJ, Fraile G, de Escalante B, Boldova R, Hurtado R, Espinosa G, REGEB Investigators; Autoimmune Diseases Study Group (GEAS). Venous thrombosis and relapses in patients with Behçet's disease. Descriptive analysis from Spanish network of Behçet's disease (REGEB cohort). Clin Exp Rheumatol. 2018;36(6):40–4.

33. Alibaz-Oner F, Ergelen R, Mutis A, Erturk Z, Asadov R, Mumcu G, Ergun T, Direskeneli H. Venous vessel wall thickness in lower extremity is increased in male patients with Behçet's disease. Clin Rheumatol. 2019;38:1447–51.

34. Batu ED. Neutrophil-mediated thrombosis and NETosis in Behçet's disease: a hypothesis. J Korean Med Sci. 2020;35(29):e213.

35. Kanakis MA, Vaiopoulos AG, Vaiopoulos GA, Kaklamanis PG. Epididymo-orchitis in Bechet's disease: a review of the wide spectrum of the disease. Acta Med Austriaca. 2017;55:482–5.

36. Kaklamani VG, Vaiopoulos G, Markomichelakis N, Kaklamanis P. Recurrent epididymo-orchitis in patients with Behçet's disease. J Urol. 2000;163:487–9.

37. Al-Ani Z, Suut S, Huasen B. Serial ultrasonography assessments of a testicular infarction mimicking testicular tumor in a Behcet disease patient. Urol Case Rep. 2014;2:45–7.

38. Akpolat T, Akpolat I, Kandemir B. Behcet's disease and AA-type amyloidosis. Am J Nephrol. 2000;20:68–70.

39. Kessel A, Vadasz Z, Toubi E. Cogan syndrome–pathogenesis, clinical variants and treatment approaches. Autoimmun Rev. 2014;13:351–4.

40. Grasland A, Pouchot J, Hachulla E, Blétry O, Papo T, Vinceneux P, Study Group for Cogan's Syndrome. Typical and atypical Cogan's syndrome: 32 cases and review of the literature. Rheumatology. 2004;43:1007–15.

41. Olfat M, Al-Mayouf SM. Cogan's syndrome in childhood. Rheumatol Int. 2001;20:246–9.

42. García Callejo FJ, Platero Zamarreno A, Sebastian Gil E, Orts Alborch MH, Marco AJ. Atypical Cogan syndrome. Clinical and laboratory spectrum. Report of 2 cases. Acta Otorrinolaringol Esp. 2002;53:191–8.

43. Iliescu DA, Timaru CM, Batras M, De Simone A, Stefan C. Cogan's syndrome. Rom J Ophthalmol. 2015;59:6–13.

44. Leff IL. Cogan's syndrome. N Y State J Med. 1967;67:2249–57.

45. Vollertsen RS, McDonald TJ, Younge BR, Banks PM, Stanson AW, Ilstrup DM. Cogan's syndrome: 18 cases and a review of the literature. Mayo Clin Proc. 1986;61:344–61.

46. Crawford WJ. Cogan's syndrome associated with polyarteritis nodosa; a report of three cases. Pa Med J. 1957;60:835–8.

47. Fisher ER, Hellstrom HR. Cogan's syndrome and systemic vascular disease. Analysis of pathologic features with reference to its relationship to thromboangiitis obliterans (Buerger). Arch Pathol. 1961;72:572–92.

48. Vollertsen RS. Vasculitis and Cogan's syndrome. Rheum Dis Clin N Am. 1990;16:433–9.

49. Gaubitz M, Lübben B, Seidel M, Schotte H, Gramley F, Domschke W. Cogan's syndrome: organ-specific autoimmune disease or systemic vasculitis? A report of two cases and review of the literature. Clin Exp Rheumatol. 2001;19:463–9.

50. Durtette C, Hachulla E, Resche-Rigon M, Papo T, Zénone T, Lioger B, Deligny C, Lambert M, Landron C, Pouchot J, Kahn JE, Lavigne C, De Wazieres B, Dhote R, Gondran G, Pertuiset E, Quemeneur T, Hamidou M, Sève P, Le Gallou T, Grasland A, Hatron PY, Fain O, Mekinian A, SNFMI and CRI. Cogan syndrome: characteristics, outcome and treatment in a French nationwide retrospective study and literature review. Autoimmun Rev. 2017;16:1219–23.

2.1 Microscopic Polyangiitis (MPA)

MPA is a necrotising vasculitis affecting small vessels, although arteritis of medium-sized vessels is also frequently observed. Patients often present with necrotising glomerulonephritis [1]. This type of vasculitis can affect several systems and organs such as brain, kidney, liver, gallbladder, small intestine, pancreas, heart, bronchus, prostate, spleen, and testicle. The vascular lesions produce areas of infarction in solid organs. In the testis, areas surrounding the affected intraparenchymal arteries show tubular sclerosis [2].

2.2 Granulomatosis with Polyangiitis (Wegener's Granulomatosis) (GPA)

Wegener's granulomatosis or granulomatosis with polyangiitis as it has been renamed [3] is a necrotising, multisystemic vasculitis, which, like other vasculitis such as microscopic polyangiitis, and eosinophilic granulomatosis with polyangiitis (EGPA or Churg-Strauss syndrome), belongs to disorders called anti-neutrophil-cytoplasmic-antibody (ANCA) associated vasculitis.

Wegener's granulomatosis presents with glomerulonephritis, necrotising granulomatous infla

mmation of the small- and medium-sized vessels of the upper and lower respiratory tract, and elevated ANCA levels. It is diagnosed between 45 and 60 years of age and its prevalence is estimated at 22–157 cases per million [4]. Urogenital tract involvement is exceptional (less than 1% of patients). Testicular involvement occurs in 12.5% to 36% of patients with urogenital tract involvement [5]. Clinically, it mimics orchitis. The epididymis is affected in 10% of cases with a clinical picture of epididymitis [6]; the epididymal lesion is isolated [7] or associated with that of the testis [8] and may be the only location of the disease. Arteries show fibrinoid necrosis with intense infiltration of neutrophils, epithelioid cells, and multinucleated giant cells [9, 10]. The consequence of these lesions is multiple testicular infarcts [11] (Figs. 2.1, 2.2, 2.3, 2.4, 2.5, and 2.6).

Hypogonadism with increased serum FSH and decreased testosterone levels is observed in 52.6% of patients with Wegener's granulomatosis. This hypogonadism does not seem to be related to cyclophosphamide, corticosteroid, or rituximab treatment. This observation suggests a subclinical involvement of the testes by systemic vasculitis [12]. In other cases, when Wegener's granulomatosis directly affects the pituitary gland, different hormonal deficiencies occur, resulting in hypogonadotropic hypogonadism in some cases in [13].

Fig. 2.1 Granulomatosis
with polyangiitis. In the
central part, there is an
oblique section of an
artery with dense focal
infiltrates in all layers of
the artery wall. The veins
are unchanged

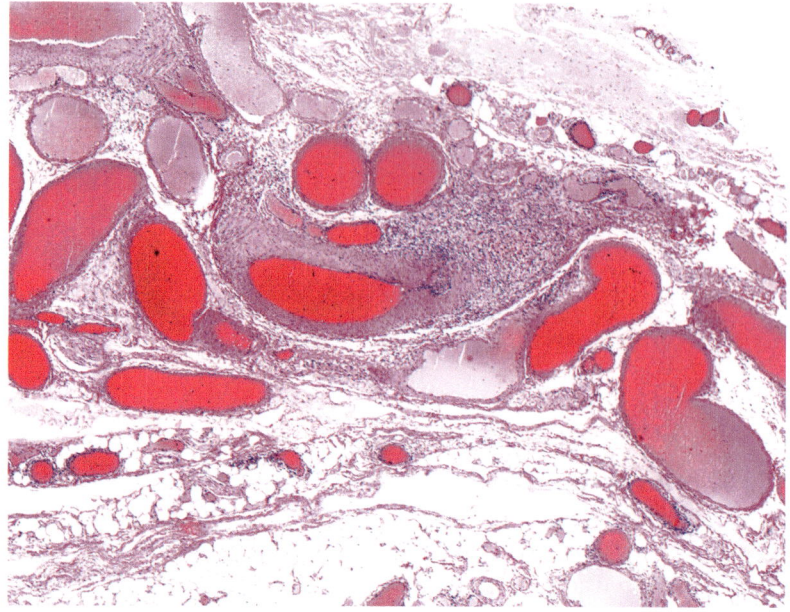

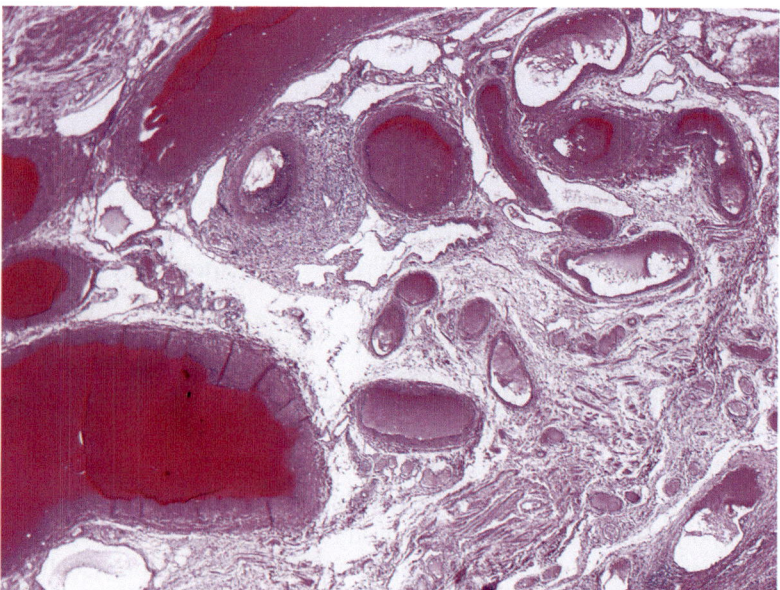

Fig. 2.2 Granulomatosis
with polyangiitis. Cross
section of the spermatic
compartment. The artery,
which is surrounded by
several veins, has a dense
crescent-shaped infiltrate
in its wall

Fig. 2.3 Granulomatosis with polyangiitis. The intima and media show necrosis and dense neutrophilic polynuclear infiltrates

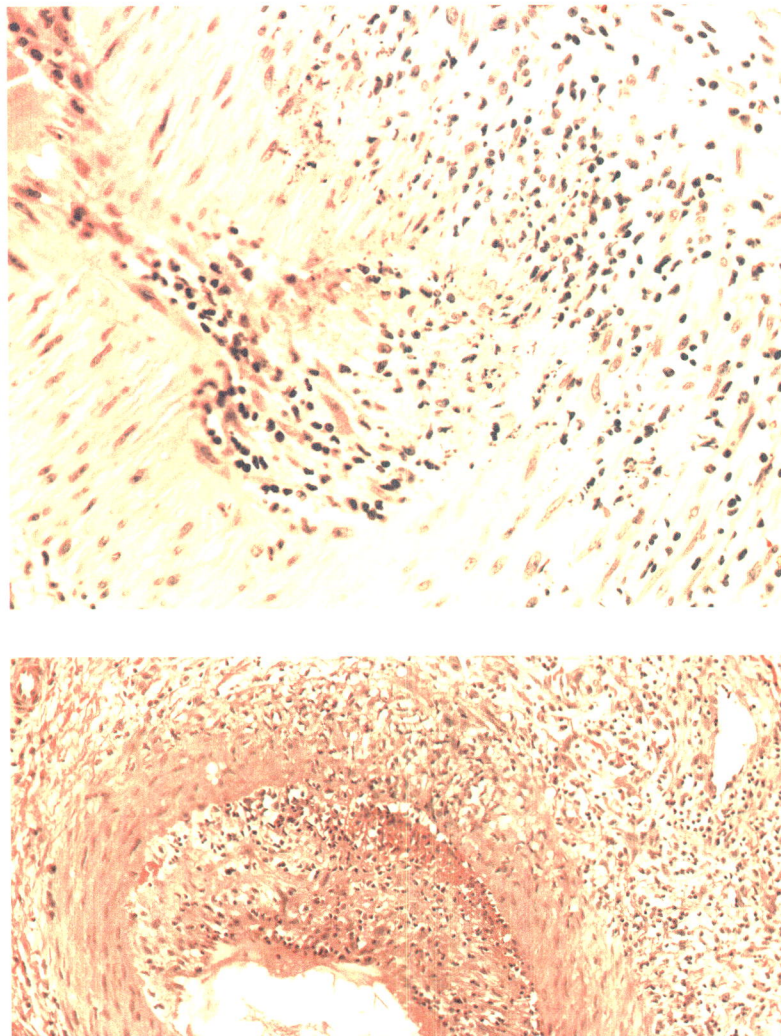

Fig. 2.4 Granulomatosis with polyangiitis. Section of an artery with partial thrombosis, segmental fibrinoid necrosis of the intima and media and non-specific inflammation of the adventitia

Fig. 2.5 Granulomatosis with polyangiitis. The vessel wall shows several granulomatous formations in the media and adventitia with a predominance of epithelioid cells in the central part and peripheral lymphocytic crowns

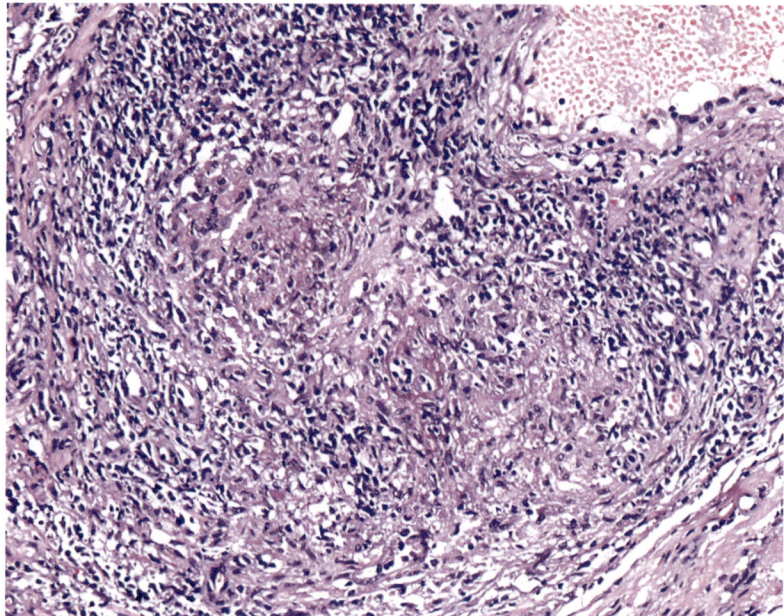

Fig. 2.6 Granulomatosis with polyangiitis. A granuloma with epithelioid cells, giant cells and lymphocytes has developed in the thickness of the vascular wall

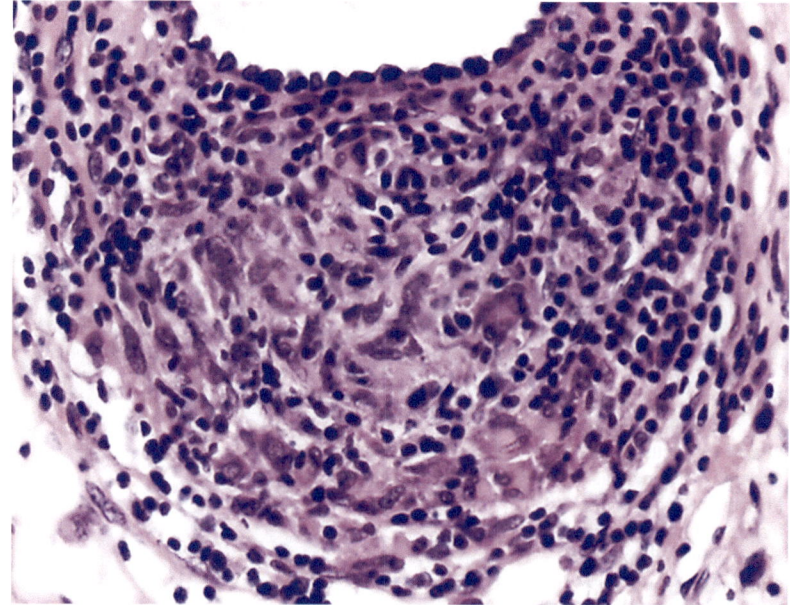

2.3   Testicular Eosinophilic Granulomatosis with Polyangiitis (EGPA) (Churg-Strauss)

EGPA (classically known as Churg-Strauss syndrome) is a systemic disorder characterized by the presence of tissue eosinophilia, necrotising granulomatous vasculitis with extravascular granulomas, asthma, fever, and eosinophilia [14]. The typical picture is the presence of asthma in an adult with chronic rhinosinusitis, pulmonary infiltrates, and more than 10% eosinophilia. Nasal polyps, otitis media, gastrointestinal disorders, and peripheral neuropathy are very frequent associated pathologies [15]. In 25% of patients, the kidney is affected, and the pathology varies from rapidly progressive glomerulonephritis to chronic kidney disease. In the same proportion, skin lesions such as purpura and nodules appear predominantly on the scalp and lower extremities [16].

Most of the affected patients are between 40 and 60 years of age. The prevalence is estimated at 2–22 cases per million people depending on the geographical area and the criteria used for its diagnosis [17]. It is ten times less frequent than granulomatosis with polyangiitis and microscopic polyangiitis [18]. The aetiology is unknown. In 30–40% of patients, vasculitis is associated with antineutrophil cytoplasmic antibodies [19]. More important than ANCA antibodies in its pathogenesis seems to be the role of TH2 type lymphocytes, which, upon expansion and activation, release substantial amounts of interleukins (IL-4, IL-5, IL-13) that stimulate B-cells, resulting in secretion of IgE and IgG4. The released eotaxin3 stimulates the extravasation of eosinophils, which infiltrate tissues and, upon degranulation, release proteins, and inflammatory mediators that cause cell damage [20–22].

Vascular lesions affect small- and medium-sized arteries and veins. They are characterized by necrotising vasculitis of small vessels (55%), fibrinoid necrosis, eosinophilic infiltration of all layers (52%), and perivascular granulomas (18%) [23]. The central part of the granulomas is formed by eosinophilic necrosis and the periphery is a palisade of histiocytes and giant cells. Lesions can be found at different evolutionary moments, making it difficult to detect all lesions in the same patient. But there is one constant fact, eosinophilic infiltrates are always present throughout the disease. Testicular involvement is exceedingly rare and is most often manifested by testicular infarcts which may or may not be associated with thrombotic lesions in other organs [24, 25].

The therapeutic approach depends on the degree of testicular involvement: when testicular lesions are focal, conservative treatment is recommended, although in many cases, the testicle will not return to normal size [26], while orchiectomy is necessary when testicular infarction is total [27].

2.4   Immunoglobulin A (IgA) Vasculitis (Henoch-Schönlein Purpura) (IgAV)

Immunoglobulin A vasculitis is a systemic immune complex-mediated leukocytoclastic vasculitis characterized by the classic tetrad of palpable non-thrombocytopenic purpura, arthritis or arthralgia, abdominal pain, and renal disease. Additional complications include gastrointestinal bleeding, orchitis, and central nervous system involvement.

It is the most common vasculitis in children but can also affect adults. It is more common in males (2:1 ratio). The annual incidence is estimated to be between 10 and 30 cases per 100,000 children [28, 29].

The incidence of involvement of the scrotum and its contents ranges from 2.4% to 38% [30, 31]. It can be uni- or bilateral. The most important clinical symptoms are pain and scrotal swelling, which are usually preceded by purpuric lesions on the skin of both extremities the week before [32, 33] but that may coincide with the skin lesions or even appear later [34].

The histology of the testicular and epididymal lesions is like that of the skin lesions. It is a leukocytoclastic vasculitis of small vessels, whether arteries, veins, or capillaries. It consists of endothelial swelling, red blood cell extravasation, and infiltration by polynuclear neutrophils with abundant signs of karyorrhexis. The IgA deposits in the vessel wall of the affected organs are pathognomonic. In rare cases, partial or total ischemic necrosis of one [26, 34–37] or both testicles [38] occurs. The pathogenesis of the disease is unknown, although it is assumed that there is a genetic basis on which environmental triggers act.

The differential diagnosis, in cases where scrotal pain is the first manifestation of the disease, is posed in all situations involving an acute scrotum and will include testicular torsion, torsion of the appendix of the testicle and epididymis, epididymitis, orchitis, hernia, hydrocele, trauma, testicular tumour, and idiopathic scrotal oedema [39]. Isotopic study with Tc99 and/or Doppler ultrasound can rule out the most severe picture, testicular ischemia due to torsion [40, 41].

Most patients with scrotal vasculitis do not require treatment. If ischaemic necrosis of the testicular parenchyma has occurred, as demonstrated by echo-Doppler scanning, the testicle should be removed. Only when the ischaemic lesions are focal conservative treatment with or without corticosteroid administration can be considered.

References

1. Han S, Rehman HU, Jayaratne PS, Carty JE. Microscopic polyangiitis complicated by cerebral haemorrhage. Rheumatol Int. 2006;26:1057–60.
2. Miyawaki Y, Katsuyama T, Sada KE, Taniguchi K, Kakio Y, Wada J. Development of intracerebral hemorrhage in the short-term clinical course of a patient with microscopic polyangiitis without neurological symptoms at diagnosis: an autopsy case. CEN Case Rep. 2016;5:173–8.
3. Jennette JC, Falk RJ, Bacon PA, Basu N, Cid MC, Ferrario F, Flores-Suarez LF, Gross WL, Guillevin L, Hagen EC, Hoffman GS, Jayne DR, Kallenberg CG, Lamprecht P, Langford CA, Luqmani RA, Mahr AD, Matteson EL, Merkel PA, Ozen S, Pusey CD, Rasmussen N, Rees AJ, Scott DG, Specks U, Stone JH, Takahashi K, Watts RA. 2012 revised international Chapel Hill consensus conference nomenclature of vasculitides. Arthritis Rheum. 2013;65:1–11.
4. Alba MA, Moreno-Palacios J, Beça S, Cid MC. Urologic and male genital manifestations of granulomatosis with polyangiitis. Autoimmun Rev. 2015;14:897–902.
5. Dufour JF, Le Gallou T, Cordier JF, Aumaître O, Pinède L, Aslangul E, Pagnoux C, Marie I, Puéchal X, Decaux O, Dubois A, Agard C, Mahr A, Comoz F, Boutemy J, Broussolle C, Guillevin L, Sève P, Bienvenu B, French Center-East Internists Group; French Vasculitis Study Group. Urogenital manifestations in Wegener granulomatosis: a study of 11 cases and review of the literature. Medicine. 2012;91:67–74.
6. Miller DC, Koss MN. Wegener granulomatosis presenting as epididymitis. Urology. 2009;73:1225–6.
7. Al-Arfaj A. Limited Wegener's granulomatosis of the epididymis. Int J Urol. 2001;8:333–5.
8. Lee SS, Tang SH, Sun GH, Yu CP, Jin JS, Chang SY. Limited Wegener's granulomatosis of the epididymis and testis. Asian J Androl. 2006;8:737–9.
9. Agraharkar M, Gokhale S, Gupta R. Wegener's granulomatosis diagnosed by testicular biopsy. Int Urol Nephrol. 2002;34:559–64.
10. Kechida M, Ktari K, Jellazi M, Mesfar R, Khochtali I, Saad H, Njim L. Simultaneous testicle and epididymis vasculitis revealing granulomatosis with polyangiitis. Clin Case Reports. 2022;10(8):e6231.
11. Aizpiri Antoñana L, Bauzá Quetglas JL, Prados Pérez E, López Brito K, Benito García P, Pieras Ayala EC. Granulomatosis with poliangiitis mimicking testicular torsion. Reumatol Clin. 2023;19:345–7.
12. Richter JG, Becker A, Specker C, Schneider M. Hypogonadism in Wegener's granulomatosis. Scand J Rheumatol. 2008;37:365–9.
13. Liu S, Xu Y, Li N, Chen S, Zhang S, Peng L, Bai W, Wang J, Gao J, Zeng X, Shi J, Wang M. Pituitary involvement in granulomatosis with polyangiitis: a retrospective analysis in a single Chinese hospital and a literature review. Int J Endocrinol. 2019;2019:2176878.
14. Churg J, Strauss L. Allergic granulomatosis, allergic angiitis, and periarteritis nodosa. Am J Pathol. 1951;27:277–301.
15. Comarmond C, Pagnoux C, Khellaf M, Cordier JF, Hamidou M, Viallard JF, Maurier F, Jouneau S, Bienvenu B, Puéchal X, Aumaître O, Le Guenno G, Le Quellec A, Cevallos R, Fain O, Godeau B, Seror R, Dunogué B, Mahr A, Guilpain P, Cohen P, Aouba A, Mouthon L, Guillevin L, French Vasculitis Study Group. Eosinophilic granulomatosis with polyangiitis (Churg-Strauss): clinical characteristics and long-term followup of the 383 patients enrolled in the French Vasculitis Study Group cohort. Arthritis Rheum. 2013;65:270–81.
16. Furuta S, Iwamoto T, Nakajima H. Update on eosinophilic granulomatosis with polyangiitis. Allergol Int. 2019;68:430–6.
17. Harrold LR, Andrade SE, Go AS, Buist AS, Eisner M, Vollmer WM, Chan KA, Frazier EA, Weller PF, Wechsler ME, Yood RA, Davis KJ, Platt R. Incidence of Churg-Strauss syndrome in asthma drug users: a population-based perspective. J Rheumatol. 2005;32:1076–80.
18. Berti A, Cornec D, Casal Moura M, Smyth RJ, Dagna L, Specks U, Keogh KA. Eosinophilic granulomatosis with polyangiitis: clinical predictors of long-term asthma severity. Chest. 2020;157:1086–99.
19. Sinico RA, Di Toma L, Maggiore U, Bottero P, Radice A, Tosoni C, Grasselli C, Pavone L, Gregorini G, Monti S, Frassi M, Vecchio F, Corace C, Venegoni E, Buzio C. Prevalence and clinical significance of antineutrophil cytoplasmic antibodies in Churg-Strauss syndrome. Arthritis Rheum. 2005;52:2926–35.
20. Zwerina J, Bach C, Martorana D, Jatzwauk M, Hegasy G, Moosig F, Bremer J, Wieczorek S, Moschen A, Tilg H, Neumann T, Spriewald BM, Schett G, Vaglio A. Eotaxin-3 in Churg-Strauss syndrome: a clinical and immunogenetic study. Rheumatology. 2011;50:1823–7.
21. Vaglio A, Buzio C, Zwerina J. Eosinophilic granulomatosis with polyangiitis (Churg-Strauss): state of the art. Allergy. 2013;68:261–73.
22. Izquierdo-Dominguez A, Cordero Castillo A, Alobid I, Mullo J. Churg-Strauss syndrome or eosinophilic granulomatosis with polyangeiitis. Sinusitis. 2015;1:24–43.

23. Sablé-Fourtassou R, Cohen P, Mahr A, Pagnoux C, Mouthon L, Jayne D, Blockmans D, Cordier JF, Delaval P, Puechal X, Lauque D, Viallard JF, Zoulim A, Guillevin L, French Vasculitis Study Group. Antineutrophil cytoplasmic antibodies and the Churg-Strauss syndrome. Ann Intern Med. 2005;143:632–8.

24. Li J, Yan M, Qin J, Ren L, Wen R. Testicular infarction and pulmonary embolism secondary to nonasthmatic eosinophilic granulomatosis with polyangiitis: a case report. J Investig Allergol Clin Immunol. 2020;30:380–1.

25. Vega Villanueva KL, Espinoza LR. Eosinophilic vasculitis. Curr Rheumatol Rep. 2020;22:5.

26. Zhang S, Wang Q, Li Z, Guo Q. Testicular ischemia associated with IgA vasculitis in a child: a case report and literature review. Front Pediatr. 2023;11:1219878.

27. Ichikawa T, Shimojima Y, Nomura S, Kishida D, Shiozaki M, Tanimura J, Sekijima Y. Testicular vasculitis in eosinophilic granulomatosis with polyangiitis: a case-based review. Clin Rheumatol. 2023;42:293–9.

28. Gardner-Medwin JM, Dolezalova P, Cummins C, Southwood TR. Incidence of Henoch-Schönlein purpura, Kawasaki disease, and rare vasculitides in children of different ethnic origins. Lancet. 2002;360:1197–202.

29. Søreide K. Surgical management of nonrenal genitourinary manifestations in children with Henoch-Schönlein purpura. J Pediatr Surg. 2005;40:1243–7.

30. Chamberlain RS, Greenberg LW. Scrotal involvement in Henoch-Schönlein purpura: a case report and review of the literature. Pediatr Emerg Care. 1992;8:213–5.

31. Tabel Y, Inanc FC, Dogan DG, Elmas AT. Clinical features of children with Henoch-Schonlein purpura: risk factors associated with renal involvement. Iran J Kidney Dis. 2012;6:269–74.

32. Ha TS, Lee JS. Scrotal involvement in childhood Henoch-Schönlein purpura. Acta Paediatr. 2007;96:552–5.

33. Sakanoue M, Higashi Y, Kawai K, Sugita S, Kanekura T. Henoch-Schönlein purpura with epididymitis in an adult. J Dermatol. 2011;38:620–2.

34. Ma Y, Zhang S, Chen J, Kong H, Diao J. Henoch-Schönlein purpura with scrotal involvement: a case report and literature review. J Pediatr Hematol Oncol. 2021;43:211–5.

35. Zhao L, Zheng S, Ma X, Yan W. Henoch-Schönlein purpura with testicular necrosis: sonographic findings at the onset, during treatment, and at follow-up. Urology. 2017;107:223–5.

36. Hu JJ, Zhao YW, Wen R, Luo YY, Zhou WG, Liu YH, Qin F, Liu C, He TQ. Immunoglobulin a vasculitis with testicular/epididymal involvement in children: a retrospective study of a ten-year period. Front Pediatr. 2023;11:1141118.

37. Yaseen K. Testicular infarction in an adult patient with systemic IgA vasculitis. Clin Rheumatol. 2023;42:1213–4.

38. Toushan M, Atodaria A, Lynch SD, Kanaan HD, Yu L, Amin MB, Tahhan M, Zhang PL, Kellerman PS, Swami A. Bilateral testicular infarction from IgA vasculitis of the spermatic cords. Case Rep Nephrol. 2017;2017:9437965.

39. Verim L, Cebeci F, Erdem MR, Somay A. Henoch-Schönlein purpura without systemic involvement beginning with acute scrotum and mimicking torsion of testis. Arch Ital Urol Androl. 2013;85:50–2.

40. Huang LH, Yeung CY, Shyur SD, Lee HC, Huang FY, Wang NL. Diagnosis of Henoch-Schönlein purpura by sonography and radionuclear scanning in a child presenting with bilateral acute scrotum. J Microbiol Immunol Infect. 2004;37:192–5.

41. Güneş M, Kaya C, Koca O, Keles MO, Karaman MI. Acute scrotum in Henoch-Schönlein purpura: fact or fiction? Turk J Pediatr. 2012;54:194–7.

3.1 Isolated Arteritis of the Testis, Epididymis, and Spermatic Cord

With the same testicular symptomatology as observed in systemic vasculitis (tumour, infection, or torsion of the spermatic cord) [1–4], arteritis that affects only the testis and/or epididymis [5, 6] or spermatic cord [7] have been reported. The testicle is the most frequently affected organ, followed by the epididymis and, less frequently, the spermatic cord. In some cases, both testicles and epididymides are involved, usually in a metachronous manner [8, 9] (Figs. 3.1, 3.2, 3.3, 3.4, and 3.5).

Histologically, the vascular lesions of the most frequent isolated testicular, epididymal or spermatic cord arteritis are similar to those of PAN, while most of the remaining lesions correspond to lesions like those of granulomatosis with polyangiitis (Wegener's disease). There are minor differences between isolated testicular PAN and testicular involvement in systemic PAN: a lack of thrombosis and the formation of aneurysms or the development of infarcts in the testicular parenchyma [10, 11]. In rare cases, testicular parenchymal necrosis can affect both testicles [12] and only organs of the urogenital tract such as the testis and bladder [13]. Also rarely, there may be recurrent testicular involvement [14].

The aetiology of localized arteritis is unknown, although the possibility that isolated arteritis represents a local type III hypersensitivity reaction has been seriously considered. This isolated arteritis may also affect other organs such as the appendix, gall bladder, breast, pancreas, uterus, uterine cervix, synovium, kidney, skeletal muscle, and seminal vesicle. In any case, if there is histological evidence of arteritis affecting the testis or epididymis, the necessary clinical, haematological, and biochemical studies must be performed in order to exclude a systemic disease such as PAN or granulomatosis with polyangiitis. The prognosis of isolated testicular arteritis is excellent even without steroid treatment [15, 16].

Fig. 3.1 Isolated testicular vasculitis. A 42-year-old patient with pain and swelling of the left cryptorchid testicle. The artery below the albuginea has fibrinoid necrosis of the wall and a circumferential infiltrate around it. The seminiferous tubules are hyalinized or contain only Sertoli cells

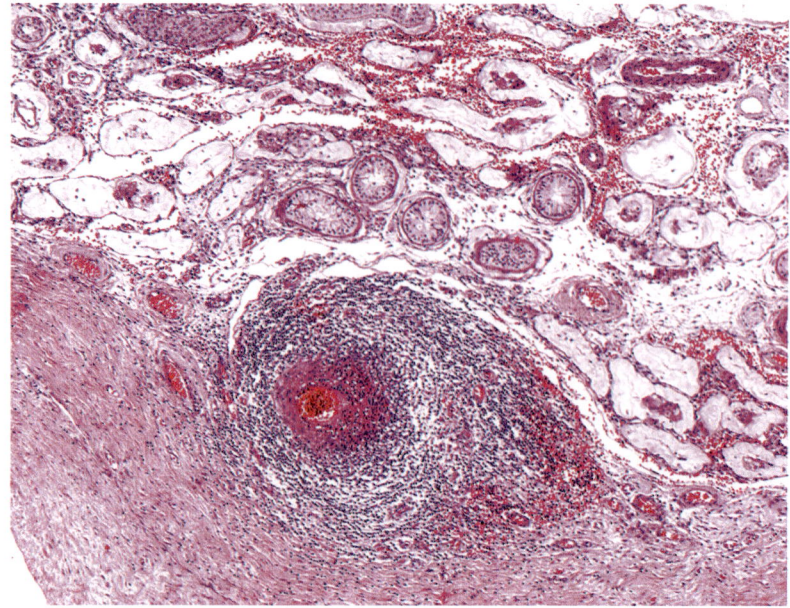

Fig. 3.2 Isolated testicular vasculitis. Intraparenchymal arteriole with fibrinoid necrosis of the wall and perivascular lymphoid infiltrates. The seminiferous tubules are completely sclerosed

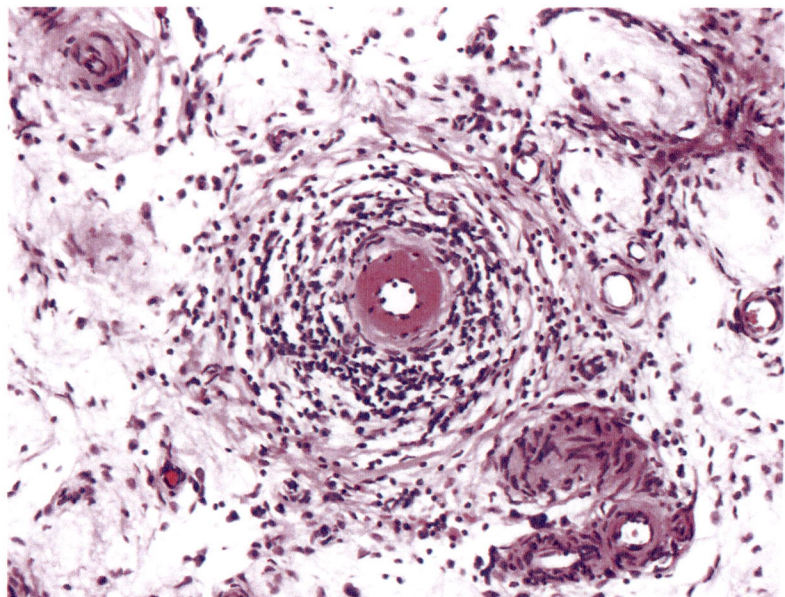

Fig. 3.3 Isolated
vasculitis of the
epididymis. In the area
opposite the section of
the epididymal duct
there is a small arteriole
with fibrinoid necrosis
of the wall surrounded
by lymphoid infiltrates

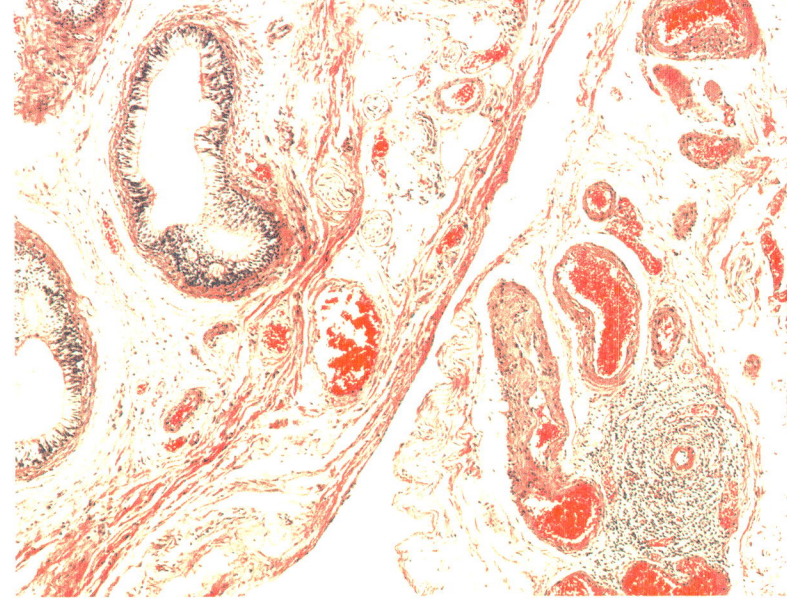

Fig. 3.4 Isolated
vasculitis of the
spermatic cord. The
arteriole shows a small
lumen and multiple
areas of fibrinoid
necrosis in the intima
and media layers. In the
thickened adventitia
there are lymphoid
infiltrates

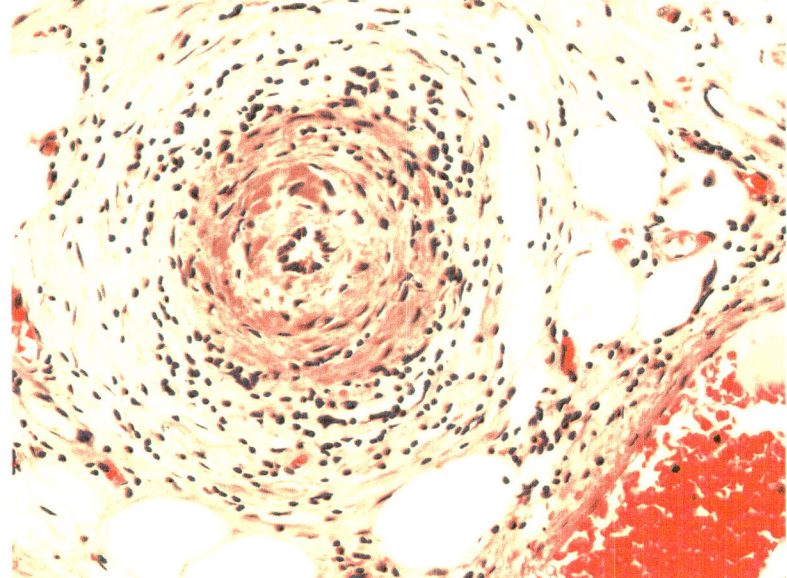

Fig. 3.5 Isolated vasculitis of the spermatic cord. In the connective tissue surrounding the cremaster muscle, there is a dense inflammatory infiltrate surrounding two arterioles with fibrinoid necrosis of their wall

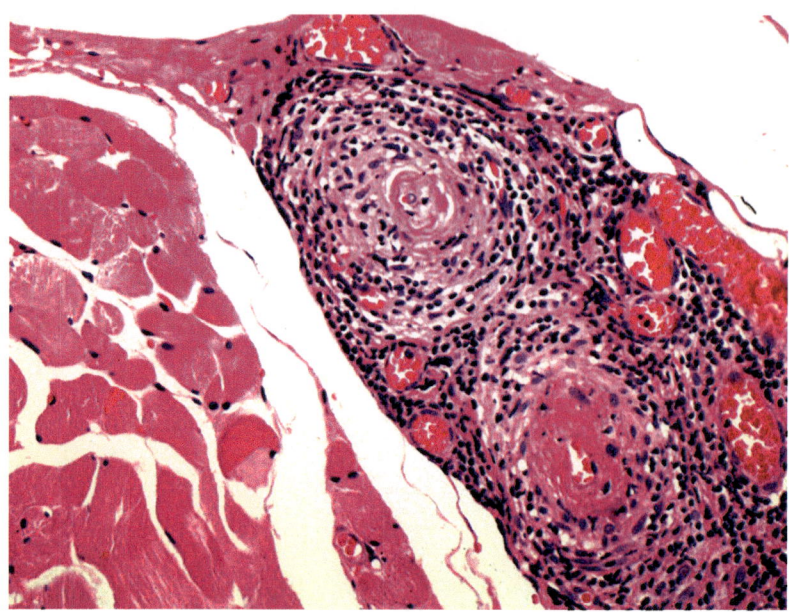

3.2 Testicular Vasculitis Associated with Germ Cell Tumour

The association of isolated vasculitis of the male genital tract with extragenital malignant tumours has been observed in rare cases of prostate adenocarcinoma, hepatocellular carcinoma, and acute myeloid leukaemia [17, 18]. In all three situations, the arterial lesions were similar to that of panarteritis nodosa.

The association of isolated vasculitis of the testis, epididymis, and spermatic cord with a testicular tumour, although reported only once in the literature [19] is not that exceptional in our experience. Vasculitis of the spermatic cord, epididymal or intratesticular vessels was reported in six cases, in patients with both seminomatous and nonseminomatous tumours. The vascular lesions strongly resemble those of Wegener's disease (granulomatosis with polyangiitis) in patients with pure seminoma or with a seminoma component in a mixed tumour as well as those of PAN in patients with nonseminomatous tumours.

3.2.1 Testicular Granulomatosis Polyangiitis-Like Granulomatosis Associated with Seminoma

The presence of granulomas in the testicle is generally associated with an infectious process (mycobacteria, fungi), autoimmune (idiopathic granulomatous orchitis) or germ cell tumours such as seminoma. In four cases, that is two pure seminomas and two other tumours with a combined seminomatous component, granulomatous vasculitis was observed, both in intratumoural vessels and in vessels at the periphery of the tumour, and in one case in epididymal arteries. The lesions were centred on a small-sized artery with very marked thickening of the medial layer and intense stenosis of the lumen. Lesions in some vessels were transmural but were more often preferentially located in the media and adventitia. The inflammatory infiltrate in some vessels was circumferential and in others focal or segmental. This infiltrate was characterized by the presence of abundant epithelioid cells and multinucleated giant cells associated with a small number of lymphocytes (Figs. 3.6, 3.7, 3.8, and 3.9). None of the patients had clinical or laboratory symptoms of Wegener's granulomatosis.

Fig. 3.6 Testicular vasculitis associated with seminoma. The artery presents stenosis of the lumen, without thrombosis, a crown of epithelioid cells surrounded by lymphocytes. Peripherally a sheet of tumour cells is observed

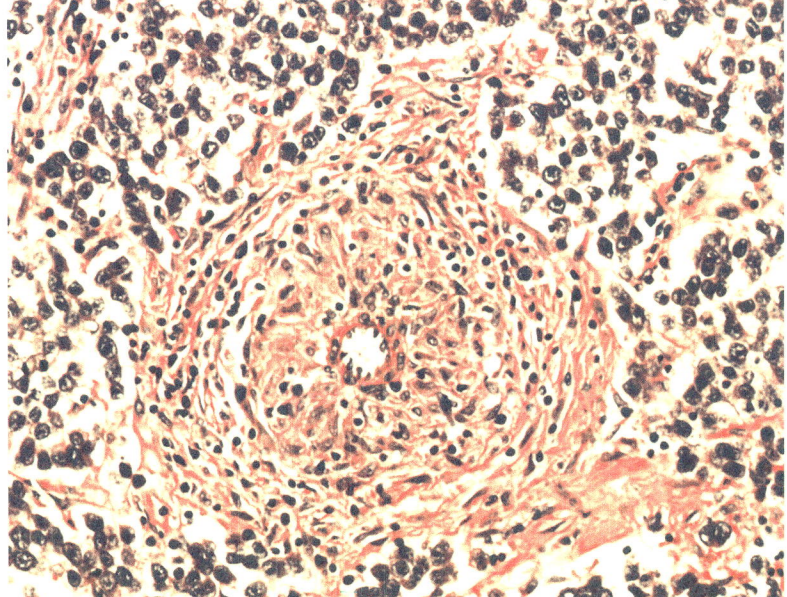

Fig. 3.7 Testicular vasculitis associated with seminoma. The arterial wall shows inflammatory infiltrates in the medial and adventitial layers. In the latter, they are more abundant and epithelioid cells predominate

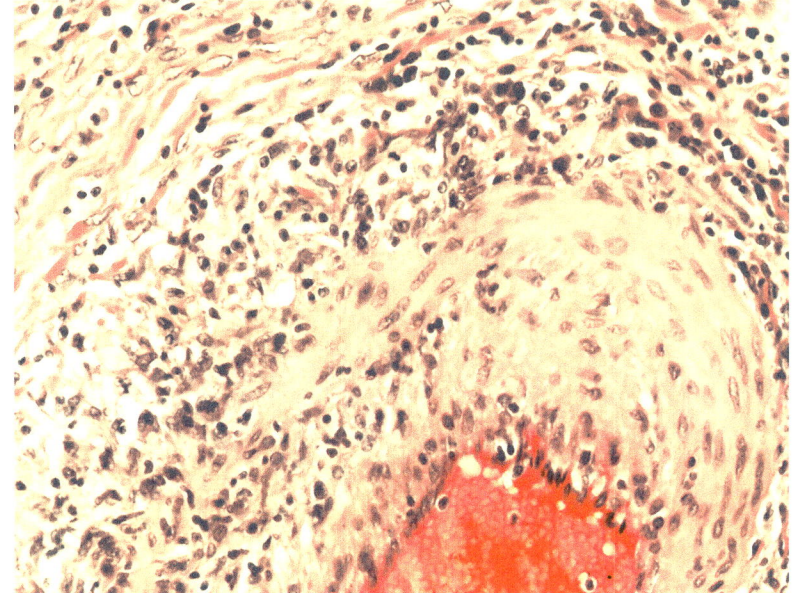

3.2.2   PAN-Like Vasculitis and Combined Nonseminomatous Germ Cell Tumour

This has been observed in patients with embryonal carcinoma alone as well as in patients in whom embryonal carcinoma is a component of mixed tumours. Patients show preferential involvement of the vessels of the spermatic cord and epididymis. The affected vessels show lesions at different evolutionary times; some of the vessels had transmural fibrinoid necrosis that could be segmental or circumferential and the infiltrates mainly consist of neutrophilic granulocytes with mononuclear cells (Figs. 3.10 and 3.11). Other vessels show reparative lesions with nonspecific infiltrates and fibrosis. It has been

Fig. 3.8 Testicular
vasculitis associated
with seminoma. Cross
section of an artery with
luminal stenosis,
hypertrophy of the
medial layer and two
granulomatous lesions in
the adventitia.
Externally, it has a
fibrous ring and
peripherally a significant
lymphoid infiltrate

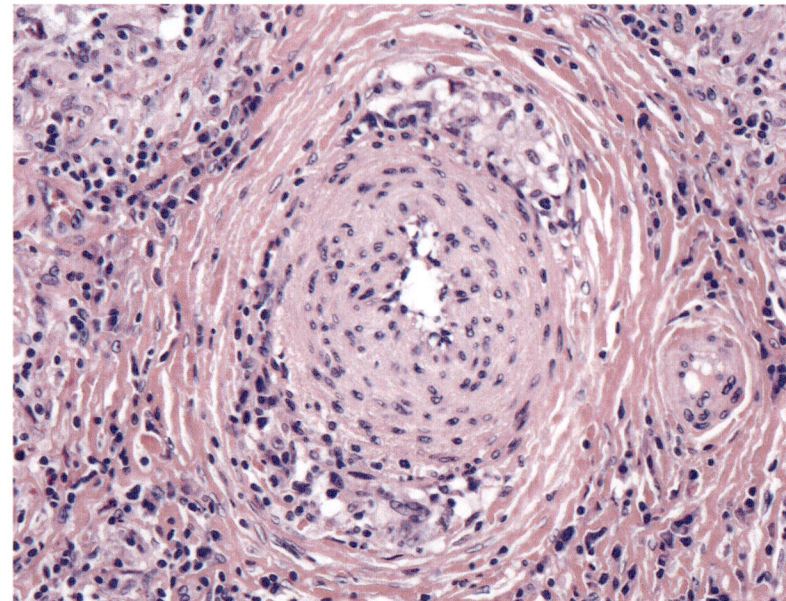

Fig. 3.9 Vasculitis of
the epididymis
associated with
seminoma. Next to the
main duct of the
epididymis, there is a
longitudinally sectioned
vessel. Note the stenosis
of the lumen and the
dense granulomatous
infiltrate in the form of a
cuff along the vessel

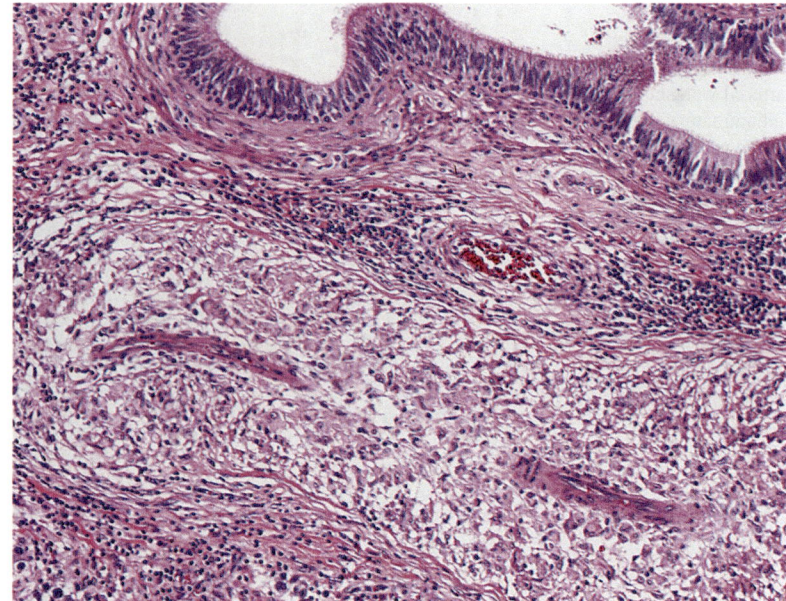

suggested that the lesions causing vascular damage are related to a cross-reaction between
tumour cell antibodies and endothelial cell antigens. The fact that only testicular vessels are
involved (in one case in the literature in which
another organ could be studied, vasculitis was not
observed in the pulmonary metastasis) is probably related to the tumoural microenvironment to
which the vessels are exposed [19].

3.2.3   Vasculitis in the Contralateral Testis

In two patients with germ cell tumour, the contralateral testicle was biopsied. In addition to
impaired spermatogenesis and absence of germ
cell neoplasia in situ (GCNIS), a small vessel
vasculitis was observed. In some vessels, it was
formed only by a dense infiltrate of T lympho-

Fig. 3.10 Vasculitis of the epididymis associated with a mixed germinal tumour with extensive areas of embryonal carcinoma. The arteriole located between the sections of the main duct of the epididymis has partial fibrinoid necrosis of the wall and lymphoid infiltrates around it

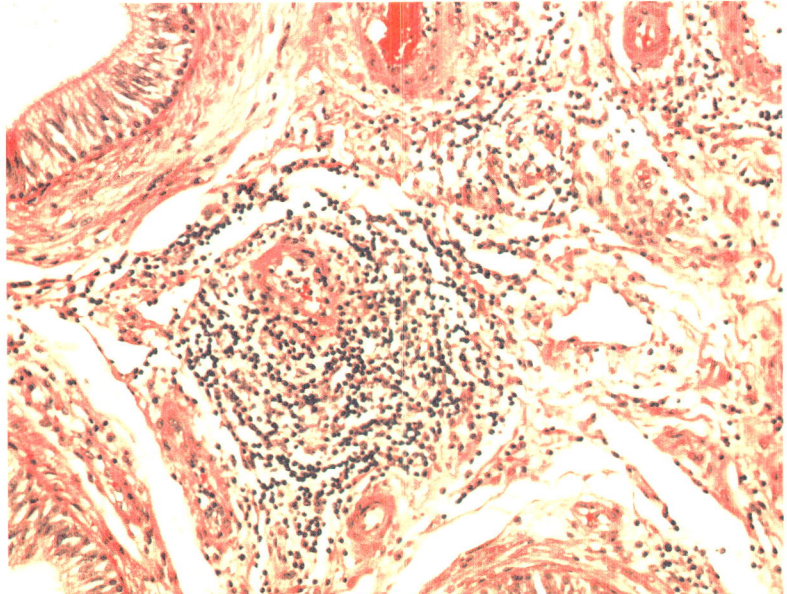

Fig. 3.11 Vasculitis of the spermatic cord associated with embryonal carcinoma. The vessel shows several areas of transmural fibrinoid necrosis. In relation to them, the inflammatory infiltrates of the intimal and adventitial layers are more intense

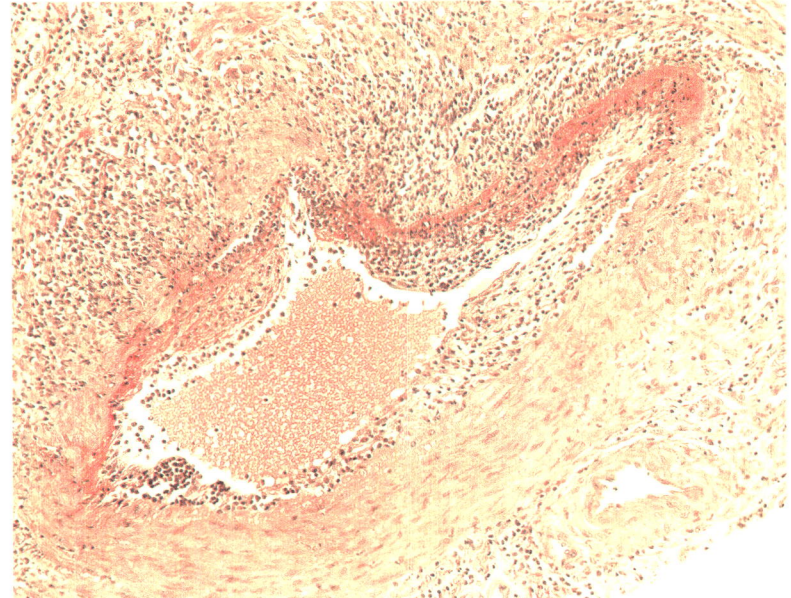

cytes in concentric rings simulating a lympho-cytic vasculitis (Fig. 3.12). In more advanced lesions, a mass of epithelioid cells was destroy-ing the vessel wall (Fig. 3.13). As both cases involved seminomas, which frequently show a significant sarcoid reaction, these vasculitis may be the result of a reaction to circulating antigens released by the tumour cells [20].

Fig. 3.12 Vasculitis in the contralateral "normal" testis in a patient with seminoma. Two non-thrombosed vessels with dense transmural and perivascular lymphoid infiltrates stand out between the seminiferous tubules

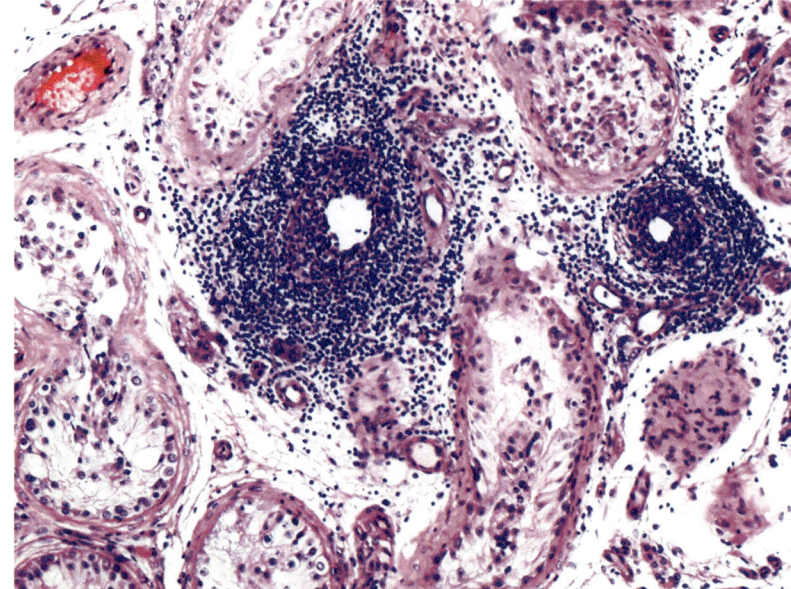

Fig. 3.13 Vasculitis in the contralateral "normal" testis in a patient with seminoma. The artery shows infiltrates in all layers. At the level of the middle layer lymphocytes predominate in some areas and in others epithelioid cells with large eosinophilic cytoplasm. The surrounding seminiferous tubules show only Sertoli cells with spherical nuclei and large eosinophilic cytoplasm

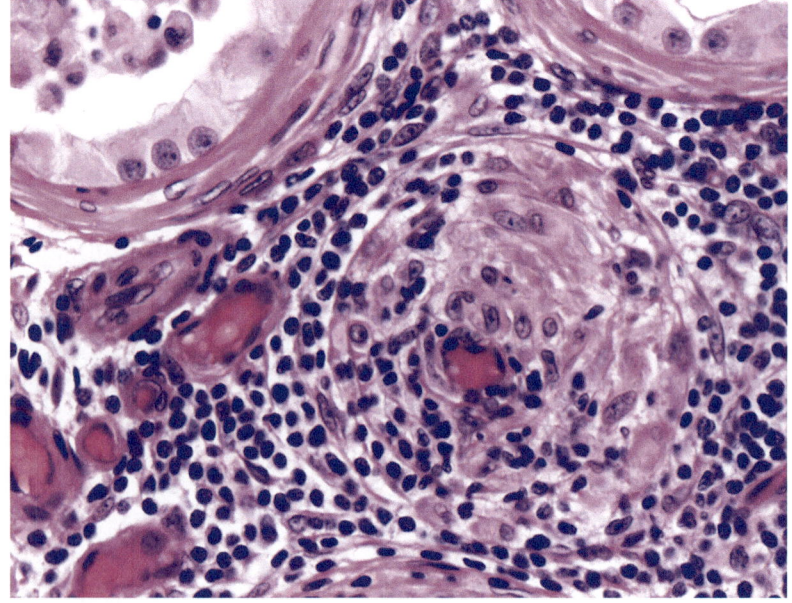

References

1. Pastor-Navarro H, Broseta-Viana L, Donate-Moreno MJ, Pastor-Guzmán JM, Lorenzo-Romero JG, Segura-Martín M, Salinas-Sánchez AS, Virseda-Rodríguez JA. Isolated testicular polyarteritis nodosa. Urology. 2007;70(1):178.

2. Atis G, Memis OF, Güngör HS, Arikan O, Saglican Y, Caskurlu T. Testicular polyarteritis nodosa mimicking testicular neoplasm. Sci World J. 2010;10:1915–8.

3. Brimo F, Lachapelle J, Epstein JI. Testicular vasculitis: a series of 19 cases. Urology. 2011;77:1043–8.

4. Islam N, Sinha D, Ghosh P, Datta C, Chatterjee U. Orchitis: an unusual presentation of polyarteritis nodosa. Indian J Pathol Microbiol. 2018;61:600.

5. Kessel A, Toubi E, Golan TD, Toubi A, Mogilner JG, Jaffe M. Isolated epididymal vasculitis. Isr Med Assoc J. 2001;3:65–6.

6. Maričić A, Stifter S, Valenčić M, Dorđević G, Markić D, Spanjol J, Sotošek S, Fučkar Z. Primary testicular necrotizing vasculitis clinically presented as neo-

plasm of the testicle: a case report. World J Surg Oncol. 2011;9:63.

7. Claeys E, Schockaert O. A funny case of Funiculitis. Acta Clin Belg. 2021;76:232–5.

8. Saito K, Washino S, Hirai M, Matuzaki A, Nokubi M, Terai C, Kobayashi Y. A case of isolated polyarteritis nodosa appeared in bilateral epididymides with asynchronous onset. Nihon Hinyokika Gakkai Zasshi. 2013;104:22–5.

9. Kechida M, Ktari K, Jellazi M, Mesfar R, Khochtali I, Saad H, Njim L. Simultaneous testicle and epididymis vasculitis revealing granulomatosis with polyangiitis. Clin Case Reports. 2022;10(8):e6231.

10. Muhammad SS, Epstein JI. Testicular vasculitis: implications of systemic disease. Hum Pathol. 1987;19:186–9.

11. Garg K, Dawson L. Single organ variant of polyarteritis nodosa in epididymis. J Cancer Res Ther. 2015;11:662.

12. Bhatia S, Herrera Hernandez LP, Kamboj AK, Rieck KM. Isolated polyarteritis nodosa presenting as bilateral testicular swelling. Am J Med. 2018;131(2):e55–6.

13. Stewart M, Marcotte G, Seidman MA, Dehghan N. Polyarteritis nodosa isolated to the testis and urinary bladder in the setting of cryptorchidism: a case report and literature review. J Med Case Rep. 2019;13:236.

14. Tanuma Y, Oda T, Yokoo A, Ito S, Takeuchi K. Recurrent polyarteritis nodosa limited to the testis. J Urol. 2003;170:1953.

15. Fraenkel-Rubin M, Ergas D, Sthoeger ZM. Limited polyarteritis nodosa of the male and female reproductive systems: diagnostic and therapeutic approach. Ann Rheum Dis. 2002;61:362–4.

16. Hernández-Rodríguez J, Tan CD, Koening CL, Khasnis A, Rodríguez ER, Hoffman GS. Testicular vasculitis: findings differentiating isolated disease from systemic disease in 72 patients. Medicine. 2012;91:75–85.

17. Shurbaji MS, Epstein JI. Testicular vasculitis: implications for systemic disease. Hum Pathol. 1988;19:186–9.

18. Lie JT. Isolated polyarteritis of testis in hairy-cell leukemia. Arch Pathol Lab Med. 1988;112:646–7.

19. Fleischmann A, Studer UE. Isolated polyarteritis nodosa of the male reproductive system associated with a germ cell tumor of the testis: a case report. Cardiovasc Pathol. 2007;16:354–6.

20. Nistal M, González-Peramato MP. Atlas on the human testis. In: Jezek D, editor. Vascular testis pathology. London: Springer; 2013. p. 243–51.

4.1 Cytomegalovirus-Associated Vasculitis of Testis and Epididymis

Human cytomegalovirus (HCMV) infection is very common in all countries. In developed countries, the proportion of adults with specific IgG antibodies approaches 60% and is nearly 90% in many developing countries. Infection is more prevalent in poorer socioeconomic countries and those with non-Caucasian backgrounds [1]. HCMV infection is the most frequent and the most serious opportunistic infection in immunocompromised patients such as those undergoing solid organ transplantation, haematopoietic stem cell transplantation, and individuals with HIV [2, 3]. It can sometimes present as a mild, self-limited syndrome, manifesting as retinitis or colitis or with severe involvement in the form of pneumonitis, hepatitis, or bone marrow suppression [4].

Cytomegalovirus-associated vasculitis is a rare manifestation that can affect any organ [5]. Cytomegalovirus-associated cutaneous vasculitis is considered the most severe and often lethal complication. Although most cases have been observed in immunocompromised patients, often transplant recipients or the HIV infected, it has also been observed in patients without these underlying conditions [6].

Vasculitis of the testis and epididymis may occur in the context of systemic HCMV involvement in immunocompromised patients and is often only an autopsy finding. It is a small vessel vasculitis, with segmental necrosis of the vascular wall, associated with two facts, a poor inflammatory reaction, and the presence of cytomegalovirus-related inclusion bodies in endothelial cells. Lesions can be observed in both the small vessels of the testis and epididymis (Figs. 4.1, 4.2, 4.3, 4.4, 4.5, and 4.6). The repercussions of vascular lesions on the testicular parenchyma, except for the presence of focal tubular atrophies, which could be secondary to ischemia, are difficult to determine, since they could also be attributed to the gonadotoxicity of the drugs used.

In general, treatment of HCMV-associated vasculitis includes early initiation of antiviral treatment and reduction of the immunosuppressive regimen as much as possible, including steroid therapy in cases where this therapy is being administered.

Fig. 4.1 Vasculitis
associated with
cytomegalovirus in a
hemophilic patient with
AIDS. Venule with
endothelial intranuclear
inclusion surrounded by
a characteristic clear
halo

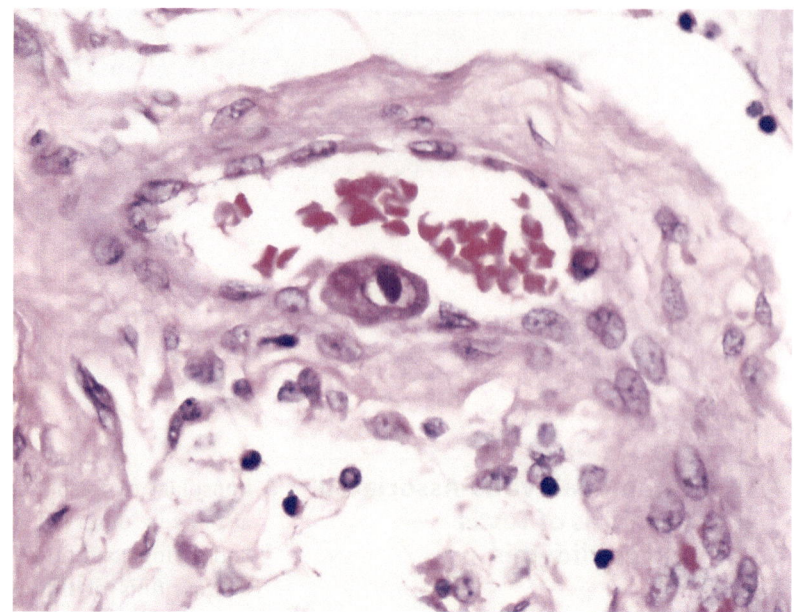

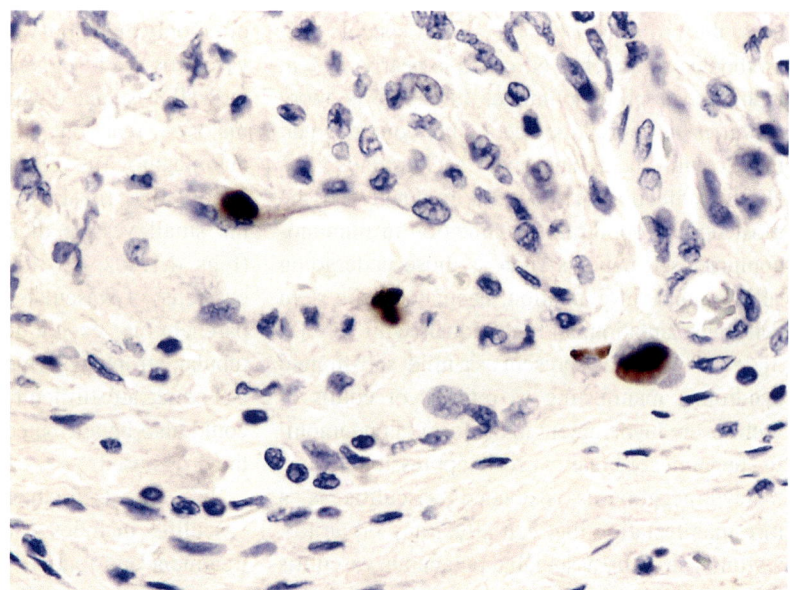

Fig. 4.2 Vasculitis
associated with
cytomegalovirus. Intense
positivity of the
endothelial intranuclear
inclusions to specific
antibodies

Fig. 4.3 Vasculitis associated with cytomegalovirus. Oblique section of an intraparenchymal vein. Focal destruction of the wall by an infiltrate of mostly polynuclear cells and some lymphocytes

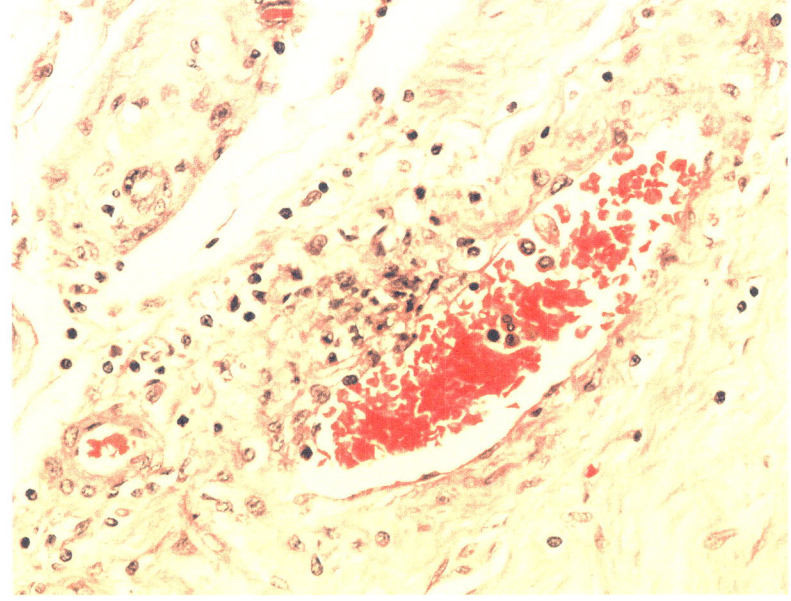

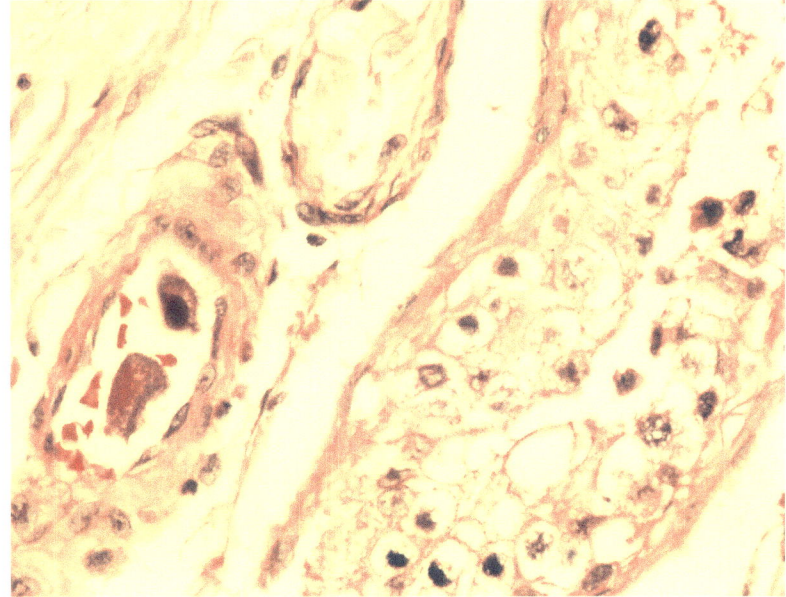

Fig. 4.4 Vasculitis associated with cytomegalovirus. Endothelial cell with a desquamated nuclear inclusion inside a vessel. The neighbouring seminiferous tubule shows only Sertoli cells as well as isolated spermatogonia and spermatocytes

Fig. 4.5 Vasculitis associated with cytomegalovirus. Intense positivity of the endothelial intranuclear inclusion with cytomegalovirus immunostaining in a vein. All seminiferous tubule cells are negative

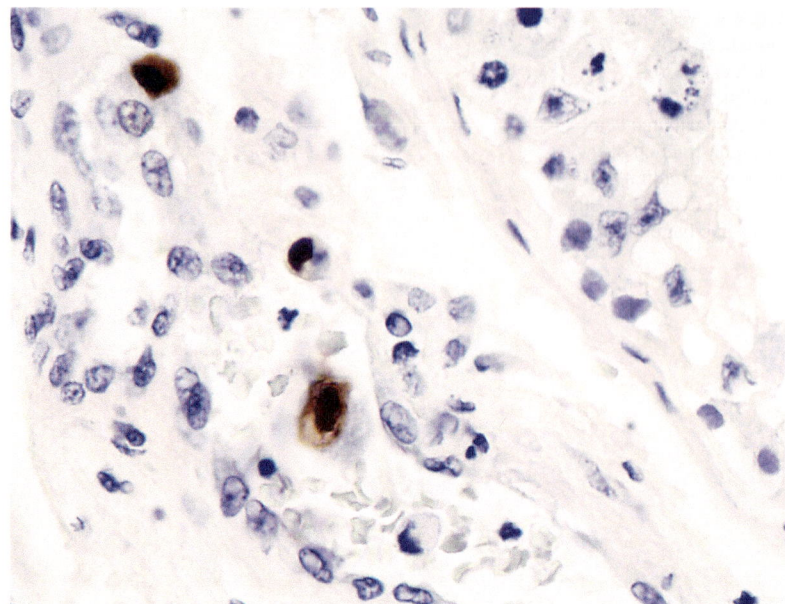

Fig. 4.6 Vasculitis associated with cytomegalovirus. In most of the small vessels of the epididymis, there are some endothelial cells with intranuclear inclusions (immunostaining for cytomegalovirus)

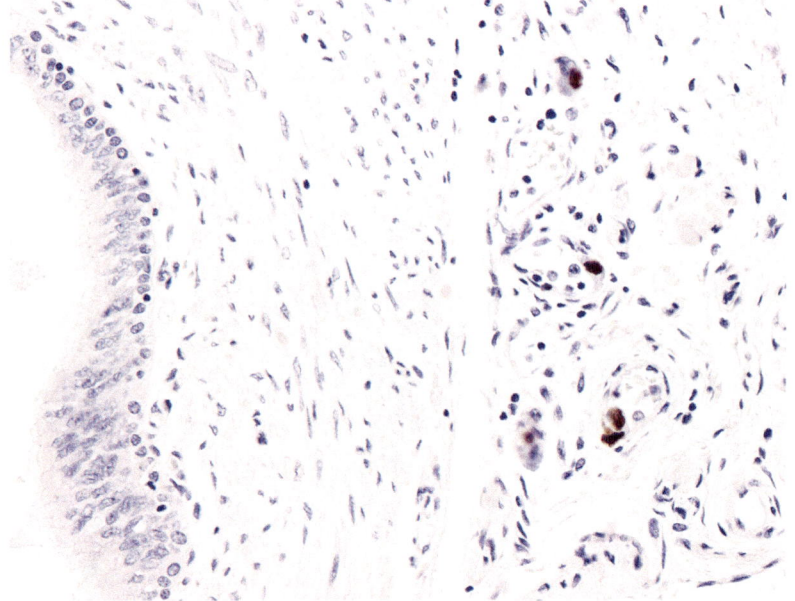

4.2   SARS-Cov-2-Associated Vasculitis of the Testis and Epididymis

Among the undesirable effects of the vaccines used in COVID-19 are among others orchioepidididymitis, thrombotic phenomena, thrombopenia and vasculitis. Vasculitis have been observed in other viriasis following vaccination (influenza) [7], affecting in most cases small vessels. SARS-Cov-2 is believed to induce a systemic small vessel vasculitis similar to that seen in IgA vasculitis (Henoch-Schönlein purpura) [8, 9] and less frequently necrotizing medium vessel vasculitis, ANCA negative with lesions similar to those of polyarteritis nodosa [10].

4.3   Necrotizing Vasculitis in Whipple's Disease

Whipple's disease is an infectious, multisystemic disease caused by the bacterium *Tropheryma whipplei*. It is a ubiquitous bacterium in sewage or stagnant water. It preferentially affects males aged 40–50 years of Caucasian descent. The most frequent symptoms are quite unspecific: fever, arthralgias, abdominal pain, diarrhoea, and weight loss [11]. Resistance to the usual treatments or repeated recurrence of diarrhoea, weight loss, and malabsorption are strongly suggestive of the infection [12–14]. Intestinal biopsy findings are pathognomonic (Fig. 4.7). In less than half a dozen cases, cutaneous manifestations appear early in the disease; the urticaria, hyperpigmentation erythroderma, and subcutaneous nodules are non-specific and are related to malnutrition. The histology of dermal lesions is varied, ranging from panniculitis [15, 16] to eosinophilic vasculitis [17].

Vascular involvement in Whipple's disease preferentially affects the media of the coronary arteries and the small hepatic and intestinal arteries [18]. Less frequently, it affects arteries of the spleen and kidney and, even less frequently, the small arteries of the lung and exceptionally, large vessels like the aorta [19, 20]. In the study of coronary arteries, there are three patterns that have the peculiarity of being focal and presenting different histological patterns along the course of the artery [21]. These patterns are: (1) Extensive invasion of the medial layer and, to a lesser degree the intimal layer, by PAS-positive bacilli, first free, then intracellular, with few inflammatory signs. (2) Panarteritis of variable intensity with or without bacilli. (3) Reparative fibrosis.

The involvement of testicular vessels has not been reported in the literature. In the autopsy of a case from our department, we found vascular lesions in all the structures, as already mentioned in the literature, except the skin, together with intestinal and lymph node involvement, preferably retroperitoneal. In our study of the testis, we observed marked tubular atrophy with wall thickening and ischemic areas in which all testicular structures had disappeared (Fig. 4.8). The contents of the tubules were reduced to spermatogonia and Sertoli cells or only Sertoli cells. The cytoplasm of these cells contained multiple refractile granulations that were identified by PAS as large accumulations of bacilli and confirmed by electron microscopy (Figs. 4.9, 4.10, 4.11, and 4.12). The interstitium showed sparse Leydig cells, small clusters of macrophages with numerous PAS-positive bacilli, and diffuse lymphocytic infiltrates (Fig. 4.13).

The most striking finding was in the small vessels, mostly arterioles. They showed a focal,

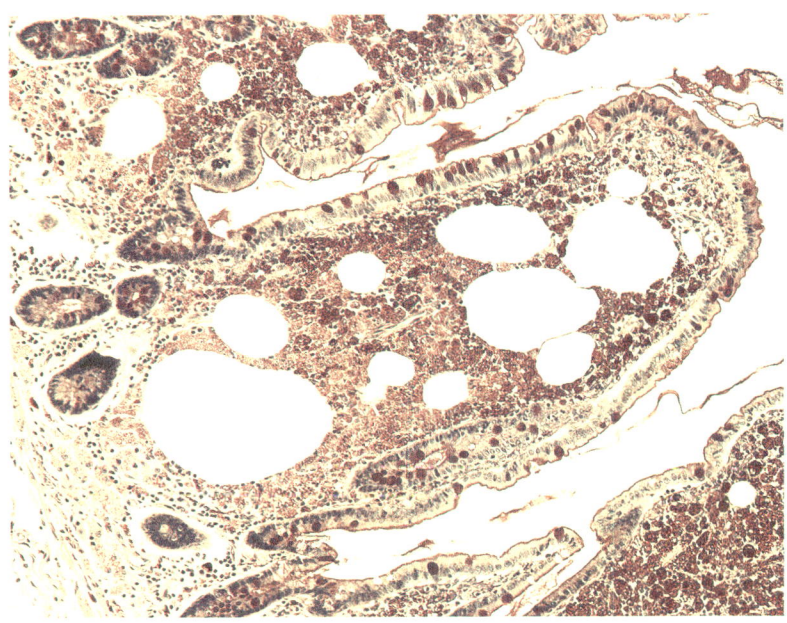

Fig. 4.7 Testicular necrotizing vasculitis in Whipple's disease. Young patient with cachexia who died without diagnosis. The intestinal villi show the alterations in the lamina propria characteristic of Whipple's disease: large accumulations of PAS-positive macrophages and optically empty spaces

Fig. 4.8 Testicular necrotizing vasculitis in Whipple's disease. Extensive ischemic atrophy of the testicular parenchyma. Some preserved seminiferous tubules are recognized only under the albuginea

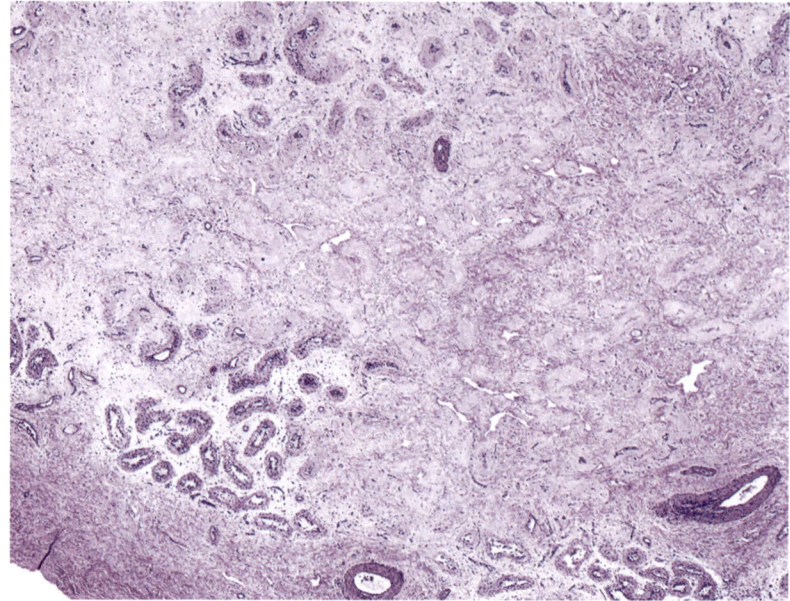

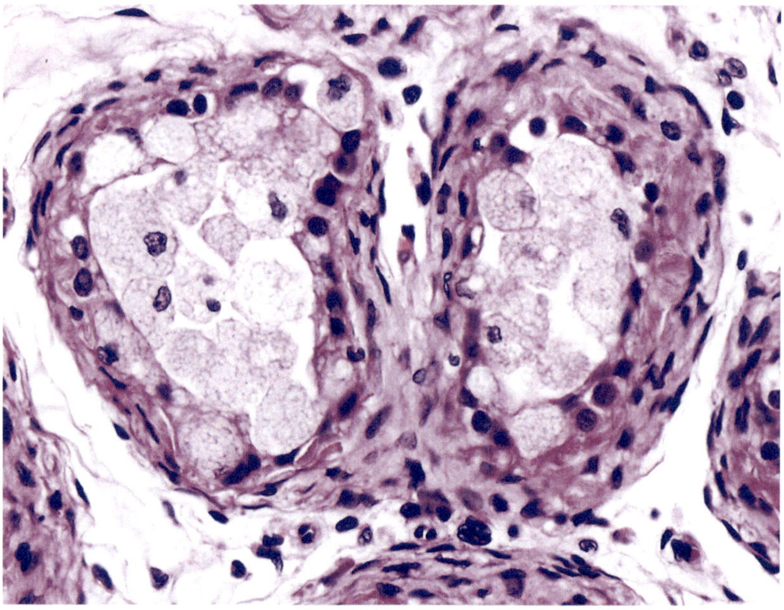

Fig. 4.9 Testicular necrotizing vasculitis in Whipple's disease. Cross section of two seminiferous tubules. Both show wall thickening, absence of lumen and a seminiferous epithelium consisting of isolated spermatogonia and Sertoli cells. These cells have a globular microvacuolated cytoplasm

necrotic lesion of the wall that affected all the layers. The only inflammatory cells present were some polynuclear cells with leukocytoclasia, isolated eosinophils, and lymphocytes (Figs. 4.14 and 4.15). No bacilli were recognizable/identified at this level. Most of the lesions were at the same evolutionary stage. The patient had not received previous treatments, so a relationship of the vasculitis with Whipple's disease seems very possible.

Whipple's disease has also been described in association with a necrotizing granulomatous arteritis with giant cells, located in the upper pole of the epididymis. PAS-positive bacilli were not observed in the vasculitis. The possibility of a common aetiology, either infectious or immune, and perhaps mediated by circulating immune complexes, has been suggested [22].

Fig. 4.10 Testicular necrotizing vasculitis in Whipple's disease. Sections of several small caliber seminiferous tubules showing intense PAS positivity of the Sertoli cell cytoplasm

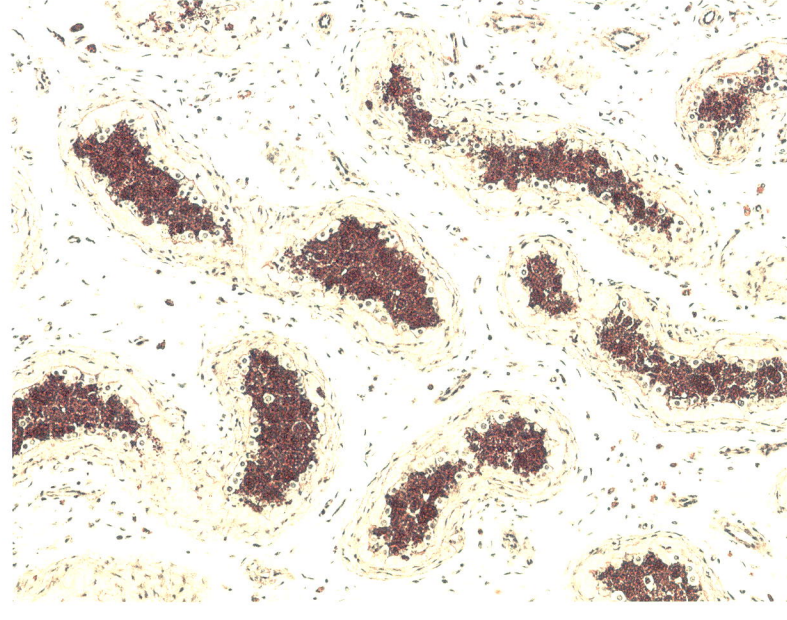

Fig. 4.11 Testicular necrotizing vasculitis in Whipple's disease. Longitudinal section of a seminiferous tubule. Of note is the presence of large accumulations of PAS-positive bacilli in the cytoplasm of the Sertoli cells. The spermatogonia and tubular wall cells appear free of bacteria

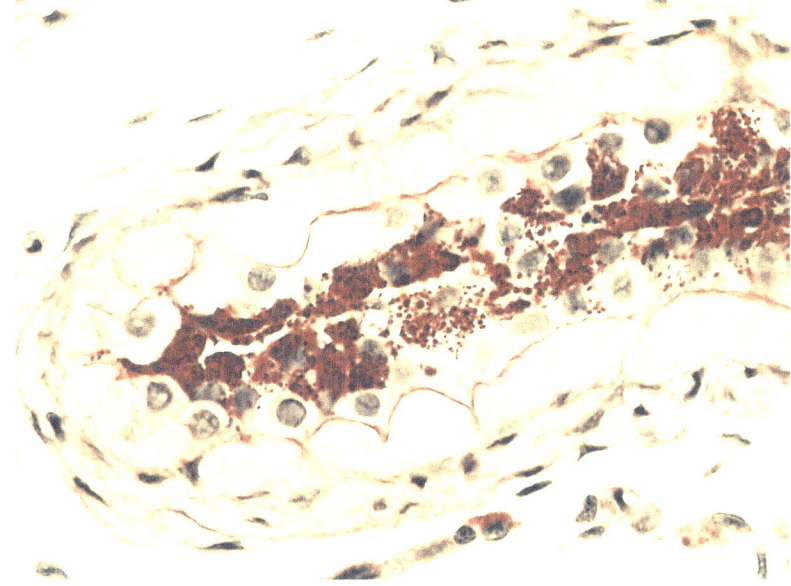

Fig. 4.12 Testicular necrotizing vasculitis in Whipple's disease. Transverse and oblique sections of a cluster of bacilli in the cytoplasm of a Sertoli cell seen under the electron microscope

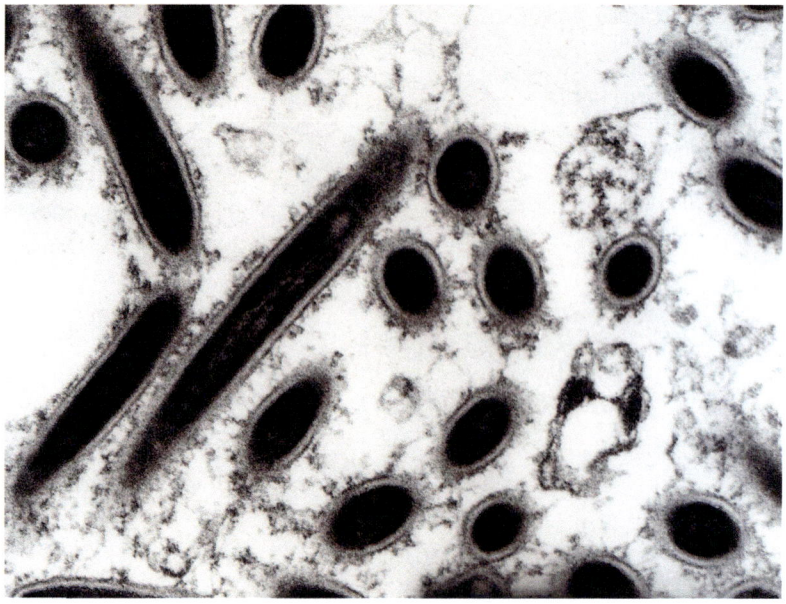

Fig. 4.13 Testicular necrotizing vasculitis in Whipple's disease. In the edematous interstitium, there are abundant macrophages and some lymphocytes. The macrophages are large and show eosinophilic and granular inclusions, some of which are PAS positive

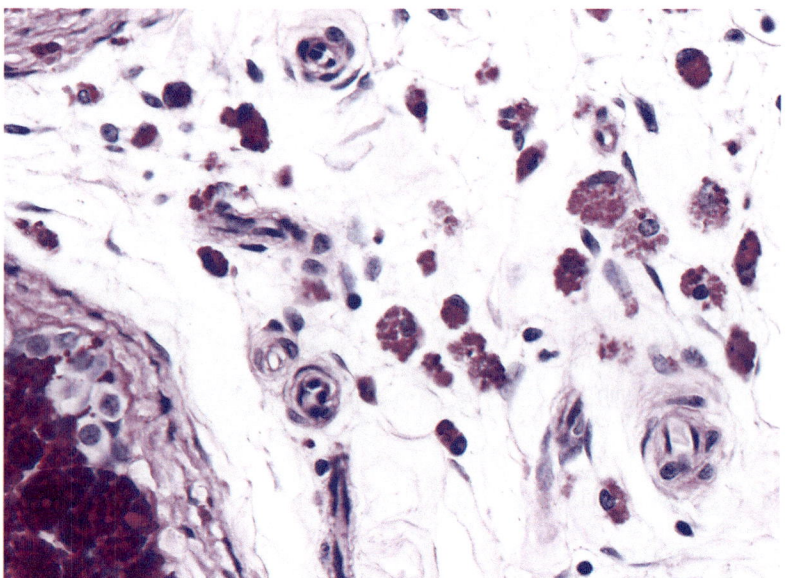

Fig. 4.14 Testicular necrotizing vasculitis in Whipple's disease. Focal necrosis of the wall of an arteriole associated with a polynuclear infiltrate. Peripherally, lymphocytes are also observed in the wall and in the interstitium

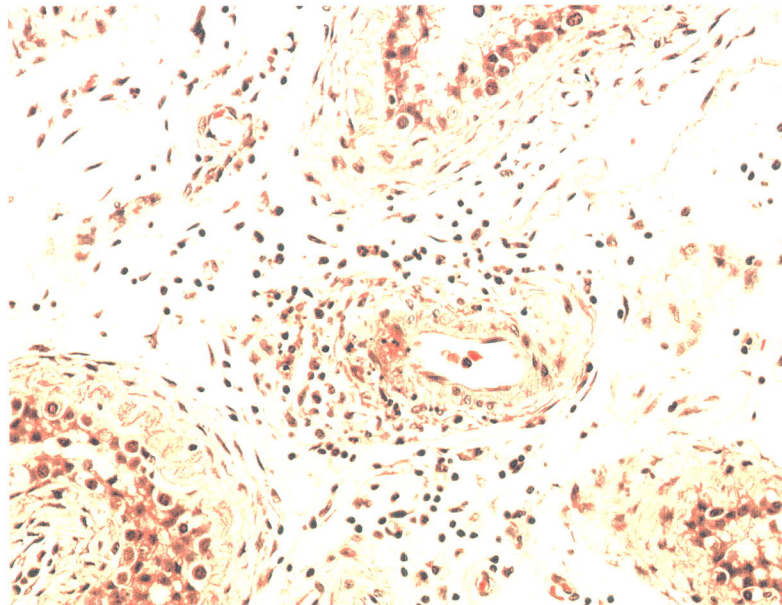

Fig. 4.15 Testicular necrotizing vasculitis in Whipple's disease. In the wall of the arteriole, there is an area of necrosis with polynuclear, karyorrhexis, and lymphocytes. The seminiferous tubules show only Sertoli cells and spermatogonia

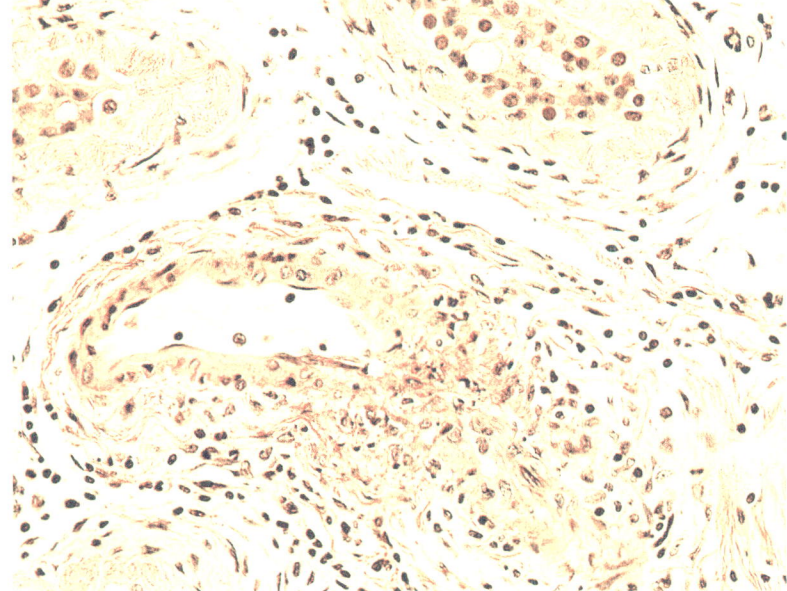

References

1. Zuhair M, Smit GSA, Wallis G, Jabbar F, Smith C, Devleesschauwer B, Griffiths P. Estimation of the worldwide seroprevalence of cytomegalovirus: a systematic review and meta-analysis. Rev Med Virol. 2019;29(3):e2034.

2. Boeckh M, Nichols WG. The impact of cytomegalovirus serostatus of donor and recipient before hematopoietic stem cell transplantation in the era of antiviral prophylaxis and preemptive therapy. Blood. 2004;103:2003–8.

3. Deayton JR, Prof Sabin CA, Johnson MA, Emery VC, Wilson P, Griffiths PD. Importance of cytomegalovirus viraemia in risk of disease progression and death in HIV-infected patients receiving highly active antiretroviral therapy. Lancet. 2004;363:2116–21.

4. Griffiths P, Reeves M. Pathogenesis of human cytomegalovirus in the immunocompromised host. Nat Rev Microbiol. 2021;19:759–73.

5. D'Alessandro M, Buoncompagni A, Minoia F, Coccia MC, Martini A, Picco P. Cytomegalovirus-related necrotising vasculitis mimicking Henoch-Schönlein syndrome. Clin Exp Rheumatol. 2014;32(3):73–5.

6. Golden MP, Hammer SM, Wanke CA, Albrecht MA. Cytomegalovirus vasculitis. Case reports and review of the literature. Medicine. 1994;73:246–55.
7. Bonetto C, Trotta F, Felicetti P, Alarcón GS, Santuccio C, Bachtiar NS, Brauchli Pernus Y, Chandler R, Girolomoni G, Hadden RD, Kucuku M, Ozen S, Pahud B, Top K, Varricchio F, Wise RP, Zanoni G, Živković S, Bonhoeffer J; Brighton Collaboration Vasculitis Working Group. Vasculitis as an adverse event following immunization - Systematic literature review. Vaccine. 2016;34:6641–51.
8. Prabhahar A, Naidu GSRSNK, Chauhan P, Sekar A, Sharma A, Sharma A, Kumar A, Nada R, Rathi M, Kohli HS, Ramachandran R. ANCA-associated vasculitis following ChAdOx1 nCoV19 vaccination: case-based review. Rheumatol Int. 2022;42:749.
9. Grossman ME, Appel G, Little AJ, Ko CJ. Post-COVID-19 vaccination IgA vasculitis in an adult. J Cutan Pathol. 2022;49:385–87.
10. Ohkubo Y, Ohmura SI, Ishihara R, Miyamoto T. Transient Pneumonitis as a Possible Adverse Reaction to the BNT162b2 COVID-19 mRNA Vaccine in a Patient with Rheumatoid Arthritis: A Case Report and Review of the Literature. Case Rep Rheumatol. 2022;2022:3124887.
11. Lagier JC, Lepidi H, Raoult D, Fenollar F. Systemic Tropheryma whipplei: clinical presentation of 142 patients with infections diagnosed or confirmed in a reference center. Medicine. 2010;89:337–45.
12. Fleming JL, Wiesner RH, Shorter RG. Whipple's disease: clinical, biochemical, and histopathologic features and assessment of treatment in 29 patients. Mayo Clin Proc. 1988;63:539–51.
13. Durand DV, Lecomte C, Cathébras P, Rousset H, Godeau P. Whipple disease. Clinical review of 52 cases. The SNFMI Research Group on Whipple Disease. Société Nationale Française de Médecine Interne. Medicine. 1997;76:170–84.
14. Arnold CA, Moreira RK, Lam-Himlin D, De Petris G, Montgomery E. Whipple disease a century after the initial description: increased recognition of unusual presentations, autoimmune comorbidities, and therapy effects. Am J Surg Pathol. 2012;36:1066–73.
15. Tarroch X, Vives P, Salas A, Moré J. Subcutaneous nodules in Whipple's disease. J Cutan Pathol. 2001;28:368–70.
16. Friedmann AC, Perera GK, Jayaprakasam A, Forgacs I, Salisbury JR, Creamer D. Whipple's disease presenting with symmetrical panniculitis. Br J Dermatol. 2004;151:907–11.
17. Al-Hamoudi W, Habbab F, Nudo C, Nahal A, Flegel K. Eosinophilic vasculitis: a rare presentation of Whipple's disease. Can J Gastroenterol. 2007;21:189–91.
18. Lopes A, Santos AF, Alvarenga MJ, Mello E, Silva A. Whipple's disease: a rare case of malabsorption. BMJ Case Rep. 2018;2018:bcr2017222955.
19. Razanamahery J, Humbert S, Gil H, Bouiller K, Magy-Bertrand N. Tropheryma Whipplei infection mimicking giant cell arteritis flare in a patient treated with interleukin-6 receptor blocker tocilizumab. Clin Exp Rheumatol. 2020;124:245–6.
20. Depascale R, Pizzi M, Padoan R. Whipple's aortitis. Rheumatology. 2022;61(9):e294.
21. James TN, Haubrich WS. De subitaneis mortibus. XIV. Bacterial arteritis in Whipple's disease. Circulation. 1975;52:722–31.
22. Middlekauff HR, Fang MA, Hahn BH. Polyarteritis nodosa of the epididymis in a patient with Whipple's disease. J Rheumatol. 1987;14:1193–5.

5.1 Vasculitis Associated with Treatment with Oestrogens and Antiandrogens in Patients with Gender Identity Dysphoria

The action of oestrogens on the testicular parenchyma has been known for a long time, especially noted in studies of hormonal treatment of patients with prostate carcinoma [1–3], but without histological studies referring to vascular alterations. It has been known for decades that oestrogens can protect against the development of cardiovascular diseases [4], but it has also been observed that these hormones can participate in the development of arteriosclerosis [5, 6]. Oestrogens have been classically related to the development of varicose veins [7, 8], and, particularly, to venous thromboembolism as the use of combined oral contraceptives is responsible for 22,000 cases each year in Europe [9]. This pathology is facilitated by the changes produced by oestrogens in the levels of coagulation factors. It increases procoagulant factors, decreases anticoagulant factors, and alters fibrinolysis [10]. All this has instigated strategies to obtain new formulations that reduce the risk of venous thromboembolism [11]. Oestrogens have also been related to hepatic vascular disorders, such as vasculitis and peliosis [12], and with triggering strokes and myocardial infarctions [13]. Only a minority of patients develop systemic vasculitis [14].

Currently, treatment with oestrogens and antiandrogens is part of the transition process from male to female, so every day more and more people request hormone therapy despite the side effects of these treatments [13, 15, 16]. Prolonged treatment with high doses of oestrogens associated or not with antiandrogens has been especially studied by our group in a series of 62 bilateral orchiectomy specimens in patients with gender identity disorders, all of them asymptomatic. Apart from the logical changes of tubular atrophy, loss of spermatogenesis and Leydig cell atrophy caused by these treatments, the most surprising fact is the development of vascular lesions [17].

Forty percent of patients presented vascular lesions both in vessels of the spermatic cord or epididymis and intratesticular vessels. The affected vessels showed different types of lesions. In larger ones, arteriosclerosis predominates, and in small ones vasculitis (Fig. 5.1). Leaving aside arteriosclerosis, which will be discussed in another section, vasculitis was observed in nine cases. The histological pattern of vasculitis was highly variable. Sometimes it affected only one sector of the wall, involving all the layers of the vessel, without associated necrosis. Lymphocytes predominated in the infiltrates in all cases. Specifically in small vessels, preferably arteri-

Fig. 5.1 A 37-year-old patient with gender identity disorder and a history of treatment with oestrogens and antiandrogens for years. Vessels of the tunica vasculosa. The transversely sectioned artery has fibrous wall thickening, the most deeply situated artery shows fibrinoid necrosis with transmural inflammatory infiltrates. The veins show no alterations. The seminiferous tubules are sclerosed. Masson trichrome staining

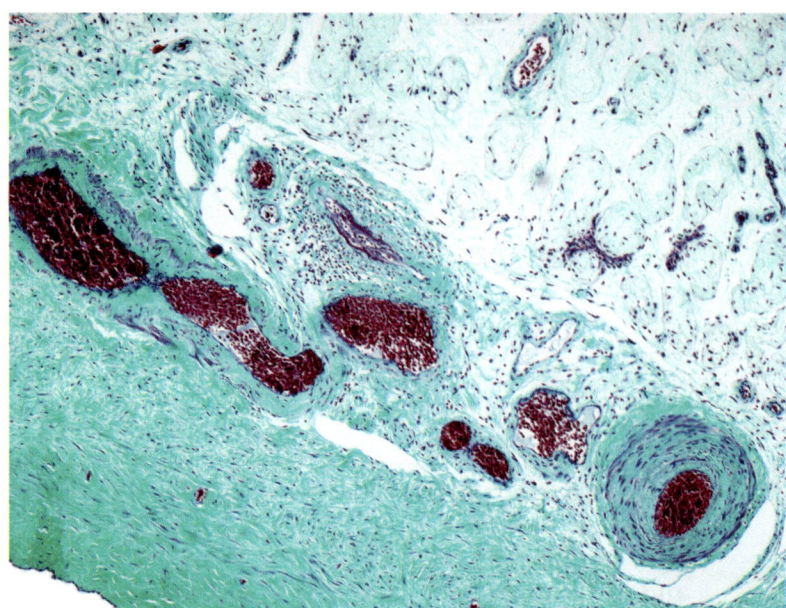

Fig. 5.2 Vasculitis and oestrogen therapy. Several sections of a small intraparenchymal artery with circumferential fibrinoid necrosis and abundant lymphoid infiltrates in the medial and adventitial layers. It is surrounded by sclerosed seminiferous tubules

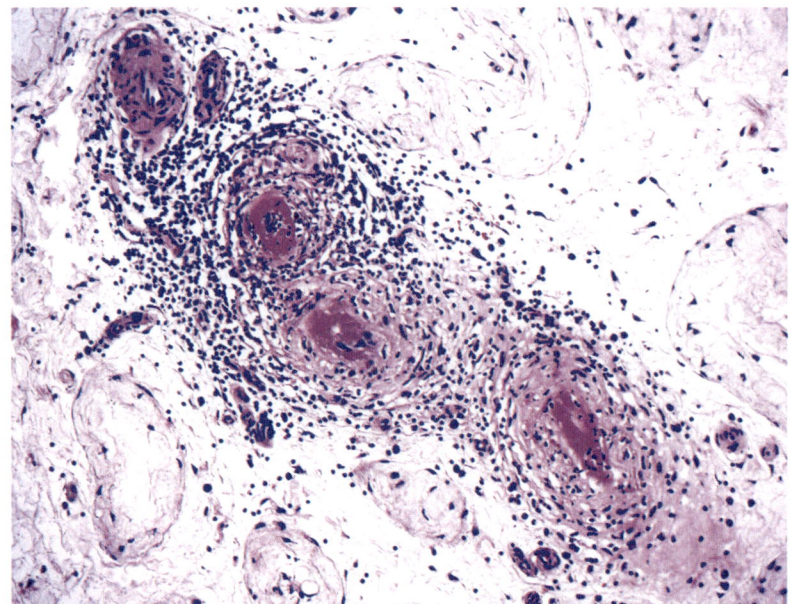

oles, the predominant lesions were like those of PAN, showing vasculitis with fibrinoid necrosis of the wall, either segmental or circumferential, and a marked lymphocyte infiltrate in the adventitia (Fig. 5.2).

The lesions of the capillaries and venules mainly consisted of endothelial swelling and perivascular lymphoid rings (Fig. 5.3). The lesions were observed in two cases in parates-

ticular structures (vaginal, epididymis, and spermatic cord vessels) (Figs. 5.4, 5.5, and 5.6). This fact seems of special importance, since, if we remember that isolated testicular vasculitis is only present in 0.003% of all surgical specimens [18, 19], this group of patients presents vasculitis in more than 9% of cases. Therefore, it cannot be excluded that in some cases there is a systemic vasculitis.

Fig. 5.3 Vasculitis and oestrogen therapy. Subalbugineal venule with segmental involvement of the wall consisting of endothelial swelling and accumulation of lymphoid cells in the media and adventitia

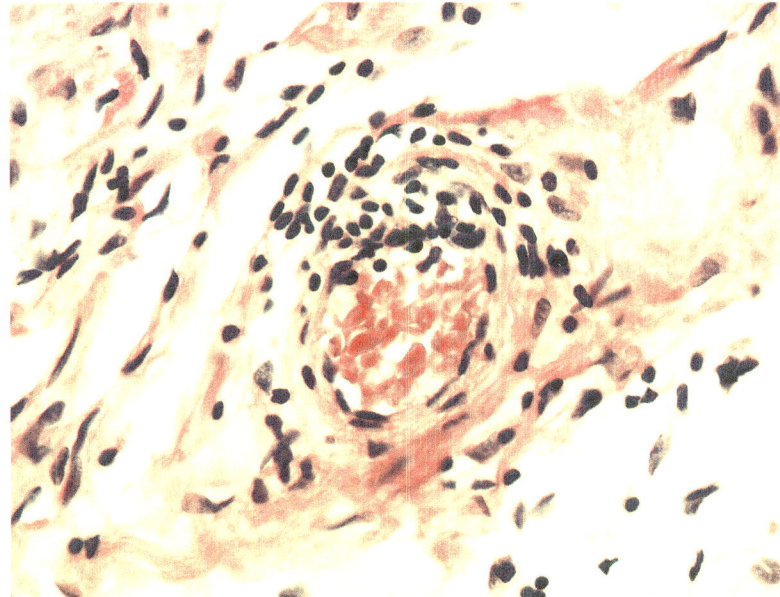

Fig. 5.4 Vasculitis and oestrogen therapy. Testicular vaginal layer. Cross sections of arteries and veins can be seen on the parietal sheet. The smaller caliber artery is barely recognizable due to the abundance of lymphoid infiltrates in its wall

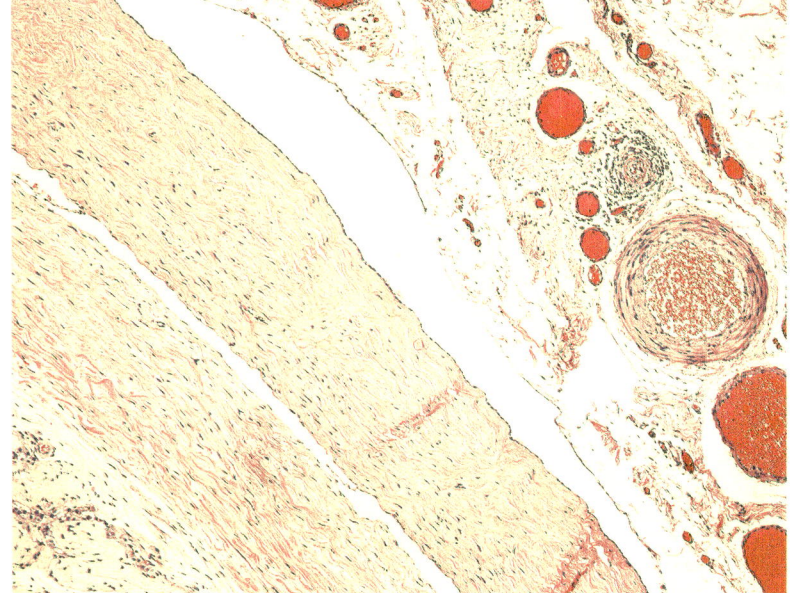

It is difficult to establish a relationship between the degree of testicular atrophy and the time of appearance of the vasculitis since many variables may be involved such as age at the start of treatment, treatment duration, and the doses used. Added to these difficulties are self-medication, intermittent therapeutic adherence, and the fact that the patients studied were of 13 different nationalities. The intimate mechanism of vascular lesions and the possible involvement of other organs is unknown. In any case, the data seem to have sufficient consistency to justify further study in two aspects: (1) determining whether the vascular lesions are limited to the genital sphere or affect other organs and (2) searching for the most effective treatment association that will ensure the required degree of feminization with low doses.

Fig. 5.5 Vasculitis and oestrogen therapy. The section of the medium caliber artery shows no alterations. The small-caliber one has luminal stenosis, a circumferential inflammatory infiltrate in all layers, predominantly in the tunica adventitia. Detail of the previous figure

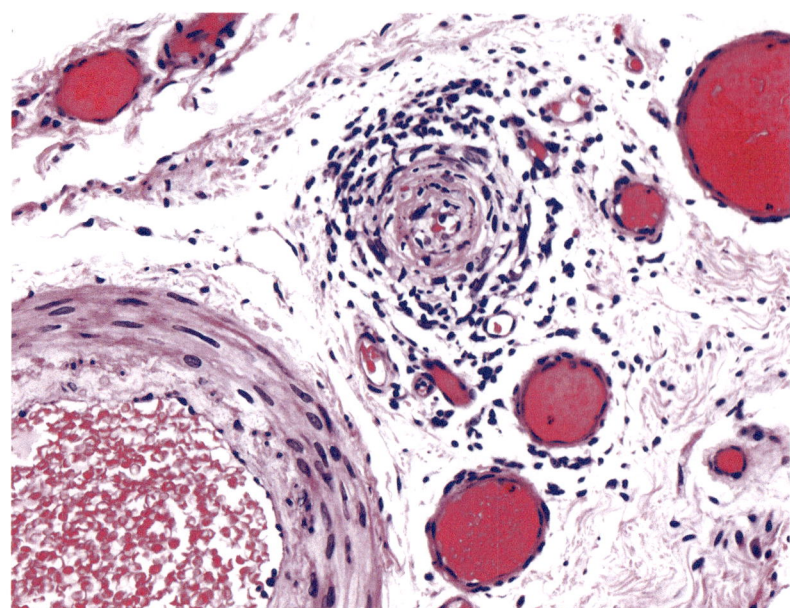

Fig. 5.6 Vasculitis and oestrogen therapy. Most of the arterioles of the cremaster muscle have fibrinoid necrosis of the wall and preferentially circumferential lymphoid infiltrates

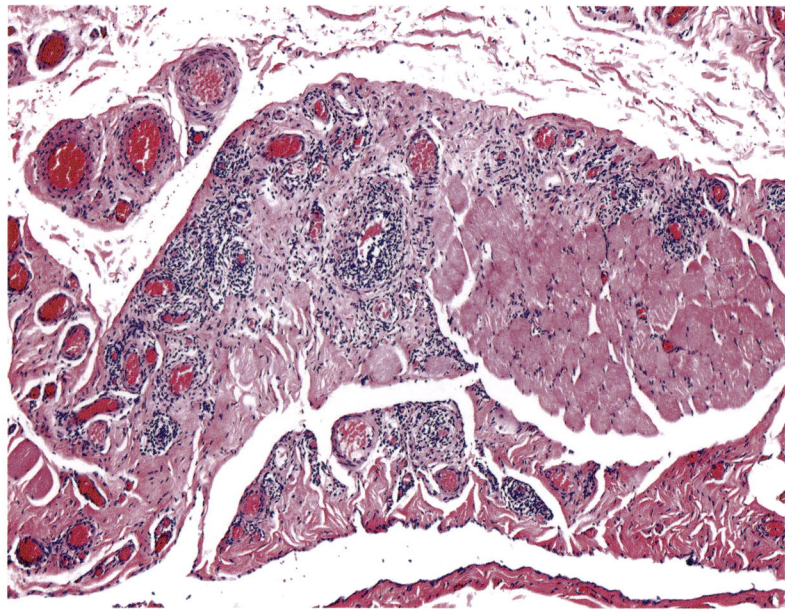

5.2   Bilateral Vasculitis Associated with Testosterone Treatment

The main indication for testosterone replacement therapy is male hypogonadism in which androgen deficiency is the main cause of clinical symptoms. These conditions include primary hypogonadism, hypothalamic-pituitary hypogonadism (secondary hypogonadism), late-onset hypogonadism (LOH), and secondary hypogonadism that can appear in chronic diseases such as thalassemia, sickle cell disease, alcoholism, hemochromatosis, and DAX-1 mutations, among others [20].

Clinical treatment with testosterone has well-known contraindications such prostate cancer, severe lower urinary tract symptoms, severe untreated sleep apnoea, poorly controlled severe heart failure, or a haematocrit >50%. Treatment with testoterone is usually a safe therapy [21]; however, among the reported risks of treatment with testosterone are thrombosis of the portal vein and superior mesenteric vein [22], pulmonary thromboembolism, myocardial infarction, cerebrovascular stroke or worsening of acne in female-to-male transgender adults [23].

Arterial vessel thrombosis is rare but has been described in cases of renal infarction due to renal artery thrombosis [24], myocardial infarction due to occlusive thrombus in the left anterior descending artery [25], and dermal and epidermal infarctions due to small vessel thrombosis [26]. No cases of vasculitis have been described to our knowledge.

Testicular vasculitis, which has been observed in our series, affected an adult patient, DSD 47XY,

treated with testosterone for hypogonadism, who underwent orchiectomy due to the impossibility of descending the testicle. Vascular involvement involved numerous vessels, both in the testis and in the epididymis. Most of the lesions met the characteristics of a leukocytoclastic vasculitis: involvement of small vessels, preferably postcapillary veins. In the initial stages, the most notable observations were the infiltration of the vascular wall by neutrophils and degeneration of the neutrophils (leukocytoclasia) with nuclear dust (karyorrhexis), fibrinoid necrosis of the vascular wall, the vessel being unrecognizable, extravasation of red blood cells, and the presence of eosinophils (Figs. 5.7, 5.8, 5.9, 5.10, and 5.11). In the most advanced lesions, the prominent observation was the abundant perivascular lymphocytic infiltrate (Fig. 5.12). The presence of eosinophilic infiltrates suggests that it is a drug-induced vasculitis.

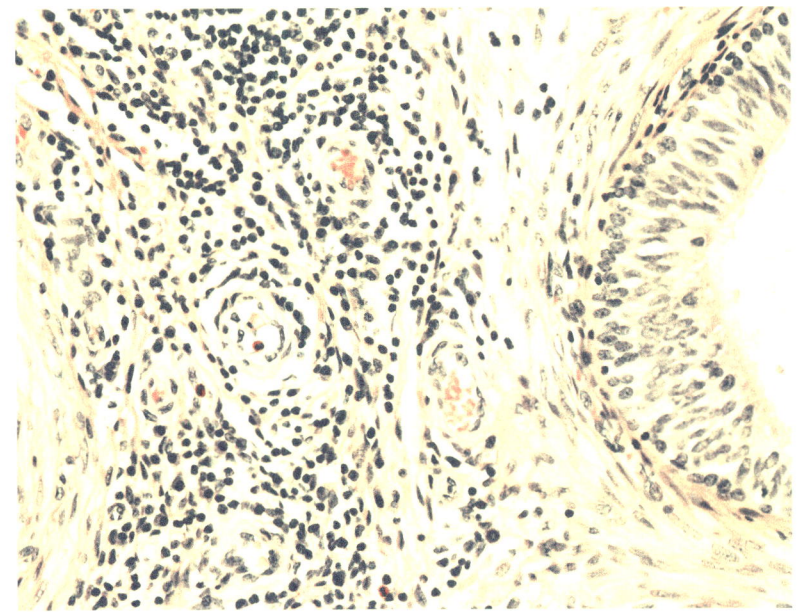

Fig. 5.7 A 21-year-old patient with DSD and hypogonadotropic hypogonadism treated with testosterone. Intense lymphoid infiltrate around small vessels in the epididymis

Fig. 5.8 Vasculitis and testosterone treatment. Cross section of two small veins of the epididymis. In one, abundant polynuclear cells are observed in the tunica intima and media, in the other, crescent-shaped lymphocyte infiltrates, located preferably in the adventitia

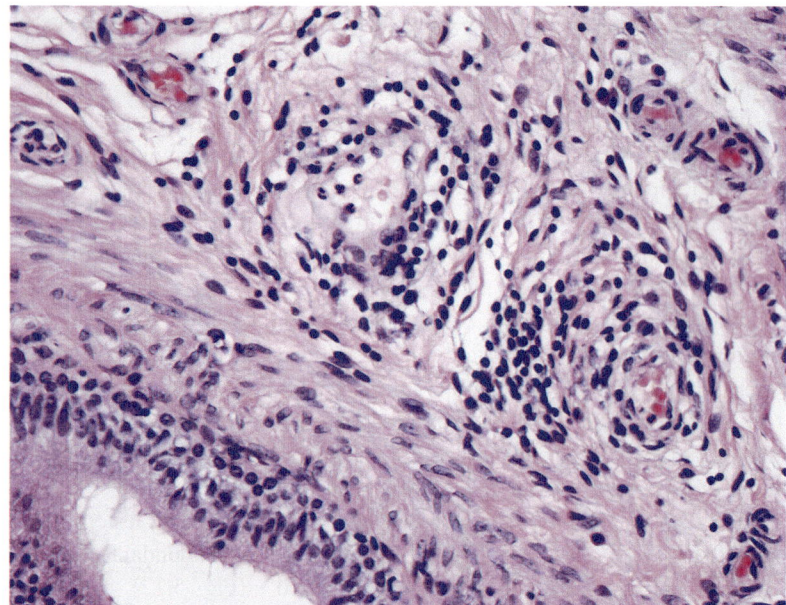

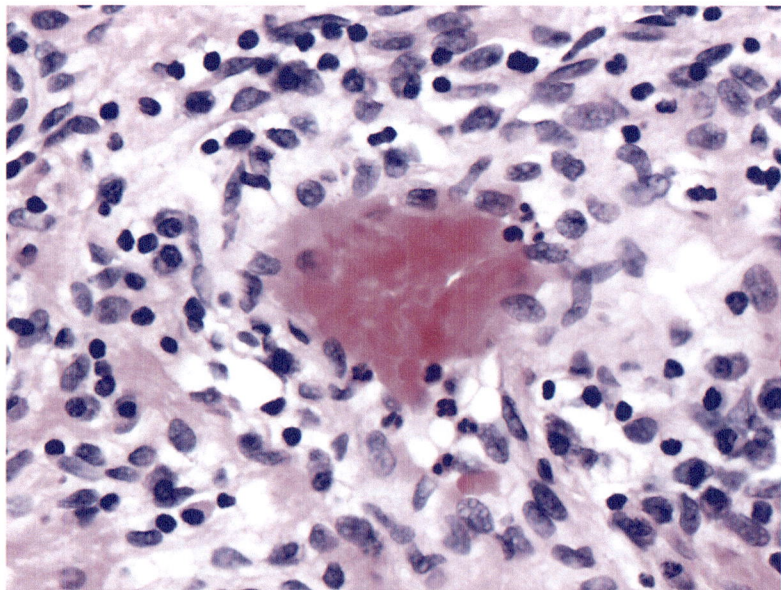

Fig. 5.9 Vasculitis and testosterone treatment. Fibrinoid necrosis of the wall of a small epididymal vessel surrounded by abundant polynuclear cells and peripherally by other lymphoid cells

Fig. 5.10 Vasculitis and testosterone treatment. Postcapillary vein with endothelial swelling, initial fibrinoid necrosis with isolated polynuclear neutrophils. Abundant lymphoid infiltrates in the intertubular tissue of the epididymis

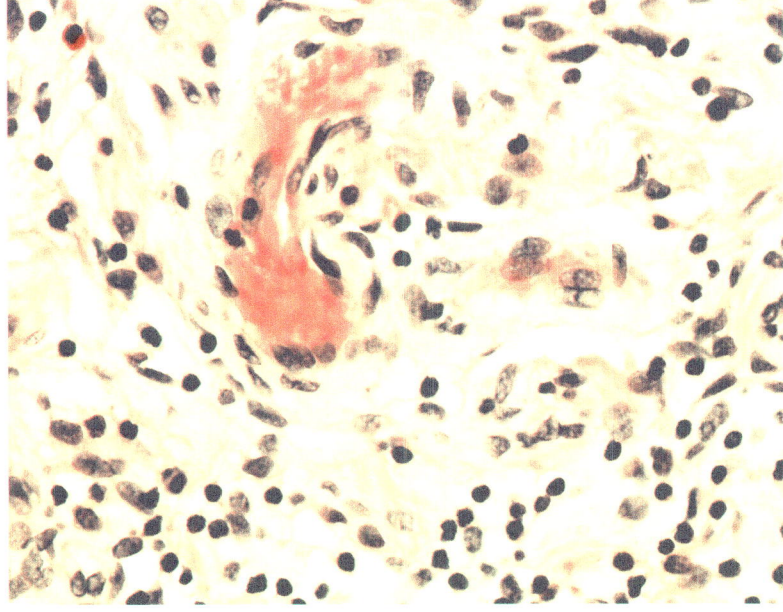

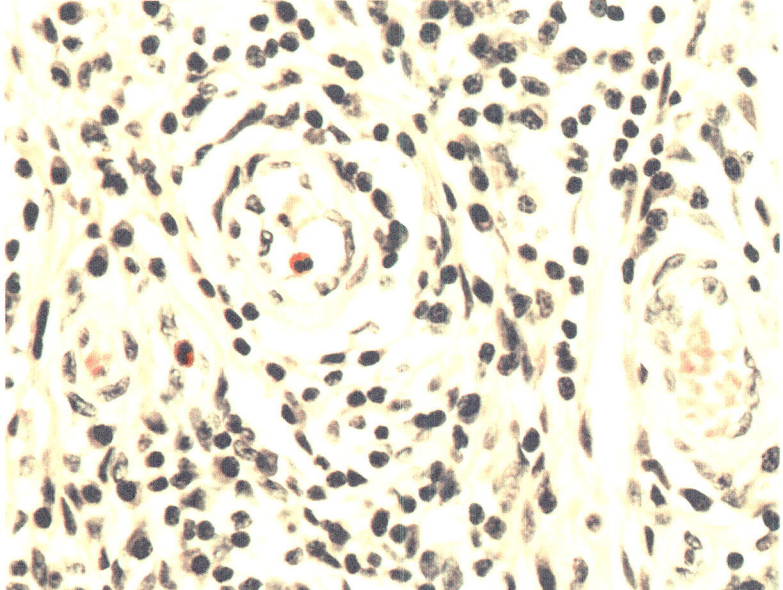

Fig. 5.11 Vasculitis and testosterone treatment. Vein with endothelial swelling, and lymphoid infiltrates in the wall and in the interstitial tissue. The presence of eosinophils both in the lumen and in this interstitial infiltrate stands out

Fig. 5.12 Vasculitis and testosterone treatment. Perivascular lymphoid infiltrates following the path of small veins between the seminiferous tubules. The seminiferous tubules show decreased size, thickening of the wall, absence of lumen and atrophy of the seminiferous epithelium, which is represented by spermatogonia and Sertoli cells. Intense decrease in Leydig cells

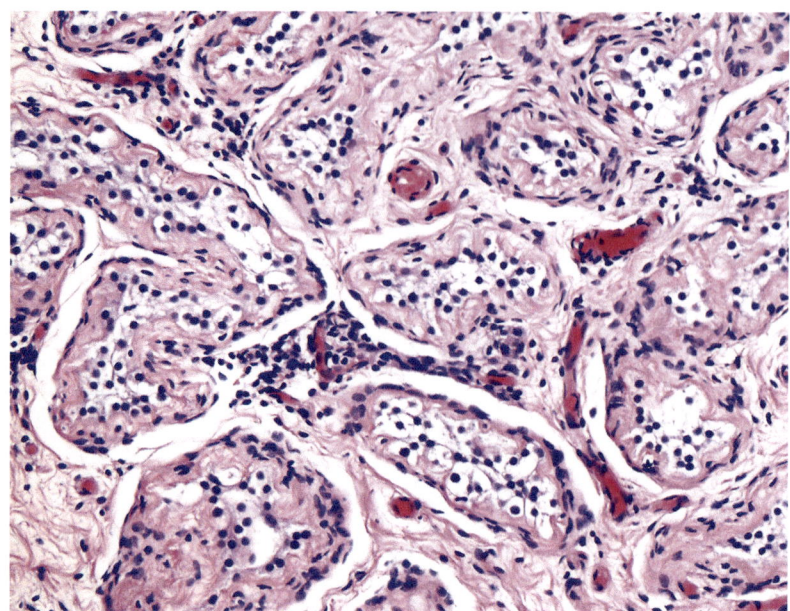

References

1. De la Balze FA, Mancini RE, Bur GE, Irazu J. Morphologic and histochemical changes produced by estrogens on adult human testes. Fertil Steril. 1954;5:421–36.
2. Turo R, Smolski M, Esler R, Kujawa ML, Bromage SJ, Oakley N, Adeyoju A, Brown SC, Brough R, Sinclair A, Collins GN. Diethylstilboestrol for the treatment of prostate cancer: past, present and future. Scand J Urol. 2014;48:4–14.
3. Condappa A, Gossell-Williams M, Aiken W. Favourable response of serum prostate-specific antigen to conjugated oestrogen in castrate-resistant prostate cancer in Jamaica. Ecancermedicalscience. 2018;12:829.
4. Dai-Do D, Espinosa E, Liu G, Rabelink TJ, Julmy F, Yang Z, Mahler F, Lüscher TF. 17 beta-estradiol inhibits proliferation and migration of human vascular smooth muscle cells: similar effects in cells from postmenopausal females and in males. Cardiovasc Res. 1996;32:980–5.
5. Murakami H, Harada N, Sasano H. Aromatase in atherosclerotic lesions of human aorta. J Steroid Biochem Mol Biol. 2001;79:67–74.
6. Haffner SM, Valdez RA, Stern MP, Katz MS. Obesity, body fat distribution and sex hormones in men. Int J Obes Relat Metab Disord. 1993;17:643–9.
7. Brand FN, Dannenberg AL, Abbott RD, Kannel WB. The epidemiology of varicose veins: the Framingham Study. Am J Prev Med. 1988;4:96–101.
8. Guido C, Perrotta I, Panza S, Middea E, Avena P, Santoro M, Marsico S, Imbrogno P, Andò S, Aquila S. Human sperm physiology: estrogen receptor alpha (ERα) and estrogen receptor beta (ERβ) influence sperm metabolism and may be involved in the pathophysiology of varicocele-associated male infertility. J Cell Physiol. 2011;226:3403–12.
9. McDaid A, Logette E, Buchillier V, Muriset M, Suchon P, Pache TD, Tanackovic G, Kutalik Z, Michaud J. Risk prediction of developing venous thrombosis in combined oral contraceptive users. PLoS One. 2017;12(7):e0182041.
10. Douxfils J, Morimont L, Bouvy C. Oral contraceptives and venous thromboembolism: focus on testing that may enable prediction and assessment of the risk. Semin Thromb Hemost. 2020;46:872–86.
11. Morimont L, Haguet H, Dogné JM, Gaspard U, Douxfils J. Combined oral contraceptives and venous thromboembolism: review and perspective to mitigate the risk. Front Endocrinol. 2021;12:769187.
12. Radzikowska E, Maciejewski R, Janicki K, Madej B, Wójtowicz Z. The relationship between estrogen and the development of liver vascular disorders. Ann Univ Mariae Curie Sklodowska Med. 2001;56:189–93.
13. Maraka S, Singh Ospina N, Rodriguez-Gutierrez R, Davidge-Pitts CJ, Nippoldt TB, Prokop LJ, Murad MH. Sex steroids and cardiovascular outcomes in transgender individuals: a systematic review and meta-analysis. J Clin Endocrinol Metab. 2017;102:3914–23.
14. Radić M, Martinović Kaliterna D, Radić J. Drug-induced vasculitis: a clinical and pathological review. Neth J Med. 2012;70:12–7.
15. Chan KL, Mok CC. Development of systemic lupus erythematosus in a male-to-female transsexual: the role of sex hormones revisited. Lupus. 2013;22:1399–402.

16. Unger CA. Hormone therapy for transgender patients. Transl Androl Urol. 2016;5:877–84.

17. Peña Barreno C, Gonzalez-Peramato P, Nistal M. Vascular and inflammatory effects of estrogen and anti-androgen therapy in the testis and epididymis of male to female transgender adults. Reprod Toxicol. 2020;95:37–44.

18. Shurbaji MS, Epstein JI. Testicular vasculitis: implications for systemic disease. Hum Pathol. 1988;19:186–9.

19. Hernández-Rodríguez J, Tan CD, Koening CL, Khasnis A, Rodríguez ER, Hoffman GS. Testicular vasculitis: findings differentiating isolated disease from systemic disease in 72 patients. Medicine. 2012;91:75–85.

20. Tsametis CP, Isidori AM. Testosterone replacement therapy: for whom, when and how? Metabolism. 2018;86:69–78.

21. Bhasin S, Brito JP, Cunningham GR, Hayes FJ, Hodis HN, Matsumoto AM, Snyder PJ, Swerdloff RS, Wu FC, Yialamas MA. Testosterone therapy in men with hypogonadism: an endocrine society clinical practice guideline. J Clin Endocrinol Metab. 2018;103:1715–44.

22. Adams MR, Pijut KD, Uttal-Veroff KC, Davis GA. Acute portal and superior mesenteric vein thrombosis with topical testosterone therapy: an adverse drug event case report. J Pharm Pract. 2023;36:988–92.

23. Yarnell CJ, Thiruchelvam D, Redelmeier DA. Risks of serious injury with testosterone treatment. Am J Med. 2021;134(1):84–94.

24. Colburn S, Childers WK, Chacon A, Swailes A, Ahmed FM, Sahi R. The cost of seeking an edge: recurrent renal infarction in setting of recreational use of anabolic steroids. Ann Med Surg. 2017;14:25–8.

25. Tan BE, Chowdhury M, Hall C, Baibhav B. Exogenous testosterone abuse and myocardial infarction in a young bodybuilder. Am J Med. 2020;133(11):e665–6.

26. Thompson K, Osorio LG, Mughni S, Jordan J, Oyesanmi O. An interesting presentation of testosterone-induced arterial thrombosis. Cureus. 2021;13(5):e14972.

6.1 Thromboangiitis Obliterans

Thromboangiitis obliterans is a rare, non-atherosclerotic, inflammatory, segmental, and occlusive disease. It mainly affects people living in South-East Asia, Middle East Asia, the Far East, and Eastern Europe, but not in Mediterranean countries or South America, and particularly, male middle-aged heavy smokers. The initial symptoms are usually digital infarcts secondary to small vessel ischaemia or intermittent claudication when the popliteal arteries and their branches are affected. The disease is progressive and leads to gangrene of the extremities. The initial symptoms are usually intermittent claudication as the popliteal arteries and their branches are affected. The disease is progressive and leads to gangrene of the extremities. In some patients, there is obvious visceral involvement with lesions in coronary, cerebral, mesenteric, and pulmonary arteries and less frequently in vessels of the kidney, eye, and joints [1].

The aetiology is unknown, although the strong association with tobacco has suggested that TAO is a type of tobacco allergy or autoimmune-triggered response when nicotine is present [2]. Some nicotine metabolites, like cotinine, aggravate the inflammatory response in patients with TAO [3]. In non-smoking patients, a significant exposure to cold weather, fire smoke or cannabis has been reported [4, 5].

Patients with TAO usually present the five criteria proposed by Shionoya et al. [6]: an age of less than 50 years old, a smoking habit, an absence of risk factors for atherosclerosis such as hypertension, hypercholesterolemia or diabetes mellitus, phlebitis migrans or involvement of the upper extremities, and infrapopliteal arterial occlusion [6].

TAO of the spermatic vessels may present as part of a systemic involvement [7, 8], as an isolated manifestation of the disease [9–11] or mimicking a spermatic cord [12] or testicular tumour [13, 14]. Macroscopically, the lesions appear as nodular indurations along the spermatic cord.

Histopathology, in the absence of disease biomarkers, remains the gold standard for TAO diagnosis. Histologically, small- and medium-sized vessels are involved. The lesion is typically segmental. Lesions vary with the duration of the disease. In the initial lesions, a thrombus with micro-abscesses of polymorphonuclear and multinucleated giant cells is observed (Fig. 6.1). Infiltrates extend to all layers, sparing the internal elastic lamina. In the intermediate phase, there is a progressive organization of the thrombus, with the infiltrates being predominantly mononuclear, occasionally epithelioid cells with or without Langhans cells (Fig. 6.2). In late cases, the thrombus is recanalized and fibrosis of the vascular wall occurs without loss of elastic laminae. The fibrosis spreads around and entraps veins and nerves (Figs. 6.3, 6.4, 6.5, and 6.6). The adipose tissue of the spermatic cord and paratesticular structures is also affected, so ischaemic lesions,

Fig. 6.1 The artery focally shows a dense infiltrate of polymorphonuclear leukocytes extending to all layers, a characteristic feature of early lesions

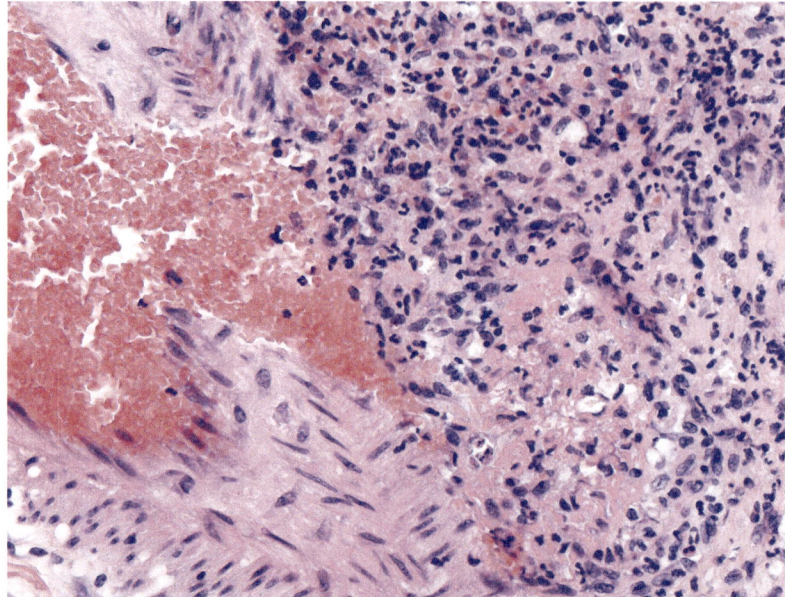

Fig. 6.2 Cross section of a vessel with organized thrombosis and adventitial fibrosis. Masson trichrome staining

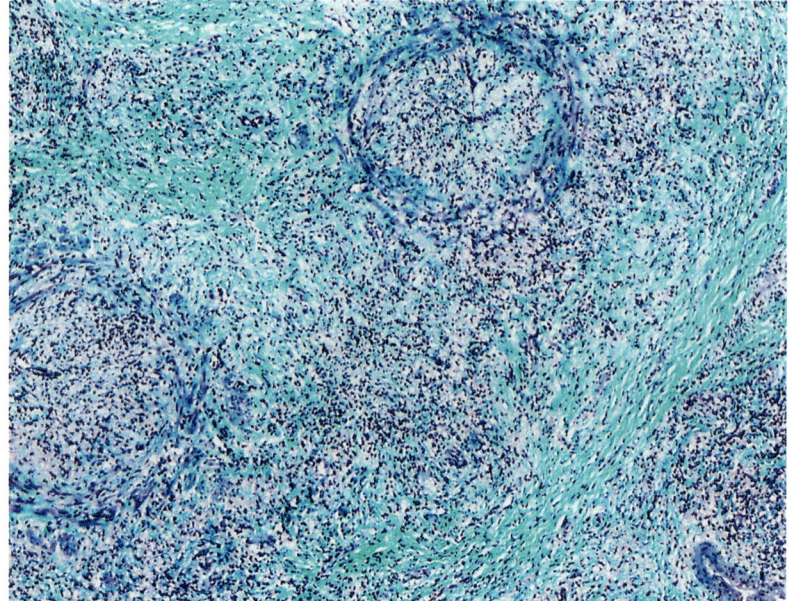

areas of steatonecrosis, lipogranulomas, and steatofibrosis are frequently observed.

The macroscopic differential diagnosis is with tumours of the paratesticular structures in some cases. Histologically, panarteritis nodosa, arteriosclerosis obliterans (ASO), and thromboembolism should be considered. Differently from panarteritis nodosa, in TAO, there is no destruction of the vascular wall, no aneurysms, and the internal elasticity of the arteries is not affected. The differential diagnosis between chronic lesions of TAO and ASO can be difficult. Onion-like-shaped recanalizing vessels in the occluded arteries, adventitial fibrosis without medial

Fig. 6.3 In old lesions several vessels of the spermatic cord with inflammatory phenomena are trapped by fibrosis. Masson trichrome staining

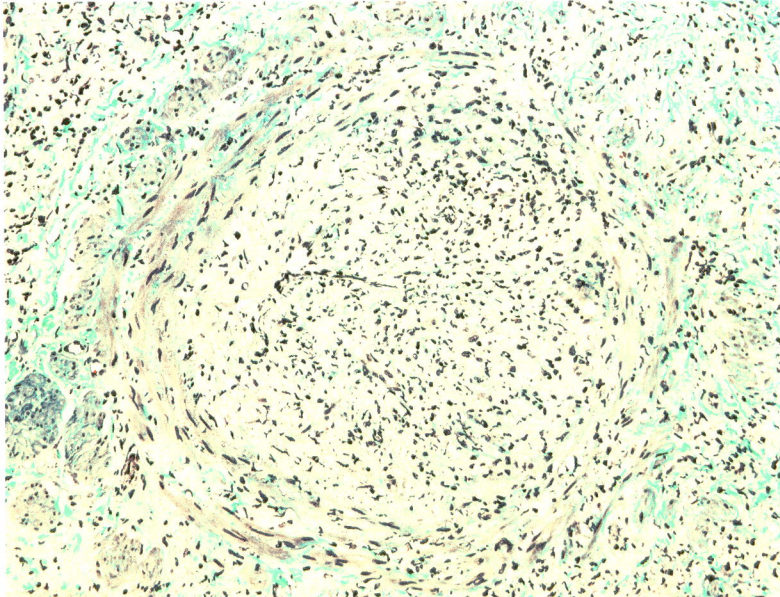

Fig. 6.4 Vessel with chronic inflammation and numerous neo-formed capillaries as a sign of recanalization

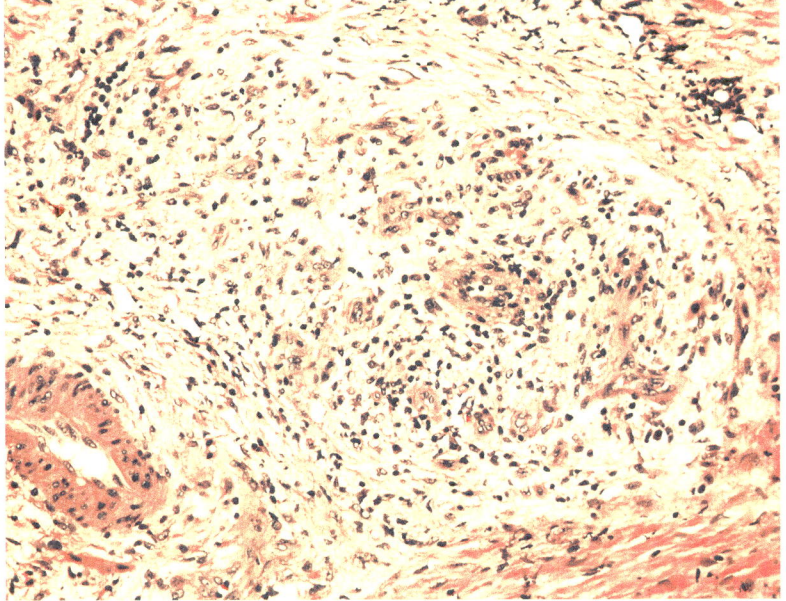

fibrosis, swelling of the endothelium of the vasa vasorum and oedema beneath the external elastic lamina are considered characteristic of TAO [15]. Thromboembolism and TAO may share intimal inflammation and medial intactness, but in thromboembolism, the inflammatory infiltrates are not significant outside the intima, and, in most cases, there is no involvement of veins and nerves.

Fig. 6.5 Transverse section of the spermatic cord showing three nerves within a fibrous tissue with chronic inflammation

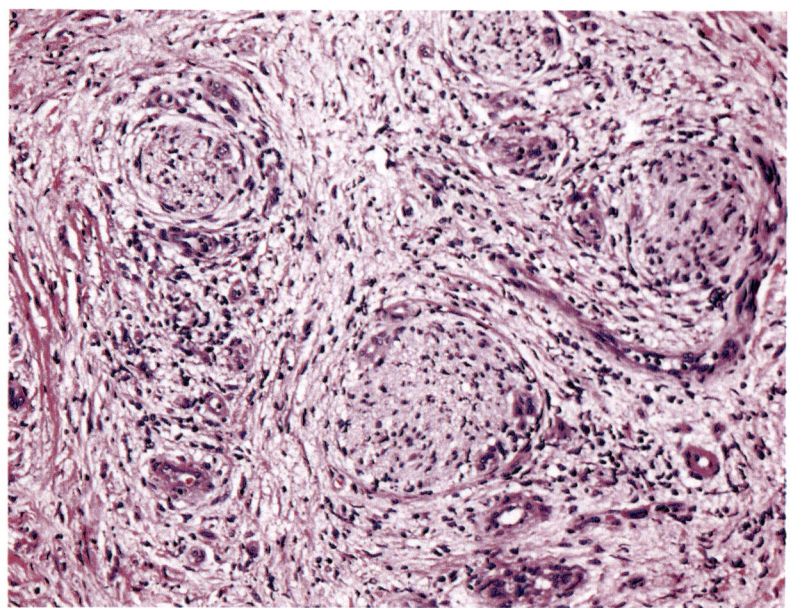

Fig. 6.6 The nerve is surrounded by incomplete rings of fibroblasts, collagen, and lymphoid cells

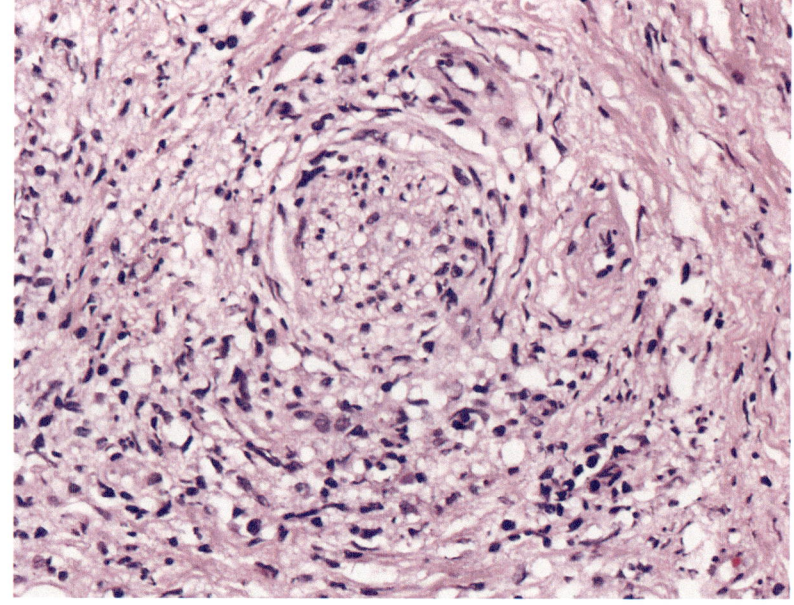

References

1. Fakour F, Fazeli B. Visceral bed involvement in thromboangiitis obliterans: a systematic review. Vasc Health Risk Manag. 2019;15:317–53.
2. Lazarides MK, Georgiadis GS, Papas TT, Nikolopoulos ES. Diagnostic criteria and treatment of Buerger's disease: a review. Int J Low Extrem Wounds. 2006;5:89–95.
3. Shi S, Song L, Liu Y, He Y. Cotinine aggravates inflammatory response in thromboangiitis obliterans through TLR-4/MyD88/NF-κB inflammatory signaling pathway. Int Angiol. 2020;39:261–2.
4. El Omri N, Eljaoudi R, Mekouar F, Jira M, Sekkach Y, Amezyane T, Ghafir D. Cannabis arteritis. Pan Afr Med J. 2017;26:53.
5. Drummer OH, Gerostamoulos D, Woodford NW. Cannabis as a cause of death: a review. Forensic Sci Int. 2019;298:298–306.

6. Shionoya S. Diagnostic criteria of Buerger's disease. Int J Cardiol. 1998;66(1):243–5; discussion 247.

7. Mathé CP. Thrombo-angiitis obliterans (Buerger's disease) of the spermatic arteries: report of a case. J Urol. 1940;44:768–70.

8. Cope E. Thrombo-angitis obliterans of the spermatic cord. S Afr Med J. 1968;42:872–3.

9. Lee McGregor A, Simson FW. Thrombo-angiitis obliterans: with special reference to a case involving the spermatic vessels. Br J Surg. 1929;16:539–41.

10. Nesbit RM, Hodgon NB. Thrombo-angiitis obliterans of the spermatic cord. J Urol. 1960;83:445–7.

11. Abercrombie GF. Thrombo-angiitis obliterans of the spermatic cord. Br J Surg. 1965;52:632–3.

12. Kuwahara M, Matsushita K, Nakamura K, Yoshinaga H, Aki M, Fujisaki N, Furihata M, Ohtsuki Y. Thromboangiitis obliterans of the spermatic cord: a case report. Hinyokika Kiyo. 1993;39:369–72.

13. Roberts JA, Meyer JP. Buerger's disease presenting as a testicular mass: a rare presentation of an uncommon disease. Urol Ann. 2016;8:249–51.

14. Harwood EA, Blazek AJ, Radio SJ, Deibert CM. Buerger's disease in the testicle: a case of testicular Thromboangiitis obliterans. Cureus. 2023;15(4):e37693.

15. Kurata A, Franke FE, Machinami R, Schulz A. Thromboangiitis obliterans: classic and new morphological features. Virchows Arch. 2000;436:59–67.

The Complexity of Testicular Lesions in Arteriosclerosis

7.1 Atherosclerosis

Atherosclerosis is a disease of the elastic arteries and large muscular arteries in which the characteristic lesion is an atheroma [1, 2]. Defined in this way, arteriosclerosis with atheromatosis is a lesion that is rarely seen in the testicular artery or its branches (Figs. 7.1 and 7.2). On the other hand, in the elderly, it is common to observe significant lesions of non-atherosclerotic arteriosclerosis, both in the testicular artery and in its branches or in the deferential artery [3]. The vessels show thickening of the wall, mainly at the expense of the intima. This layer is made up of a concentric proliferation of subendothelial cells which markedly narrow the lumen, in some cases leading to lumen thrombosis and dystrophic calcification. The internal elastic lamina is not affected. The medial layer usually shows muscle cell atrophy and fibrosis. Arterial lesions in elderly men correlate with the degree of aortic atherosclerosis [4] (Figs. 7.3, 7.4, 7.5, and 7.6).

This vascular pathology has repercussions on both the epididymis and the testicle. At the level of the epididymis, the most frequent lesions are observed in the head, a territory supplied by the superior epididymal artery. The efferent ducts are atrophied, the reduction of the lumen creates an obstacle to the passage of testicular fluid as well as a defect in its reabsorption. The consequences are cystic transformation of the rete testis and ectasia of the seminiferous tubules of some lobules.

The involvement of the intratesticular arterial branches produces two lesions: ischemic lesions and obstructive lesions (Figs. 7.7 and 7.8). Ischemic lesions are manifested not only by hyalinization of the seminiferous tubules of the irrigated parenchyma, but also by the disappearance of the Leydig cells between them and fibrosis of the interstitium. Obstructive lesions are secondary to ischemic lesions. When a segment of the seminiferous tubule atrophies, the rest of the tubule, which continues to produce testicular fluid and sperm, first dilates, and then atrophies. The disappearance of the Leydig cells is a good parameter to differentiate an atrophy with an ischemic mechanism from one of an obstructive nature. In the latter, the Leydig cells are preserved between the atrophic tubules. Other observations suggesting a post-obstructive atrophy are the frequent presence of a small central vacuole in the atrophic tubules, a remnant of the former lumen. In other cases, atrophic tubules produced by an obstructed mechanism show tubulitis. In cases where the arteriosclerosis is less severe, the decrease in testicular flow only produces diffuse lesions in spermatogenesis, which may be more related to a parallel decrease in pituitary hormones reaching the testis than to ischemia [5].

© The Author(s), under exclusive license to Springer Nature Switzerland AG 2024
M. Nistal, P. González-Peramato, *Testicular Vascular Lesions*,
https://doi.org/10.1007/978-3-031-57847-2_7

Fig. 7.1 Arteriosclerosis with atheromatosis. Next to the section of the ascending part of the epididymal tail, note the cross section of an artery showing luminal stenosis, eccentric thickening of the intima and focal calcification of the media. A 47-year-old patient undergoing hormonal treatment for sex change

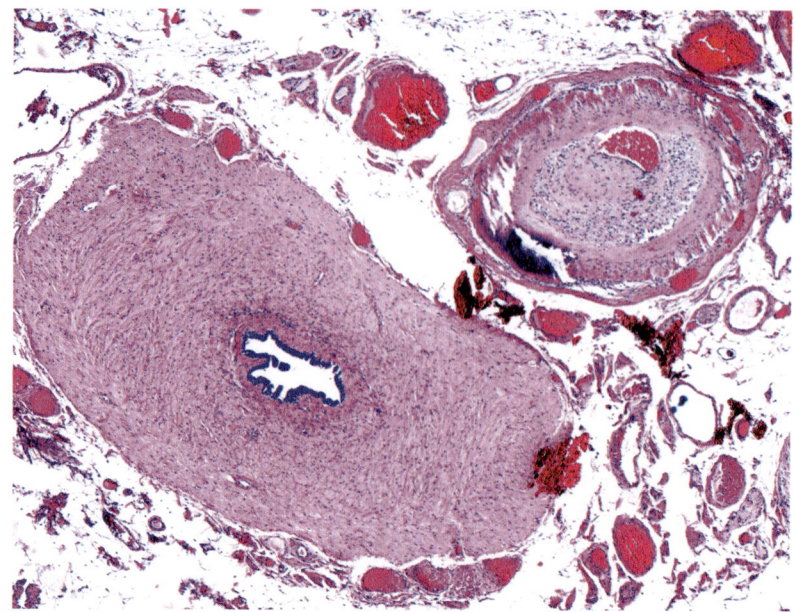

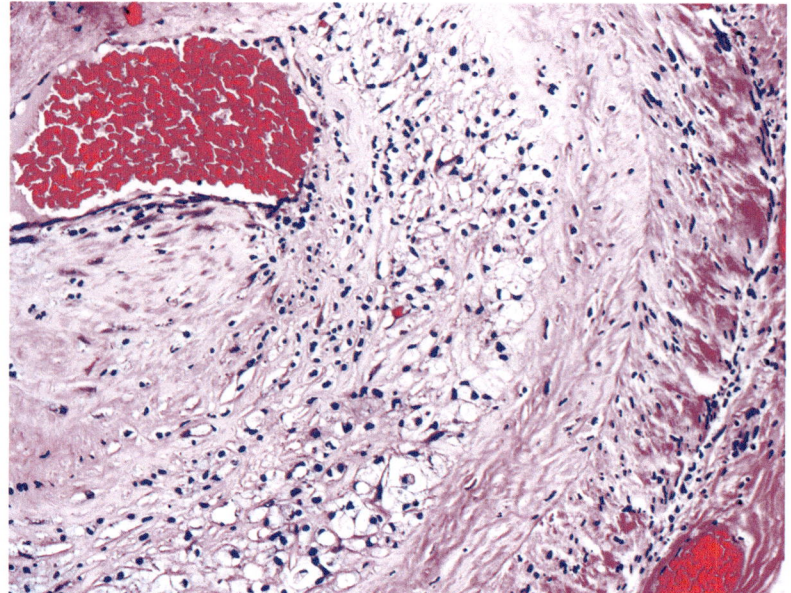

Fig. 7.2 Arteriosclerosis with atheromatosis. The intima is occupied by numerous macrophages with vacuolated cytoplasm, some lymphocytes, and an area of subendothelial fibrosis. Detail of the previous figure

Fig. 7.3 Atherosclerosis.
Cross section of the
spermatic cord in an
84-year-old patient. The
testicular artery has
luminal stenosis
secondary to concentric
hyperplasia of the intima.
The surrounding veins
show no pathology

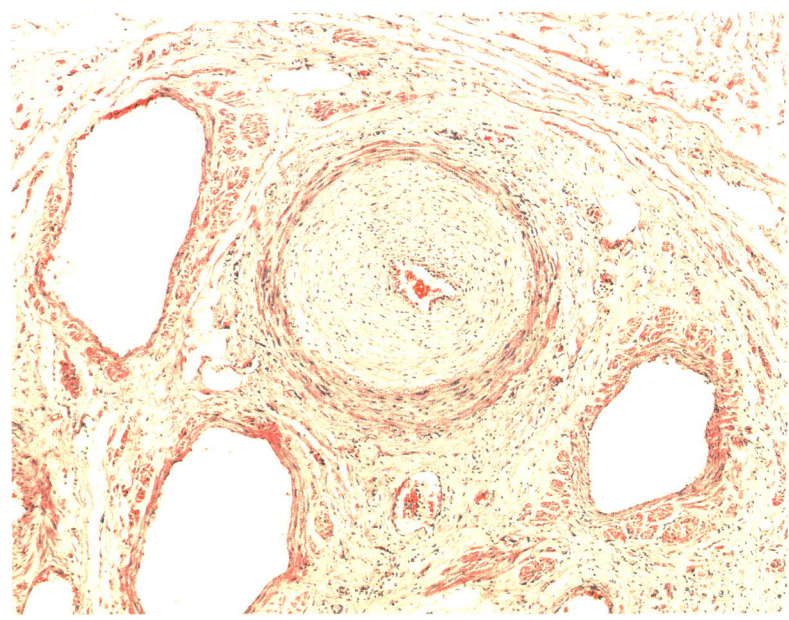

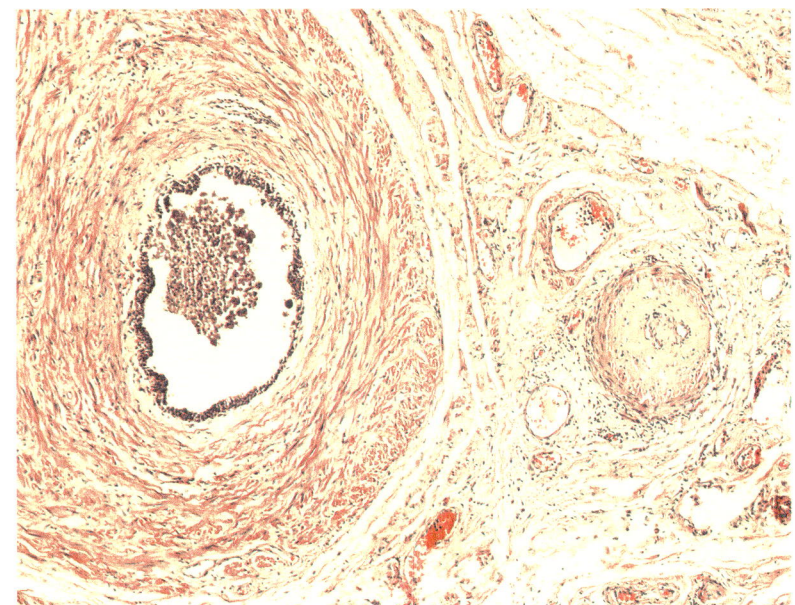

Fig. 7.4 Atherosclerosis.
The deferential artery
shows an old recanalized
thrombosis

Fig. 7.5 Atherosclerosis. Branch of the testicular artery before penetrating the albuginea with a partially calcified old thrombus

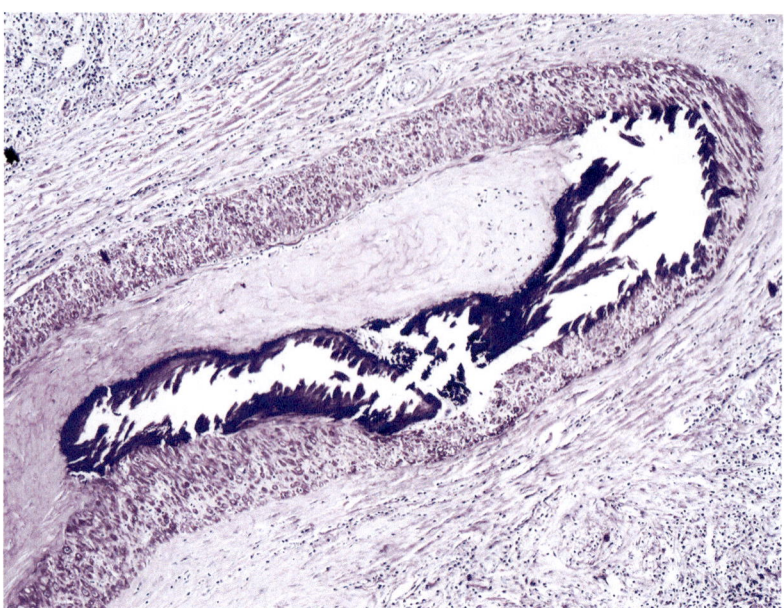

Fig. 7.6 Atherosclerosis. Arterial segments below the albuginea. All show massive fibrosis of the intima with focal fibrosis of the media. The few seminiferous tubules are completely hyalinized

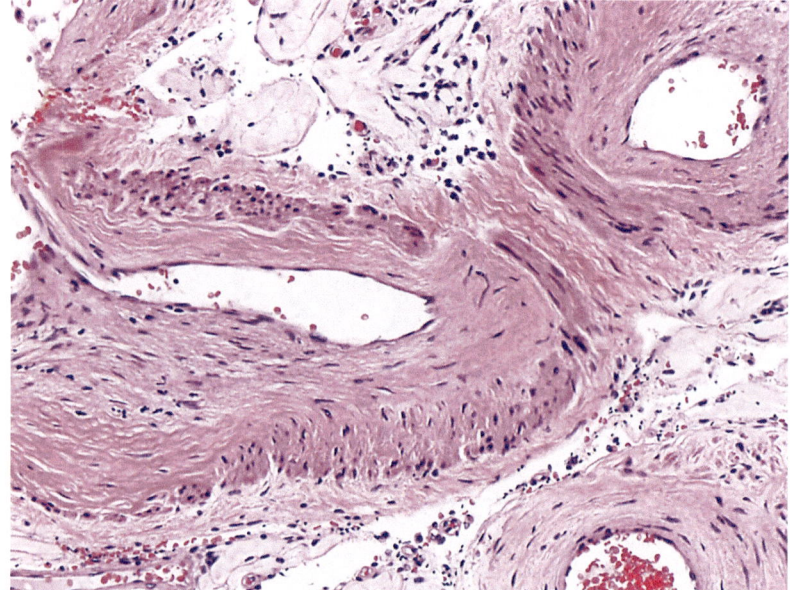

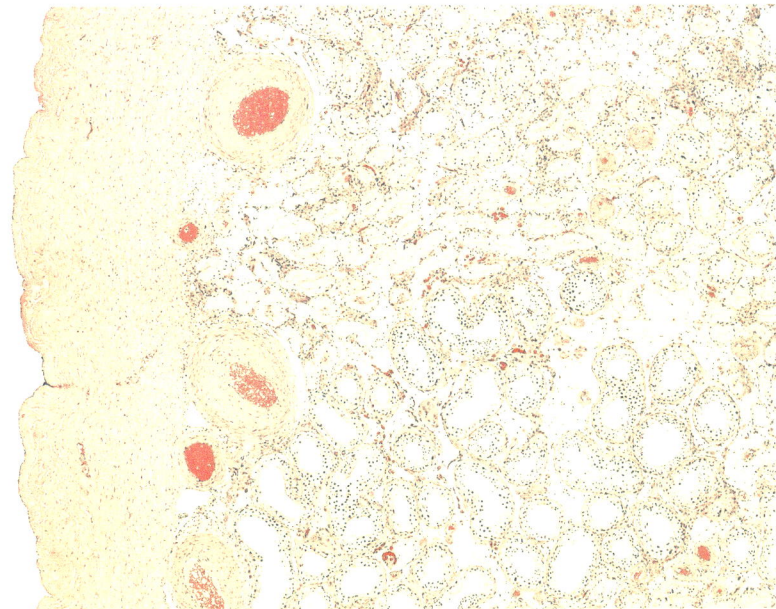

Fig. 7.7 Atherosclerosis. The testicular parenchyma has clusters of sclerosed seminiferous tubules next to others with slight lumen dilatation. Note the marked thickening of the subalbuginea arteries at the expense of the intima

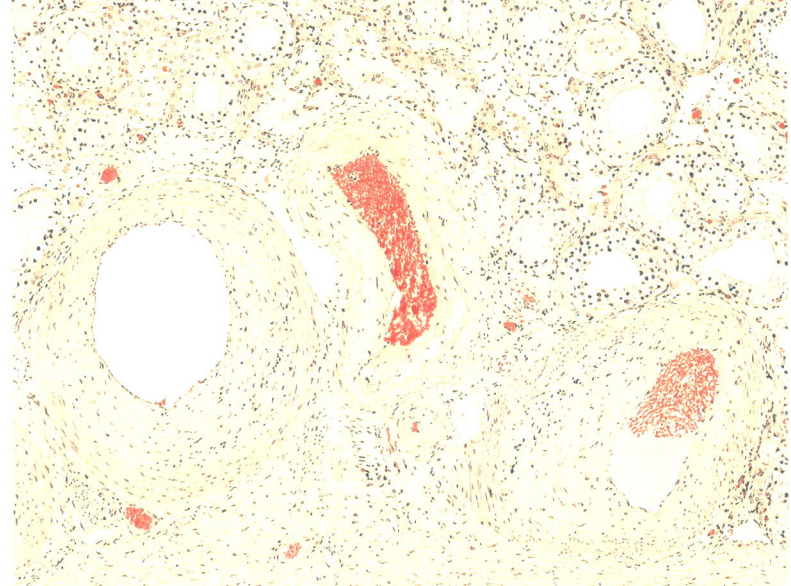

Fig. 7.8 Atherosclerosis. Spermatogenesis, in tubules that are still preserved, is represented only by spermatogonia and spermatocytes. The arteries show marked thickening of the intima

7.2 Arteriolosclerosis

Arterioles are the vascular segments between the terminal arteries and the capillaries. Their wall consists of three layers. The intima, with a continuous endothelium supported by the basement membrane, the media, consisting of the internal elastic lamina and one or two layers of smooth muscle cells, and the adventitia with isolated fibroblasts, collagen bands, extracellular matrix, and nerve fibres. The mission of the arterioles is to control resistance to blood flow. Under the action of different physiological stimuli, the muscle cells contract or relax. From their functional state they regulate two processes, blood pressure and tissue perfusion [6]. The arterioles of the testicular parenchyma are branches of the centrifugal arteries and are distributed from the apex of the testicular lobule to the periphery.

Testicular arteriolosclerosis is manifested by a thickening of the vascular wall. The two subtypes of arteriolosclerosis described in other organs [1] are also seen in the testis. In hyperplastic arteriosclerosis, there is concentric thickening with significant reduction of the arteriolar lumen due to

the increased presence of smooth muscle cells and thick basement membranes (Fig. 7.9). Alterations are similar to those seen in other organs in patients with systemic arterial hypertension with or without *diabetes mellitus*. Hyaline arteriolosclerosis is dominated by the deposition of eosinophilic material between muscle cells, which appear atrophic (Fig. 7.10). The lesions are identical to those seen in patients with sys-

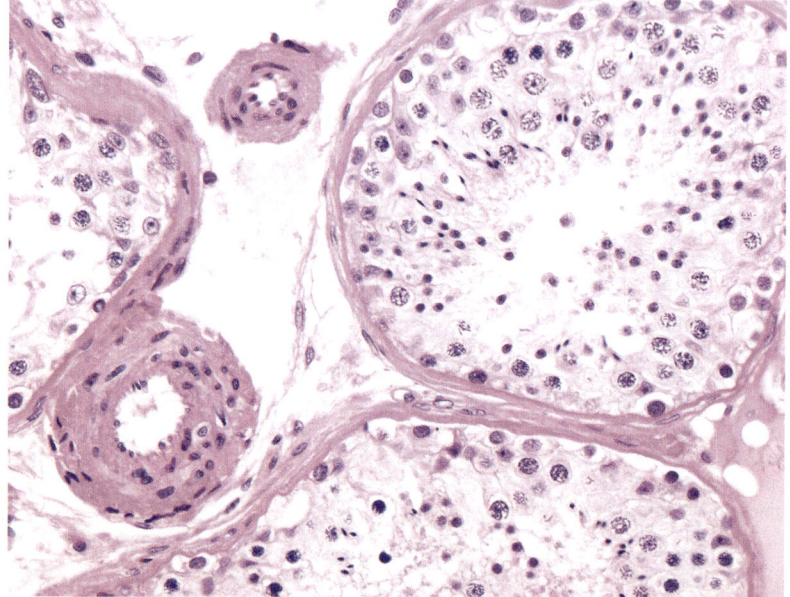

Fig. 7.9 Arteriolosclerosis. A 56-year-old patient with poorly controlled hypertension. One of the intraparenchymal arterioles shows marked thickening of the media layer due to concentric smooth muscle cell hyperplasia. The seminiferous tubules maintain complete spermatogenesis

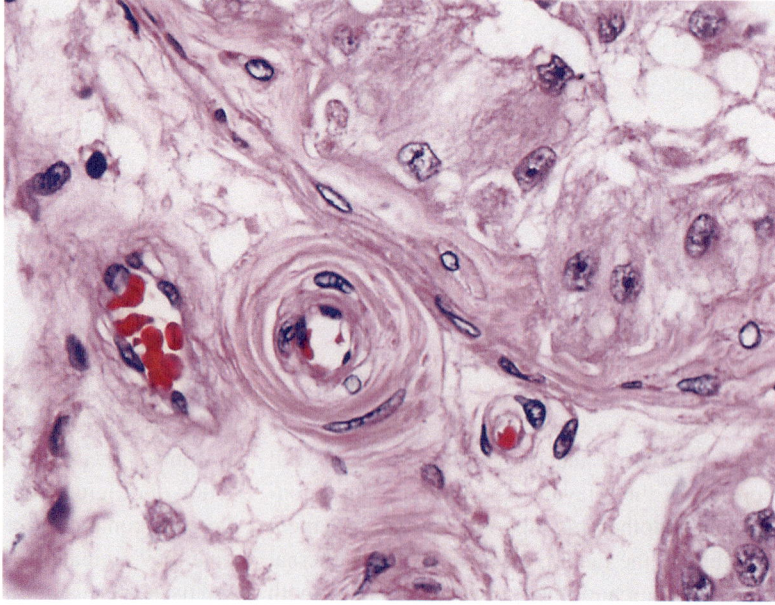

Fig. 7.10 Arteriolosclerosis. An 80-year-old patient with type II diabetes mellitus. The arteriole shows wall thickening due to of hyaline material, arranged in concentric rings. The seminiferous tubule contains only Sertoli cells

temic arterial hypertension, glomerulosclerosis, and chronic renal failure [7].

Parenchymal lesions are usually diffuse, and conditioned by the patient's accompanying pathology, such as arteriosclerosis, diabetes, renal insufficiency, or age. In some cases, only hypospermatogenesis is observed, in others there are patchy lesions of tubular sclerosis. Leydig cell clusters are decreased, and the cells contain abundant lipofuscins. Both Leydig cells and telocytes (CD34 positive interstitial cells) may show multinucleation.

7.3   Mönckeberg Medial Calcific Sclerosis

This form of arteriosclerosis was described by Mönckberg in 1903 [8] to refer to age-related calcification of the medial layer of large and medium-sized arteries without intimal involvement. It is also known as Mönckberg arteriosclerosis or other names like Mönckberg medial calcinosis and medial arterial calcification. It is associated with type II diabetes, chronic kidney disease, or pathologies such as congenital lupus erythematosus, hypervitaminosis D, osteoporosis, or chronic inflammation [9]. The radiological image is char-

acteristic: parallel and linear "railroad-track"-appearing calcifications observed along the arteries (Figs. 7.11 and 7.12). Although it is recognized that it may have a systemic distribution, it has not previously been described in the testis.

This type of arteriosclerosis was observed in a 58-year-old patient with a history of type II diabetes mellitus, who suffered amputation of the left leg due to poor circulation. Diagnosed with Mönckeber's arteriosclerosis, he developed abscessed epididymitis of the left testicle. As he did not respond to antibiotic treatment, an orchio-epididectomy was performed. The epididymitis involved only the tail and showed several abscesses with no signs of specificity. Cultures were negative (Fig. 7.13).

The testicular artery and its branches showed two associated lesions, arteriosclerosis and Mönckeberg medial calcific sclerosis. The arteriosclerosis was manifested by fibrosis of the intima and stenosis of the arterial lumen. It was diagnosed as Mönckeberg medial calcific sclerosis due to calcification of the medial layer. In this case, calcification of the internal elastic lamina, which can be seen in both processes, was not observed (Figs. 7.14, 7.15, and 7.16).

The development of Mönckeberg medial calcific sclerosis lesions has been described in four

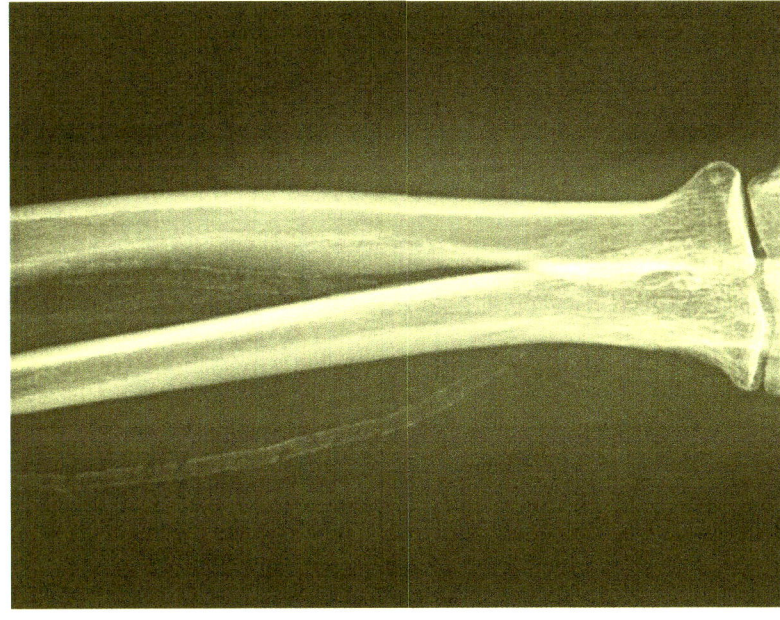

Fig. 7.11 Mönckeberg medial calcific sclerosis. Calcification simulating train tracks along the entire length of the forearm arteries

Fig. 7.12 Mönckeberg medial calcific sclerosis. Linear calcifications of the palmar digital arteries

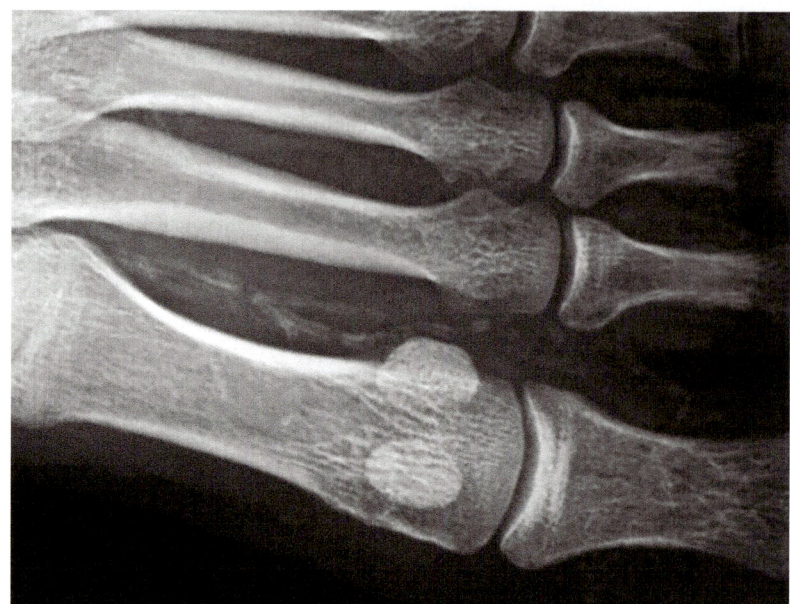

Fig. 7.13 Mönckeberg medial calcific sclerosis. A 58-year-old patient with a history of type 2 diabetes mellitus and left leg amputation due to poor vascularization. He developed abscessed epididymitis in the tail of the epididymis

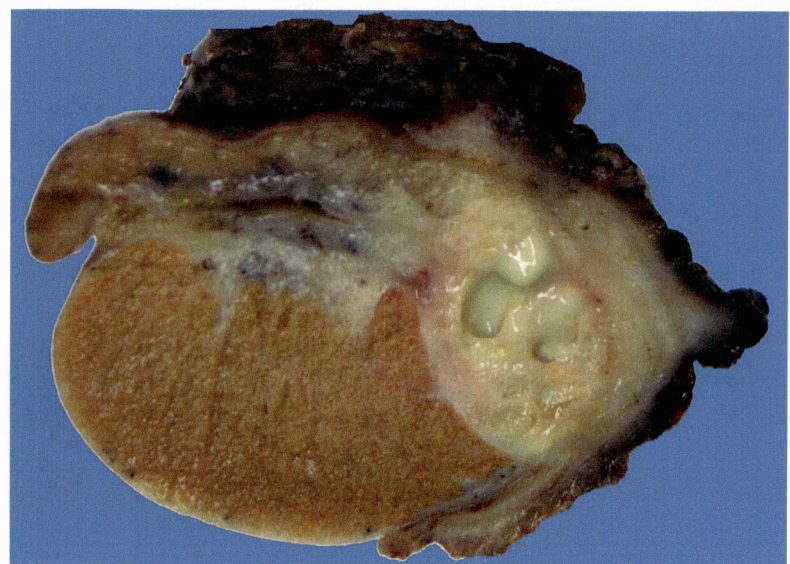

stages. In stage I, small calcium deposits are observed both inside the smooth muscle cells, in the matrix and along the internal elastic membrane. In stage II, the calcifications converge and affect three quadrants of the section extending to the full thickness of the media. In stage III, they affect the entire circumference, they may protrude into the intima and the intima shows subendothelial hyperplasia. In stage IV, there is bone and haematopoietic metaplasia of the calcifica-

tions. The deposits are formed by hydroxyapatite crystals [10]. It is rare before the age of 50 years old.

The intimate mechanism of calcification is no longer considered a passive event, and, although there are gaps in our understanding, its pathogenesis is considered an active process in which smooth muscle cells play an important role. Damage to these cells by a hostile microenvironment leads to their death or transdifferentiation, acquir-

Fig. 7.14 Mönckeberg medial calcific sclerosis. Cross section of the spermatic cord. The testicular artery shows calcification of the medial layer. In addition, the thickening of the intima suggests an atherosclerotic component

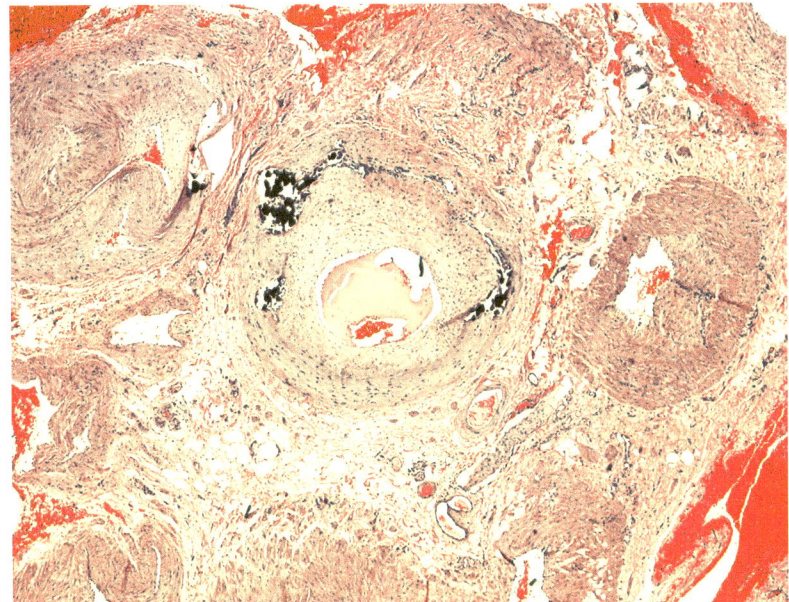

Fig. 7.15 Mönckeberg medial calcific sclerosis. Several sections of the testicular artery before entering the testis. Calcification of the medial layer is seen in all three sections of the vessel

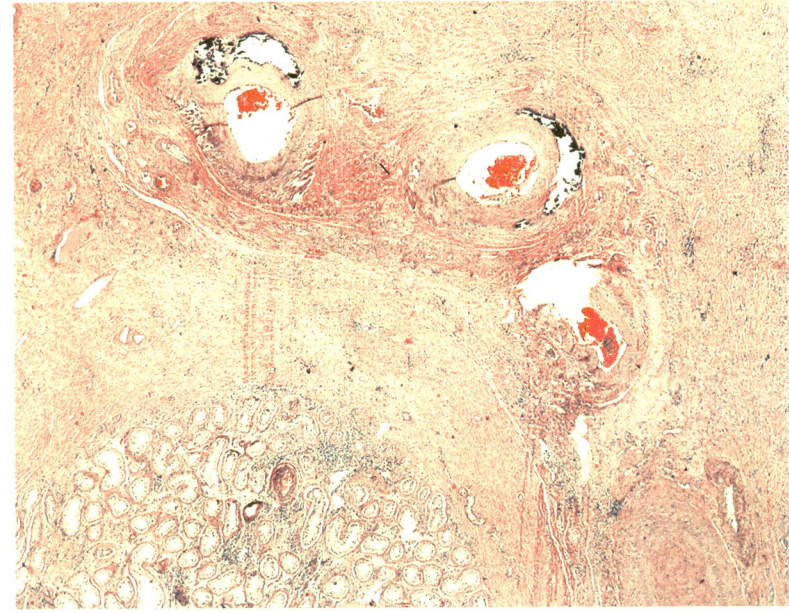

ing an osteochondrogenic phenotype that favours mineralization [11, 12]. Both benign (asymptomatic) and malignant forms have been described, depending on the clinical and histological features, and no risk factors are known to be associated with its development [13].

Fig. 7.16 Mönckeberg medial calcific sclerosis. The artery shows crescentic calcification of the media typical of Mönckeberg disease and lesions of atherosclerosis (fibrosis of the intima)

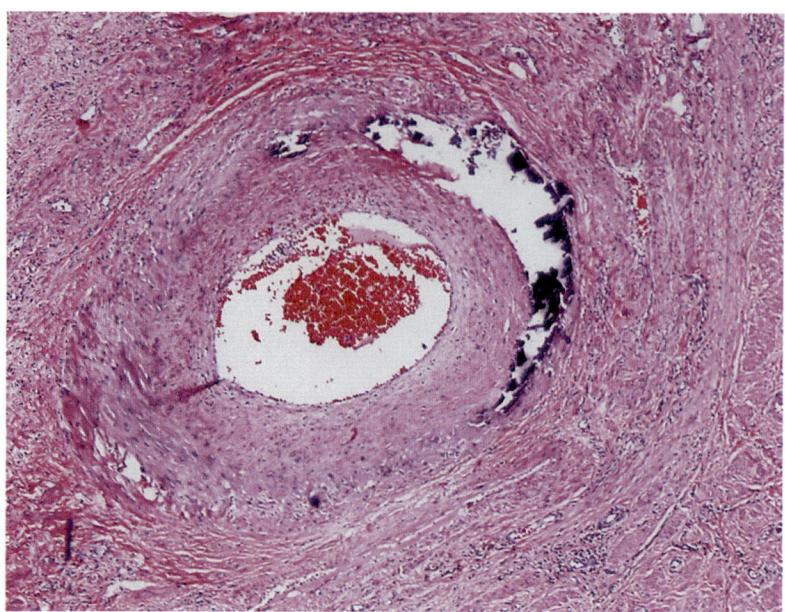

7.4 Arteriosclerosis Obliterans (ASO)

ASO is a form of atherosclerosis that preferentially affects the arteries of the lower extremities in adults over 55 years of age. Most patients have a history of hypertension, *diabetes mellitus*, and hypercholesterolemia [14]. In lesions of the testicular artery and its intraparenchymal branches, the following are observed: (a) wall thickening and lumen stenosis with or without associated thrombosis; (b) slight thickening of the intimal layer; if there is no thrombosis; (c) atrophy of the muscle cells of the medial layer; (d) significant prominence of the vasa vasorum showing swelling of the endothelial cells and abundant deposition of hyaline material around them; (e) little or no involvement of the adventitia; and (f) absence of inflammatory infiltrates (Figs. 7.17, 7.18, 7.19, 7.20, and 7.21).

The differential diagnosis can be made between ASO lesions, thromboangiitis obliterans (TAO), and thromboembolism. While the clinical symptoms of these entities are well established, the pathological anatomy is not. Many consider ASO, TAO and thromboembolism lesions to be morphologically indistinguishable. Lesions of the testicular vessels have rarely been studied and their description is based on extrapolation of what occurs in other vessels. Comparative study of the findings in the different layers of the arterial wall shows that there are two types of lesions, some characteristic of one of these three entities, others shared. The differential diagnosis can be made relatively easily when a certain type of lesion predominates, but it can be very difficult in other cases, especially when these entities may coincide in the same vessel. The fact that the long-term prognosis and survival rate of TAO is more favourable than that of ASO makes the differential diagnosis more relevant. The clinicopathological correlation is of particular importance.

ASO is characterized by the onset of clinical symptoms after the age of 50 years old, absence of *phlebitis migrans* and upper limb involvement and the presence of hypertension or hypercholesterolemia. Histologically, atrophy of the medial layer is typical, and this is not seen in either TAO or thromboembolism. However, other lesions like calcification of the media or the presence of cholesterol crystals are not pathognomonic. Calcification of the media is characteristic of Mönckeberg arteriosclerosis and cholesterol crystals can be seen in thromboembolism [15]. In TAO, the lesions are initiated by an inflammatory process affecting all layers of the arteries and

Fig. 7.17 Arteriosclerosis obliterans. A 68-year-old patient with a history of diabetes mellitus, hypertension, and hypercholesterolemia. The figures were taken from the autopsy study of the testis. The two arteries located under the albuginea show either markedly decreased lumina or absence of lumina and wall fibrosis. The seminiferous tubules have advanced sclerosis

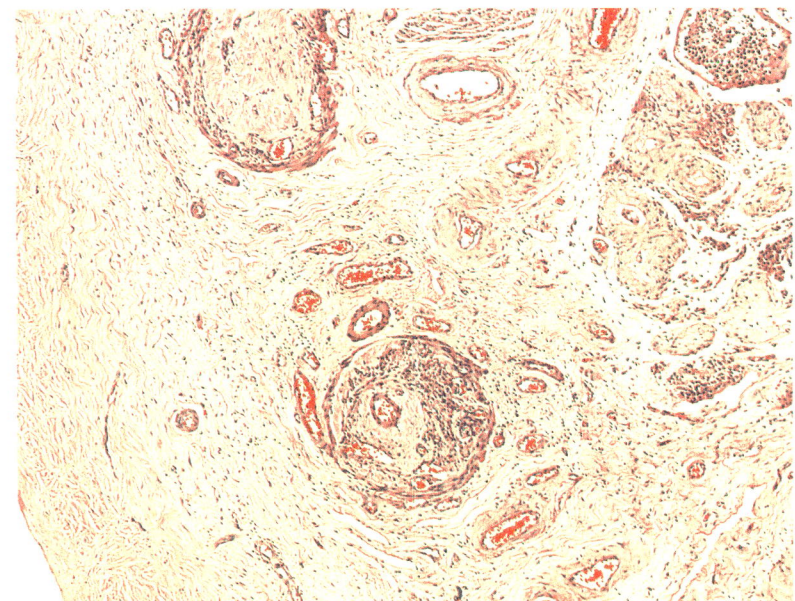

Fig. 7.18 Arteriosclerosis obliterans. The cross section of the artery shows circumferential fibrosis of the media and the focal presence of a cluster of thick-walled vasa vasorum (Masson's trichrome staining)

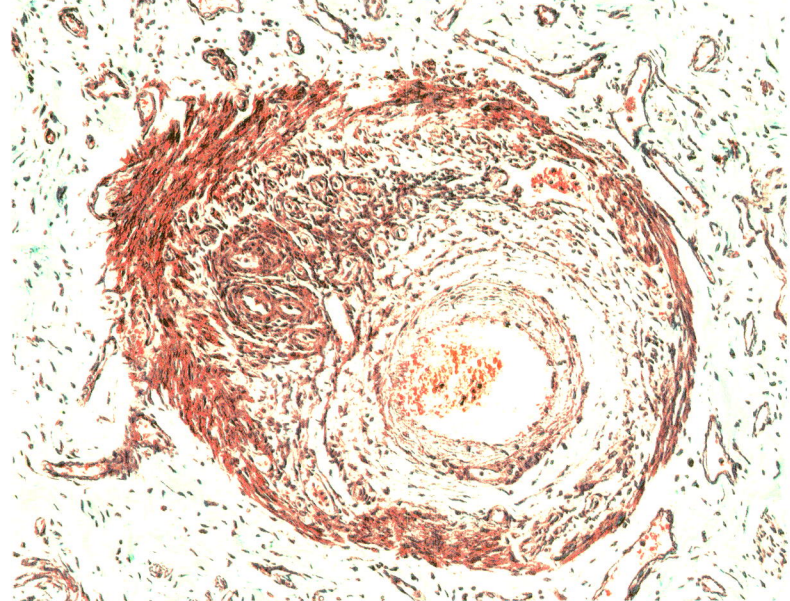

deep veins. This is associated with thrombosis, which, when organized, may eventually undergo recanalization. The middle layer shows hardly any changes. Oedema under the external elastic layer is also characteristic of TAO. The adventitia of arteries as well as veins first show inflammation and then fibrosis which may involve the accompanying nerves [16].

Fig. 7.19 Arteriosclerosis obliterans. Segment of the wall of an artery. The prominence of the vasa vasorum is notable for its thick wall and course parallel to the major axis of the vessel. These vessels are arranged in a crown in the inner part of the medial layer (Masson's trichrome staining)

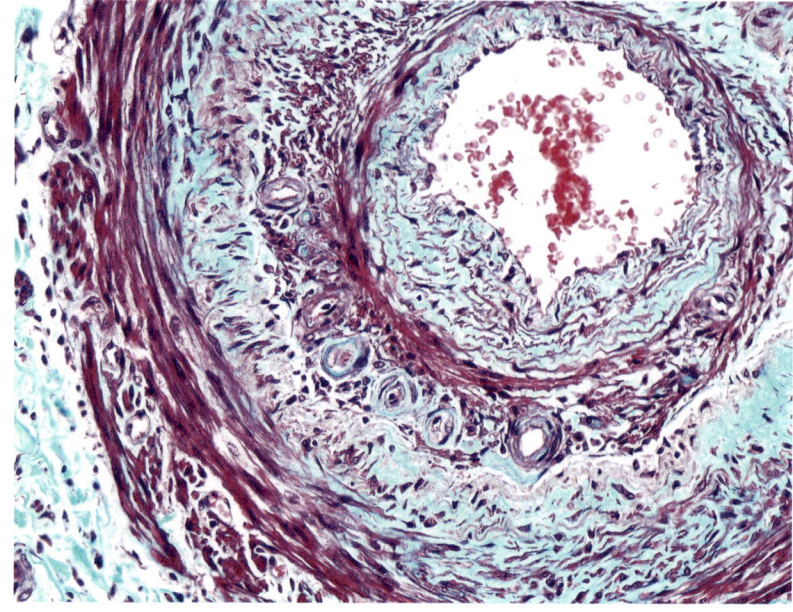

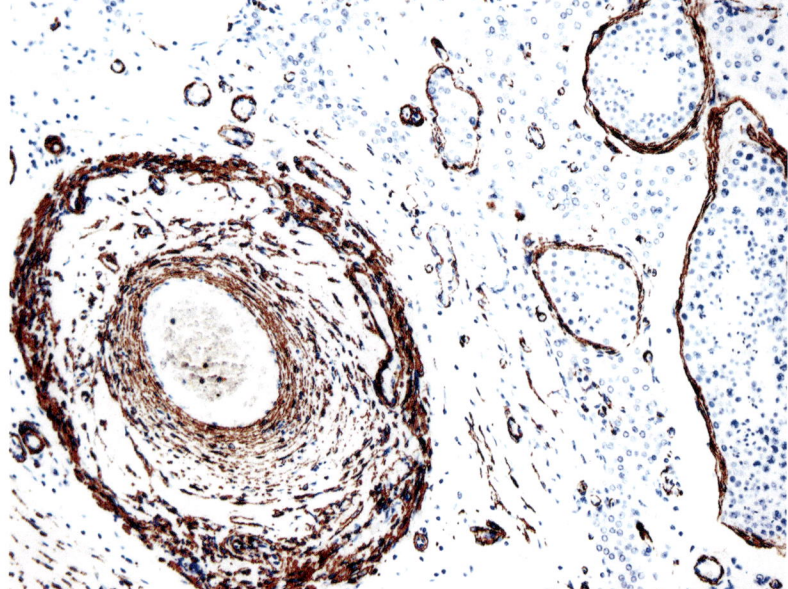

Fig. 7.20 Arteriosclerosis obliterans. Smooth muscle actin immunostaining reveals the poorly developed muscle cells in the inner medial layer. As a control, note the intense positivity of peritubular myoid cells

Fig. 7.21 Arteriosclerosis obliterans. Note the increased number and tortuosity of the vasa vasorum of the middle layer (immunostaining for desmin)

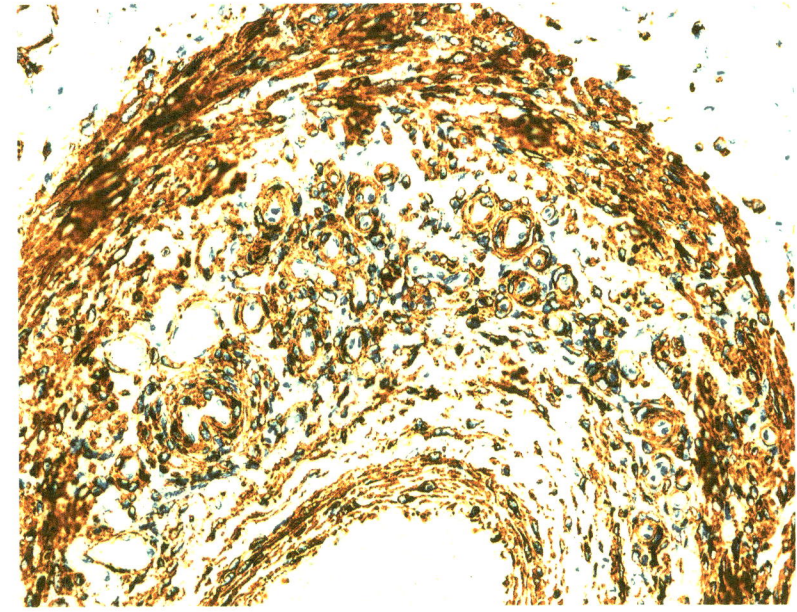

7.5   Arteriolar Hyalinosis of the Testis

Arteriolar hyalinosis is a very common physiological finding in the vessels of the spleen in both children and adults. It is common in the arterioles of the kidney, choroid, and retina in hypertensive patients or those with diabetes [17, 18] as well as in renal patients treated with calcineurin inhibitor after transplantation [19]. It is commonly seen in hepatic, pancreatic, adrenal, and lower limb arterioles in elderly patients [20].

Arteriolar hyalinosis of the testis is observed both in autopsies and in biopsies with an incidence varying from 18% to 21% depending on whether isolated arteriolar lesions or lesions diffusely affect most of these vessels. The most affected vessels are those that are between 50 and 100 microns in diameter. The age at which the lesions appear is important, it is rare in childhood, reaches a peak at the end of the third decade of life and from this age onwards it plateaus or even tends to decrease slightly [21].

This lesion is characterized by the accumulation of eosinophilic material under the endothelium of the wall of small and medium-sized arterioles. The accumulation is amorphous and not accompanied by necrosis or inflammation of the vascular wall. The deposits are eccentric, have a segmental distribution, and produce stenosis of the vascular lumen (Fig. 7.22). The deposits may contain small vacuoles, pyknotic nuclei, and atrophic smooth muscle cells. The internal elastic lamina may be missing in these areas of the wall (Fig. 7.23).

The lesions are PAS positive, diastase resistant (Fig. 7.24), Oil Red O positive (fat neutral) and Congo red negative (absence of amyloid). They show acicular crystals when examined with polarized light (cholesterol) and have deposits of different immunoglobulins (IgG, IgM), fibrin, fibrinogen, and beta-1C complement fraction [22, 23]. The type of deposition varies from vessel to vessel [24].

Under the electron microscope, the endothelial cells show no alterations except for increased thickness of the cytoplasm and abundant lipofuscins. The basement membrane in the large deposits is engulfed by them. The deposits consist of a material that is more electron dense than the basement membrane and has abundant electrodense particles of approximately 200μ. The material shows no collagen, fibrin or amyloid fibrils. While in small lesions, the material extends from the endothelial cells to the elastic laminae, in larger lesions, the latter are destroyed,

Fig. 7.22 Arteriolar
hyalinosis of the testis.
A 36-year-old patient.
Sections of several small
arteries and arterioles.
Several arterioles have
luminal stenosis, and an
accumulation of
eccentric subendothelial
hyaline material. The
seminiferous tubules are
completely hyalinized

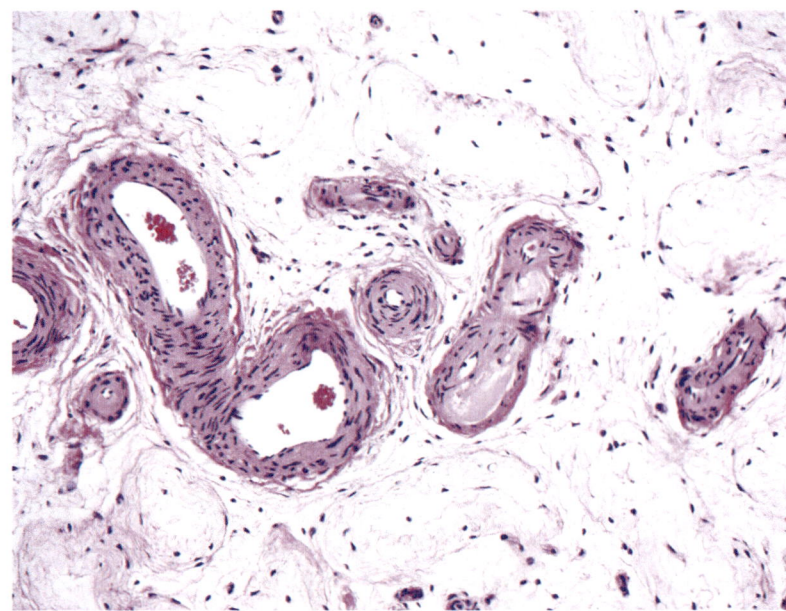

Fig. 7.23 Arteriolar
hyalinosis of the testis.
Transverse and oblique
section of two arterioles.
The hyaline deposit
causes focal destruction
of the internal elastic
lamina (orcein)

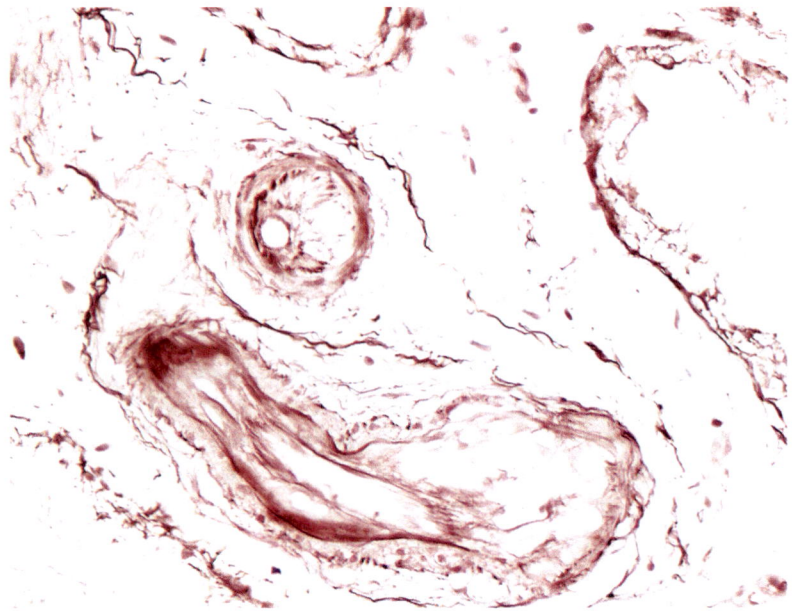

and atrophic muscle cells can be recognized within the material [25–27].

The accumulated material initially comes from the blood to which, as it accumulates, different components of the vascular wall are incorporated [28, 29]. Endothelial dysfunction induced by hemodynamic changes leads to an increase in permeability resulting in the passage of blood proteins into the subendothelial space

[22]. The accumulation of plasma proteins may be responsible for the de-differentiation of smooth muscle cells and deposition of extracellular matrix proteins as suggested by experimental studies [30].

Although arteriolar hyalinosis can be observed in testes with normal spermatogenesis, it is much more frequent in testes with pathology such as in patients with Klinefelter's syndrome, cryptorchi-

Fig. 7.24 Arteriolar hyalinosis of the testis. The arteriole has marked thickening of the intima and media due to strongly PAS positive material. Next to it, lie a lymphatic vessel and two seminiferous tubules with only containing Sertoli cells. The Leydig cells have abundant vacuolated cytoplasm

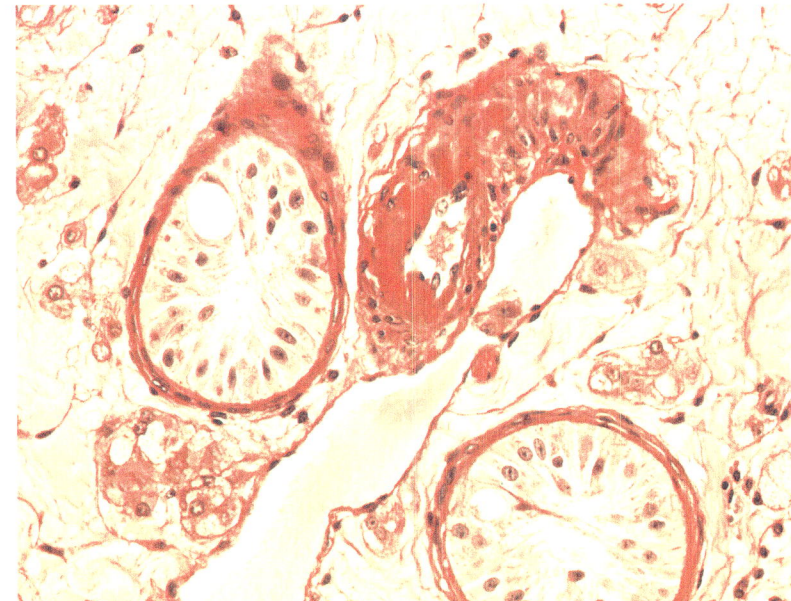

Fig. 7.25 Arteriolar hyalinosis of the testis. Cross section of an arteriole. A large part of the wall is occupied by hyaline material that produces a marked luminal stenosis. In the central part of the hyaline material a calcification with spiculated contours stands out

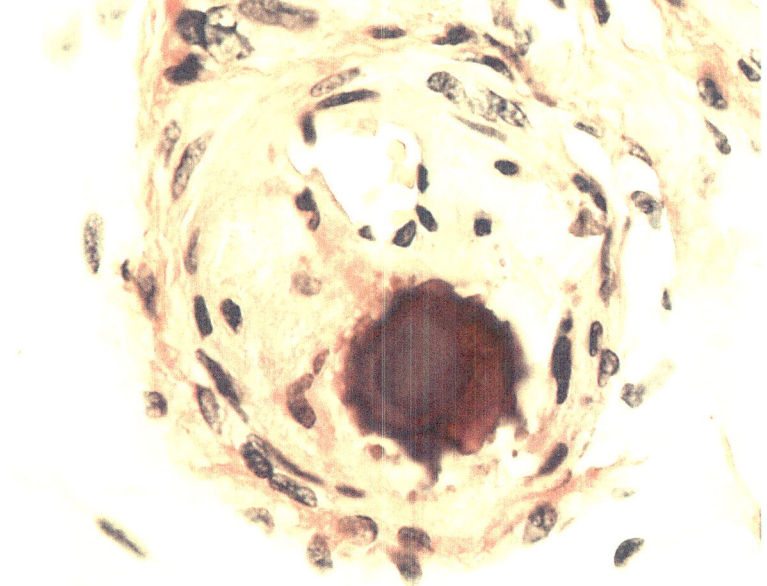

dism, diabetic, and hypertensive patients. When luminal stenosis of the arterioles is important and especially when it is associated with calcification of the vascular wall, it is logical that they produce ischemia of the parenchyma, which in mild cases is manifested by hypospermatogenesis and in more severe cases by focal sclerosis of the seminiferous tubules [31] (Figs. 7.25, 7.26, and 7.27).

Fig. 7.26 Arteriolar hyalinosis of the testis. Arteriole with hyalinosis and multiple nodular calcifications of the wall

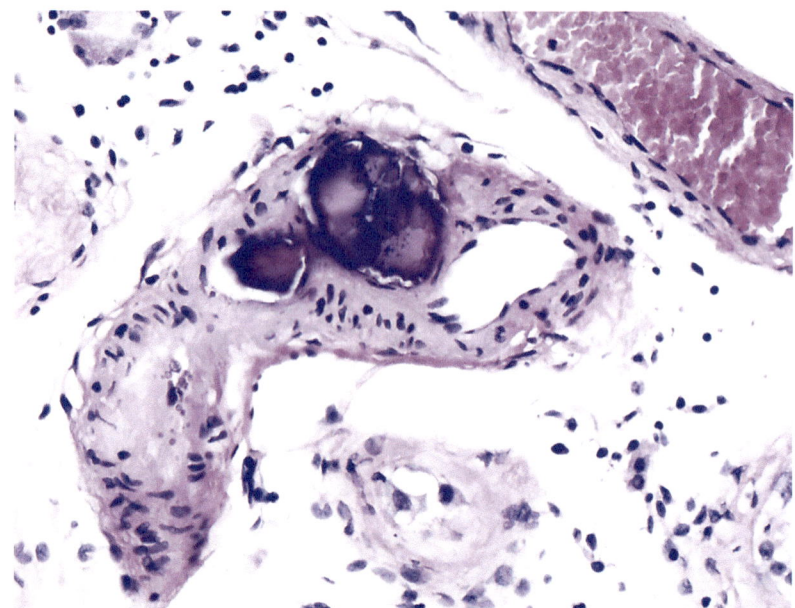

Fig. 7.27 Arteriolar hyalinosis of the testis. The central arteriole shows wall calcification

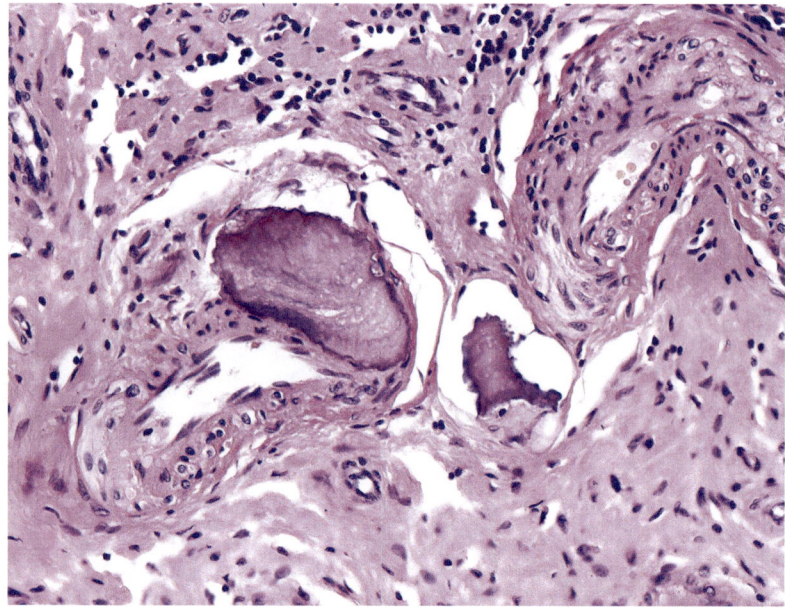

References

1. Fishbein GA, Fishbein MC. Arteriosclerosis: rethinking the current classification. Arch Pathol Lab Med. 2009;133:1309–16.
2. Dos Santos VP, Pozzan G, Castelli V, Caffaro RA. Arteriosclerosis, atherosclerosis, arteriolosclerosis, and Monckeberg medial calcific sclerosis: what is the difference? J Vasc Bras. 2021;20:e20200211.
3. Klein R, Pfitzer P. Flow cytometry of postmortem human testicular tissue in cases of atherosclerosis. Cytometry. 1984;5:636–43.
4. Regadera J, Nistal M, Paniagua R. Testis, epididymis, and spermatic cord in elderly men. Correlation of angiographic and histologic studies with systemic arteriosclerosis. Arch Pathol Lab Med. 1985;109:663–7.
5. Paniagua R, Nistal M, Saez FJ, Fraile B. Ultrastructure of the aging human testis. J Electron Microsc Tech. 1991;19:241–60.

6. Martinez-Lemus LA. The dynamic structure of arterioles. Basic Clin Pharmacol Toxicol. 2012;110:5–11.

7. Hill GS. Hypertensive nephrosclerosis. Curr Opin Nephrol Hypertens. 2008;17:266–70.

8. Mönckeberg JG. Ueber die reine Mediaverkalkung der Extremitaetenarterien und ihr Verhalten zur Arteriosklerose. Virchows Arch Pathol Anat. 1903;171:141–67.

9. Stack A, Sheffield S, Seegobin K, Maharaj S. Mönckeberg medial sclerosis. Cleve Clin J Med. 2020;87:396–7.

10. Janzen J, Bültmann B, Leitritz M, Rothenberger-Janzen K, Vuong PN. Histopathological aspects of arterial calcifications. Perfusion. 2003;16:136–40.

11. Lanzer P, Boehm M, Sorribas V, Thiriet M, Janzen J, Zeller T, St Hilaire C, Shanahan C. Medial vascular calcification revisited: review and perspectives. Eur Heart J. 2014;35:1515–25.

12. Ho CY, Shanahan CM. Medial arterial calcification: an overlooked player in peripheral arterial disease. Arterioscler Thromb Vasc Biol. 2016;36:1475–82.

13. Pisani I, De Troia A, Allegri L, Corradi D, Vaglio A. Malignant Mönckeberg medial calcific sclerosis. Intern Emerg Med. 2018;13:615–7.

14. Huang PP, Li SZ, Han MZ, Xiao ZJ, Yang RC, Qiu LG, Han ZC. Autologous transplantation of peripheral blood stem cells as an effective therapeutic approach for severe arteriosclerosis obliterans of lower extremities. Thromb Haemost. 2004;91:606–9.

15. Fazeli B, Ligi D, Keramat S, Maniscalco R, Sharebiani H, Mannello F. Recent updates and advances in Winiwarter-Buerger disease (Thromboangiitis obliterans): biomolecular mechanisms, diagnostics and clinical consequences. Diagnostics. 2021;11:1736.

16. Kurata A, Franke FE, Machinami R, Schulz A. Thromboangiitis obliterans: classic and new morphological features. Virchows Arch. 2000;436:59–67.

17. Moritz AR, Oldt MR. Arteriolar sclerosis in hypertensive and non-hypertensive individuals. Am J Pathol. 1937;13:679–728.

18. Salman L, Martinez L, Faddoul G, Manning C, Ali K, Salman M, Vazquez-Padron R. Hyaluronan inhibition as a therapeutic target for diabetic kidney disease: what is next? Kidney. 2023;4(6):e851–60.

19. Matos AC, Câmara NO, Requião-Moura LR, Tonato EJ, Filiponi TC, Souza-Durão M, Malheiros DM, Fregonesi M, Borrelli M, Pacheco-Silva A. Presence of arteriolar hyalinosis in post-reperfusion biopsies represents an additional risk to ischaemic injury in renal transplant. Nephrology. 2016;21:923–9.

20. Dustin P. Arteriolar hyalinosis. Int Rev Exp Pathol. 1962;1:73–138.

21. Hatakeyama S, Sengoku R, Takayama S. Histological and submicroscopic studies on arteriolar hyalinosis of the human testis. Bull Tokyo Med Dent Univ. 1966;13:511–30.

22. Krawczyński K. Immunohistochemical study of arteriolar (simple) hyalinosis in spleen. Am J Pathol. 1971;62:253–64.

23. Gamble CN. The pathogenesis of hyaline arteriolosclerosis. Am J Pathol. 1986;122:410–20.

24. Crawford T, Woolf N. Hyaline arteriolosclerosis in the spleen: an immuno-histochemical study. J Pathol Bacteriol. 1960;79:221–5.

25. Biava CG, Dyrda I, Genest J, Bencosme SA. Renal hyaline arteriolosclerosis. An electron microscope study. Am J Pathol. 1964;44:349–63.

26. Fisher ER, Perez-Stable E, Pardo V. Ultrastructural studies in hypertension. I. Comparison of renal vascular and juxtaglomerular cell alterations in essential and renal hypertension in man. Lab Investig. 1966;15:1409–33.

27. Frei D, Hedinger C. Arterioläre Hyalinose in Hodenbiopsien [Arteriolar hyalinosis in testicular biopsies (author's transl)]. Virchows Arch A Pathol Anat Histol. 1979;381:269–81.

28. Duguid JB, Anderson GS. The pathogenesis of hyaline arteriolosclerosis. J Pathol Bacteriol. 1952;64:519–22.

29. Still WJ, Hill KR. The pathogenesis of hyaline arteriolar sclerosis. AMA Arch Pathol. 1959;68:42–8.

30. Mencke R, Umbach AT, Wiggenhauser LM, Voelkl J, Olauson H, Harms G, Bulthuis M, Krenning G, Quintanilla-Martinez L, van Goor H, Lang F, Hillebrands JL. Klotho deficiency induces arteriolar hyalinosis in a trade-off with vascular calcification. Am J Pathol. 2019;189:2503–15.

31. Nistal M, Potenciano J, Contreras F. Arteriolar hyalinosis of the testis. Arch Esp Urol. 1973;5:481–500.

8.1 Cholesterol Thromboembolism (Atheromatous Embolism)

This refers to the presence of atherosclerotic plaque material from the aorta inside the testicular artery or, more frequently, in one of its branches. The material may be constituted only by cholesterol crystals or by macrophages with xanthomized cytoplasm (Figs. 8.1, 8.2, 8.3, 8.4, 8.5, and 8.6).

A cholesterol embolism is not as rare as classically considered, in fact, it is frequent in elderly patients with ulcerated atherosclerosis. Sometimes it appears after an iatrogenic process such as in patients who undergo vascular surgery, endovascular aneurysm repair, invasive radiological procedures, or who receive anticoagulants, but, in most cases, there is no previous history. Clinically, the clinical manifestations of testicular cholesterol thromboembolism are asymptomatic in many/most cases but, in a small number of cases, are dominated by testicular pain, leading to an initial suspicion of testicular torsion. Histologically, it may produce minimal ischemic changes and be an autopsy finding in a patient with ulcerated atheroma plaques in the aorta while, in other cases, the image is that of a segmental or global infarction.

Segmental infarction of the testicle is a rare entity with about 40 published cases. The cause is unclear in most of the reported cases, although it has been described in association with trauma, epididymitis, vasculitis, fibroplasia of the intima of the spermatic artery or haematological disorders, and most have been considered idiopathic. Cholesterol embolism produces a segmental, haemorrhagic necrosis of the testicular parenchyma that stands out macroscopically as a reddish lesion that is well-demarcated from the neighbouring parenchyma. Atheromatous detritus is observed inside the arteries [1].

Global testicular infarction is relatively frequent. It has been described secondary to spermatic cord torsion, birth trauma, epididymitis, sickle cell disease, incarcerated inguinal hernia or as idiopathic. Global testicular infarction due to cholesterol embolism is exceptional. It may present with acute testicular pain simulating testicular torsion or a malignant tumour. It has been described in several patients undergoing endovascular aneurysm repair [2, 3]. In the few cases with histological study, extensive necrosis with cholesterol crystals has been observed in the intratesticular arterial branches with a small part of testicular parenchyma in the periphery being spared. Both orchiectomy [4] and conservative treatment have been used [5].

Fig. 8.1 Atheromatous embolism. Interlobular artery surrounded by several lymphatic vessels. The lumen is occupied by parallel acicular formations. The seminiferous tubules have a decreased caliber, wall thickening and defective spermatogenesis that does not progress beyond first order spermatocytes

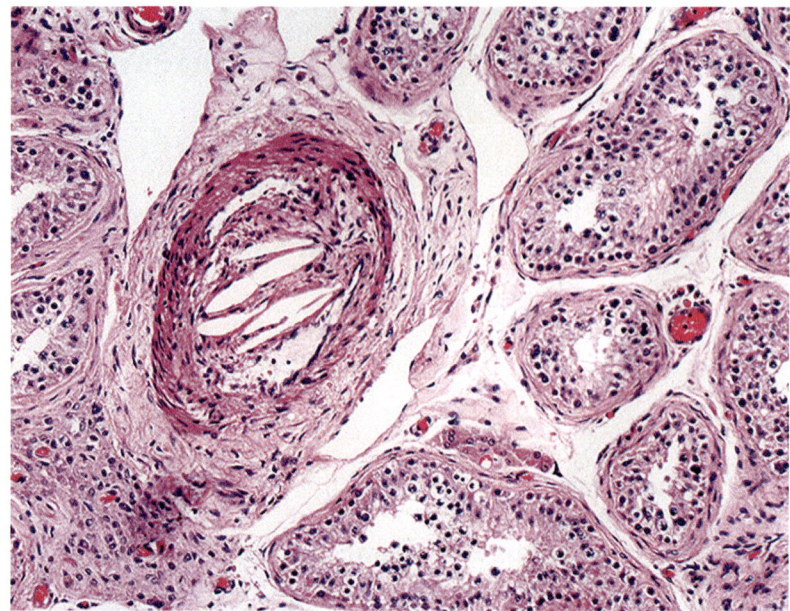

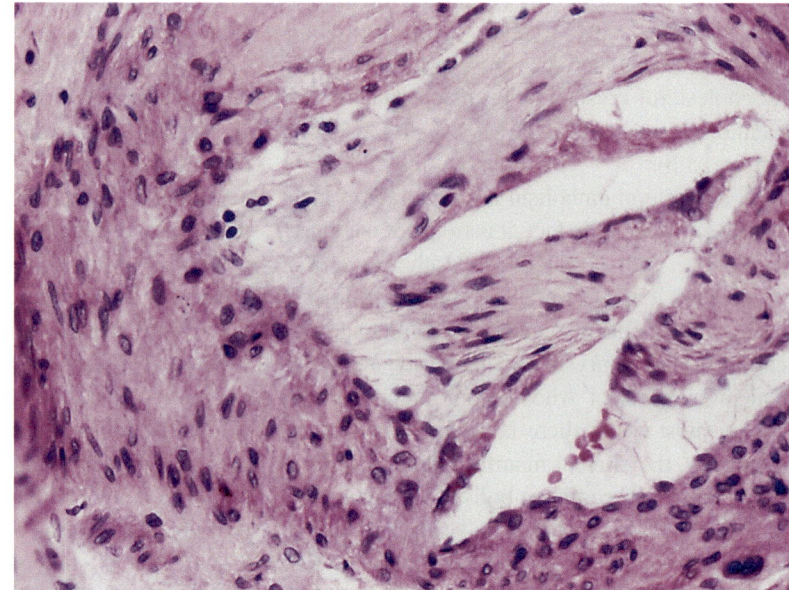

Fig. 8.2 Atheromatous embolism. The lumen of the artery is occupied by a thrombus in which several cholesterol crystals are prominent. One has perforated the intima and part of the media of the vascular wall with cholesterol clefts

Fig. 8.3 Atheromatous embolism. Most of the lumen of this intraparenchymal artery is occupied by clusters of macrophages. The surrounding seminiferous tubules have significant atrophy

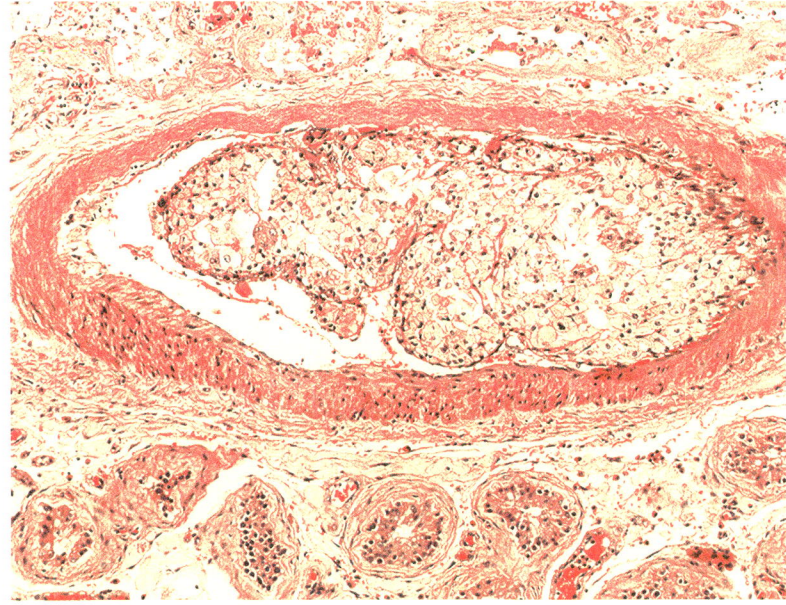

Fig. 8.4 Atheromatous embolism. In the detail of the previous figure, the xanthomized appearance of the cytoplasm of the cells of the embolus of an atheromatous plaque can be recognized

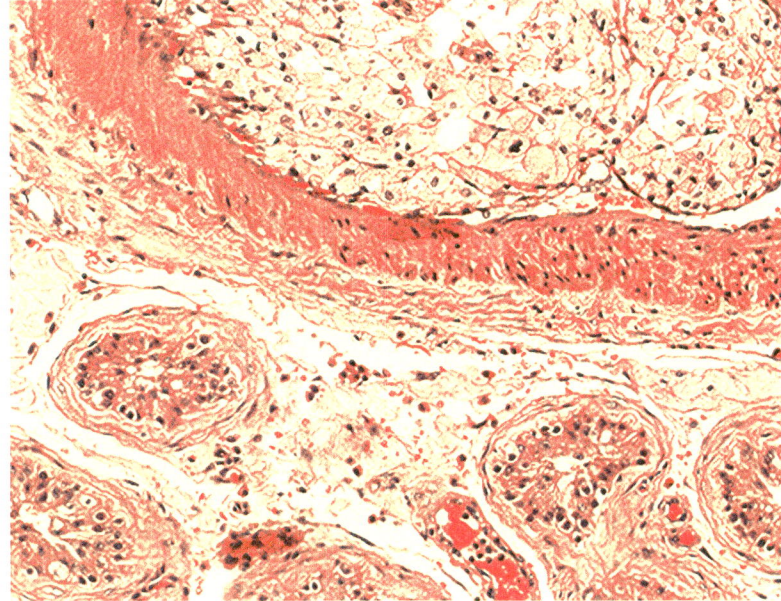

Fig. 8.5 Atheromatous embolism. The section of the arteriole shows the beginning of the organization of a thrombus. Fibrin, histiocytes in the central part and partial endothelialization of this material are observed peripherally

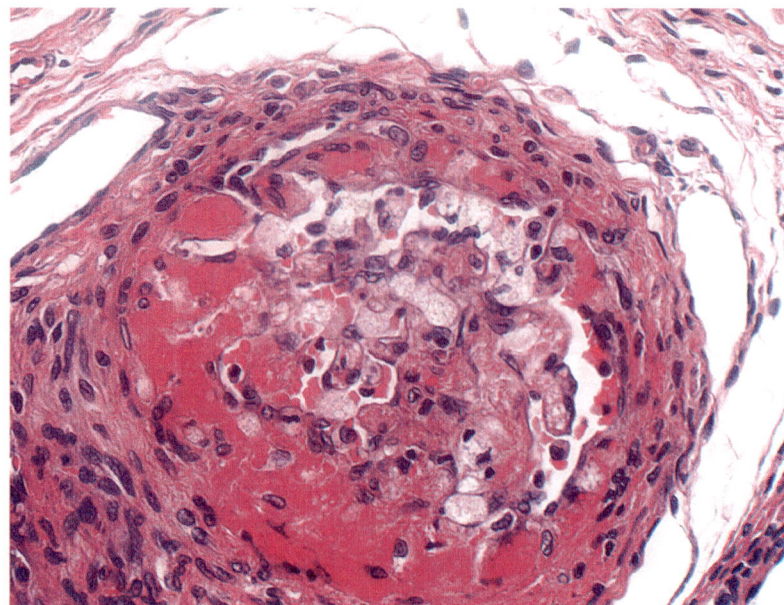

Fig. 8.6 Atheromatous embolism. Subalbuginea artery with recanalized thrombus. The thrombus material is in continuity with a markedly thickened intima

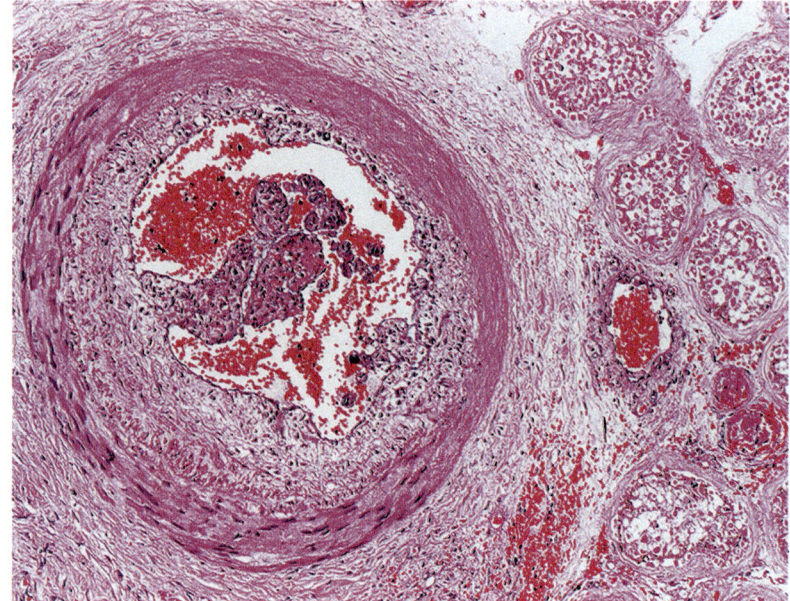

8.2 Intracavitary Nodular Polypoid Calcifying Proliferation in the Rete Testis

The presence of nodular formations with or without calcification is a characteristic lesion of the rete testis and is related to poor peripheral perfu-sion. It is characterized by the development, inside the cavities of the rete testis, of pedunculated masses of a cell-poor tissue with a tendency to calcify. The lesion is bilateral, may be associated with other lesions of the rete testis, and has been described as an autopsy finding [6].

The rete testis consists of three parts: septal rete, mediastinal rete, and extratesticular rete testis. The septal rete is constituted by the straight ductules that connect the seminiferous tubules with the mediastinal rete. The mediastinal rete is comma-shaped with the widened part towards the upper pole of the testis; it conducts spermatozoa and fluid from the seminiferous tubules to the extratesticular rete. The mediastinal rete is formed by less than a dozen cavities that are parallel to each other, and in which the 1400 straight ducts that form the septal rete perpendicularly or obliquely terminate. Normally the cavities of the mediastinal rete show hardly any content. To prevent their dilatation, the chordae tendineae are arranged inside them from one wall to the other. The chordae tendineae are similar in structure to the chordae tendineae of the heart valves. The thinner ones consist of a central axis of collagenous fibres and isolated fibroblasts with a lining from flattened cells of the epithelium of the rete testis. The thicker chordae have a capillary inside (Fig. 8.7). The extratesticular rete connects the mediastinal rete with the efferent ducts that form the head of the epididymis. It begins at perforations of the albuginea and its cavities generally present various degrees of dilatation (bullae rete) [7]. Among the functions of the rete testis are homogenization of the testicular fluid, reabsorption of potassium and, sometimes, phagocytosis of malformed spermatozoa.

The lesions described as intracavitary nodular polypoid calcifying proliferation in the rete testis are sessile or more frequently pedunculated formations, which settle directly on the chordae tendineae and protrude into the cavities of the mediastinal rete testis. Some show only a central part consisting of an eosinophilic fibrin-like material lined by the flat epithelium of the rete testis (Figs. 8.8, 8.9, and 8.10). Others have a more complex structure. The eosinophilic material constitutes several nodular formations, separated from each other by a myxoid stroma with some fibroblasts. In the acellular material, Perl-(iron) and von Kossa-(calcium) positive deposits are initiated. Finally, there are totally nodular polypoid calcified formations. These calcifications can be amorphous or annular (Figs. 8.11 and 8.12). No inflammatory cells are observed in any formation. There are no inflammatory infiltrates in the testis or epididymis.

The aetiology of these lesions is unknown, but there are several findings in the histories of these patients that are interesting: Intense arteriosclerosis, myocardial infarction, or a history of gastrointestinal bleeding. Everything suggests that at some point these patients have had one or more episodes of poor peripheral perfusion. The testicular mediastinum, in which the

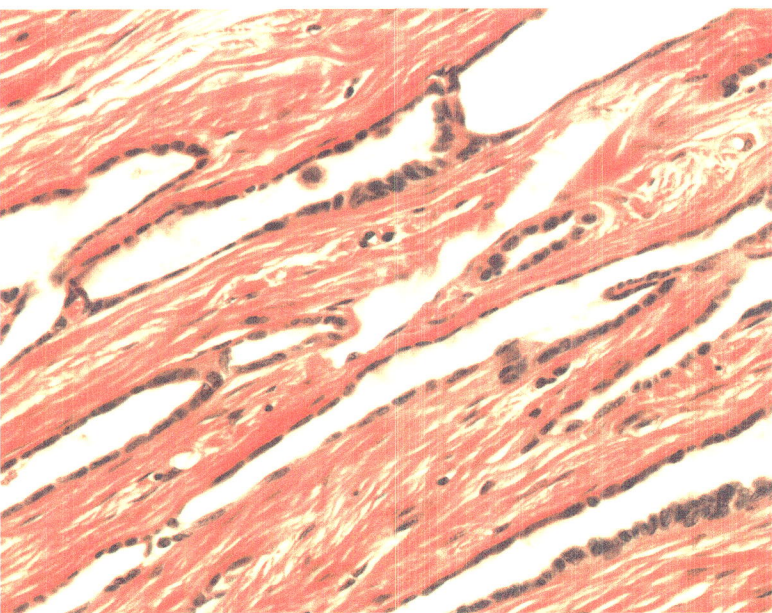

Fig. 8.7 Normal rete testis mediastinum. The cavities of the rete testis mediastinum are optically empty spaces lined by flat cells with islets of cubic or cylindrical cells. Chordae tendineae obliquely cross their interior

Fig. 8.8 Intracavitary nodular polypoid calcifying proliferation of the rete testis. Cell-depleted hyaline material in the interior of the cavities. This material is lined by the epithelial cells of the rete testis

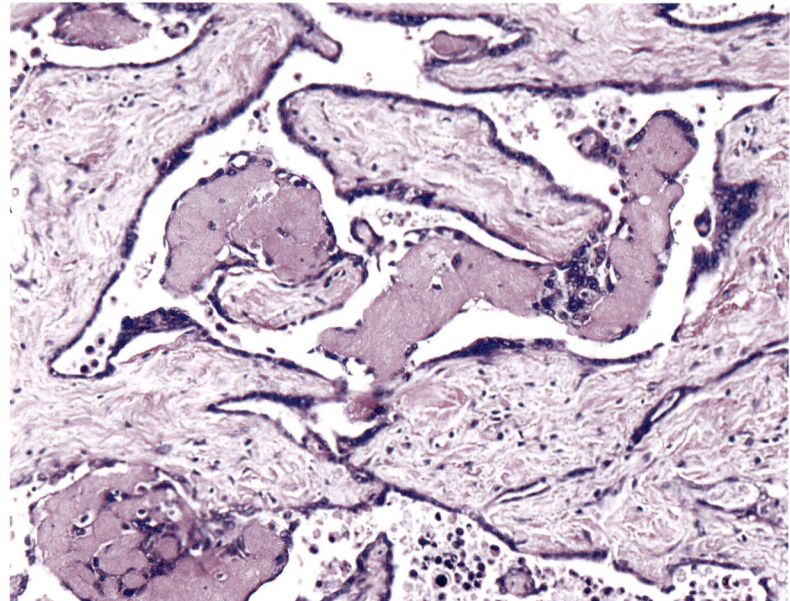

Fig. 8.9 Intracavitary nodular polypoid calcifying proliferation of rete testis. Several nodular formations within a dilated cavity of the rete testis. All are seated on a chordae tendineae

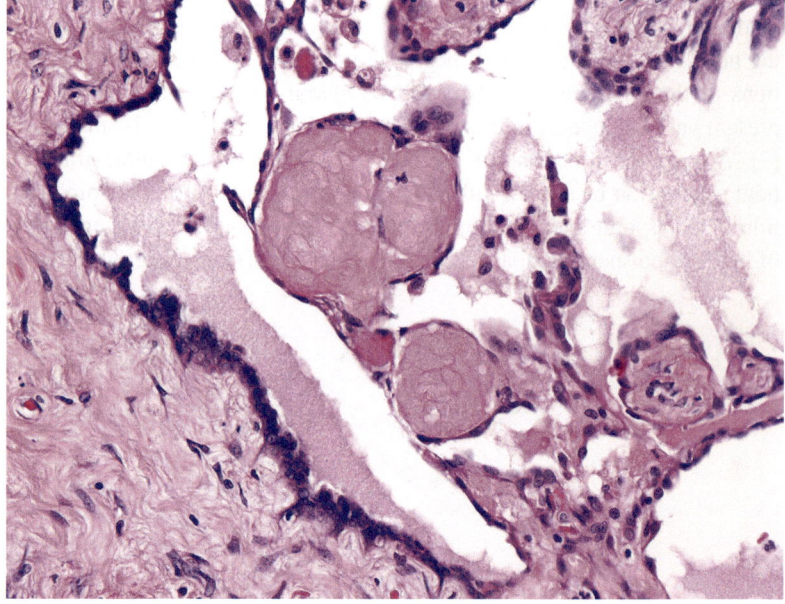

rete testis sits, is a poorly vascularized area of the testis [8, 9]. Only the thicker chordae tendineae have some capillaries. It seems quite likely that hypoxia produces changes in the permeability of endothelial cells, which could lead to accumulation of fibrin-like material, which later which would later undergo dystrophic calcification.

In the differential diagnosis, one should consider the presence of microliths in the rete testis and testicular mediastinal calcifications as in chronic renal insufficiency, and postorchitic and tumour calcifications. Microliths in the rete testis have been observed in a wide variety of processes: cystic dysplasia of the rete testis; undescended testis or associated with testicular

Fig. 8.10 Intracavitary nodular polypoid calcifying proliferation of the rete testis. Nodular proliferation consisting of a myriad of concentric nodular calcifications simulating parasite eggs

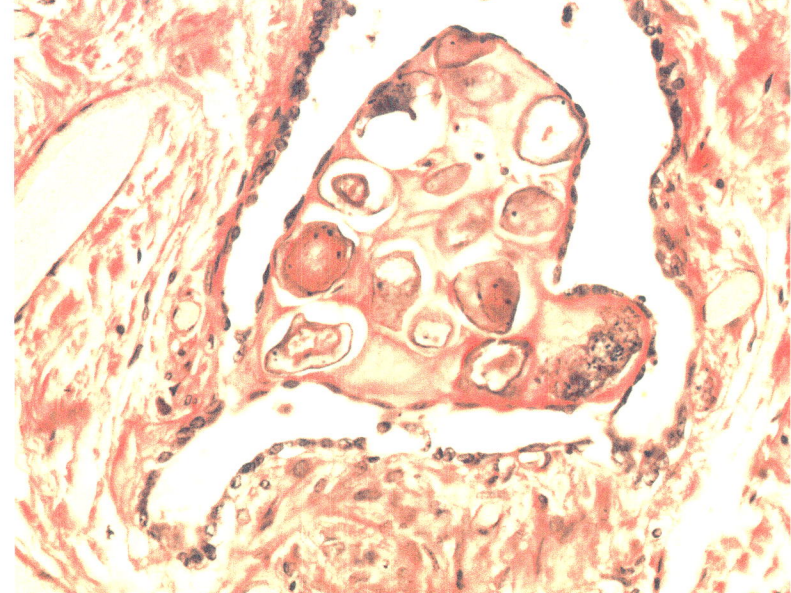

Fig. 8.11 Intracavitary nodular polypoid calcifying proliferation of the rete testis. There are large calcifications occupying a dilated cavity of the rete testis

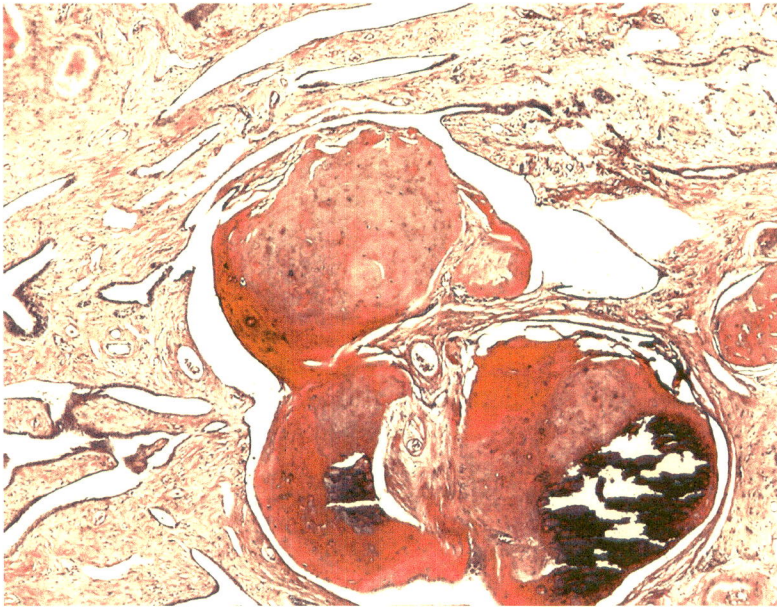

microlithiasis or malignancy. They can be single or form a morular conglomerate, they are located under the epithelium of the rete testis and do not affect the chordae tendineae, they do not usually protrude into the cavities. Their spherical structure of concentric mineralized layers is characteristic [10]. In chronic renal failure, calcifications of the rete testis are asso-ciated with other lesions typical of the disease, such as urate and oxalate deposits, a discrete inflammatory infiltrate, and the presence of foreign body giant cells [11]. The calcifications observed in some orchites [12], and in tumours are more irregular and are preferentially located in the parenchyma rather than in the testicular mediastinum [13, 14].

Fig. 8.12 Intracavitary nodular polypoid calcifying proliferation of the rete testis. Partial ossification of an intracavitary proliferation. The cells occupying the lumina are desquamated germ cells. The epithelium of the rete testis is cubic. There is no inflammatory reaction

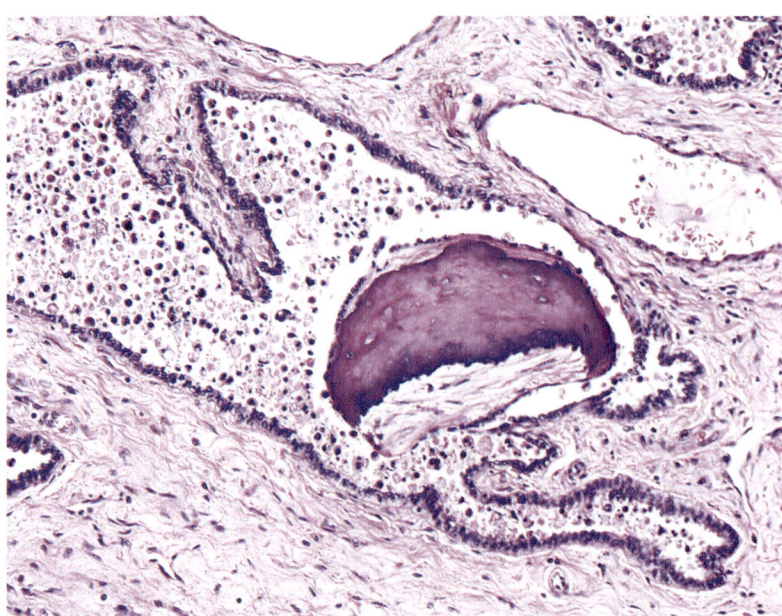

8.3 Ischemic Epididymitis

Ischemic epididymitis is a chronic, granulomatous, destructive, non-infectious, asymptomatic lesion, related to an alteration of the arterial flow of the epididymis caused either by vasculitis or arteriosclerosis. The most affected part of the epididymis is the head (Fig. 8.13).

The irrigation of the head and part of the body of the epididymis depends on the epididymal arteries, which are collateral branches of the testicular artery. Part of the epididymal body and tail is supplied by branches of the deferential artery. All the arteries run along the surface of the epididymis. There are connections between the branches of the deferential artery and the epididymal arteries, as well as branches originating from the arteries of the testicular parenchyma and the epididymal arteries. In the head of the epididymis the epididymal arteries give rise to spiral branches that penetrate into its interior following the conjunctival septa where they form arterioles [9]. The efferent ductules have a large bed of fenestrated, subepithelial, circularly arranged capillaries, whereas the more distal segments of the epididymis are much less vascularized [15].

Histologically, ischemic epididymitis is characterized by the presence of the following lesions [16]: (a) necrosis of the epithelium of the efferent ductules forming clusters that protrude into their lumen; (b) accumulation of macrophages under the epithelium whether it is necrotic or only appears atrophic; (c) presence of macrophage clusters in the tubular lumen; (d) reaction of multinucleated giant cells surrounding the necrotic ducts or inside the ducts with abundant cholesterol crystals; and (e) a lymphoid infiltrate between the most preserved tubules (Figs. 8.14, 8.15, and 8.16). These lesions are sometimes associated with other lesions such as cavitation of part of the epididymis, ceroid granulomas, sperm granulomas or epididymitis nodosa. Cavitation of the epididymis is probably the result of significant necrosis of several efferent ducts close to each other. In many cases, it is surrounded by macrophages with eosinophilic and granular cytoplasm similar to ceroid granulomas [17] (Figs. 8.17 and 8.18). Its size can be seen with the naked eye (brown patches). Epididymitis nodosa is rare and its neoformed ductules are arranged in a highly collagenized stroma.

In the main duct of the epididymis, the lesions consist of subepithelial haemorrhages in some areas and an accumulation of cholesterol crystals in the same location along a segment in which the epithelium has disappeared.

Fig. 8.13 Normal epididymis. The head of the epididymis is formed by the efferent ductules. They are arranged close to each other, in contact with their walls. The external contour is circular while the internal contour is scalloped due to the different heights of the cells lining them

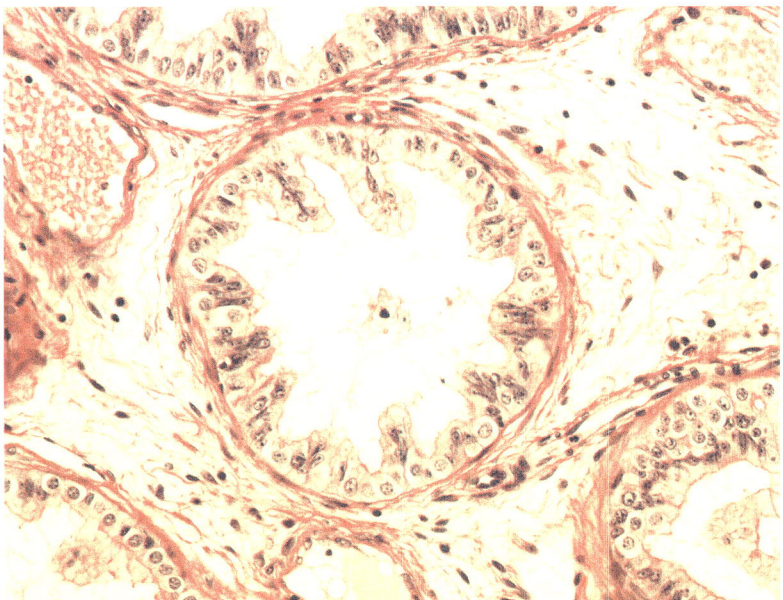

Fig. 8.14 Ischemic epididymitis. The efferent ductules show a large decrease in size and are widely separated by an inflammatory tissue

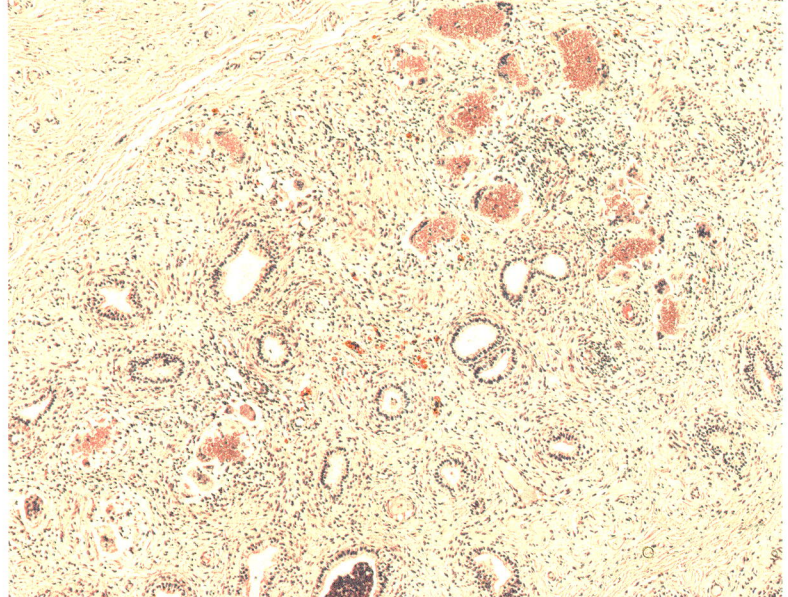

The aetiology of ischemic epididymitis is related to the age of the patient. Vasculitis is most frequent in young adults [18], while in older adults, the dominant lesions are those of arteriosclerosis [19].

Fig. 8.15 Ischemic epididymitis. Except for one atrophic efferent ductule the others have undergone necrosis. A dense inflammatory infiltrate occupies the intertubular interstitium

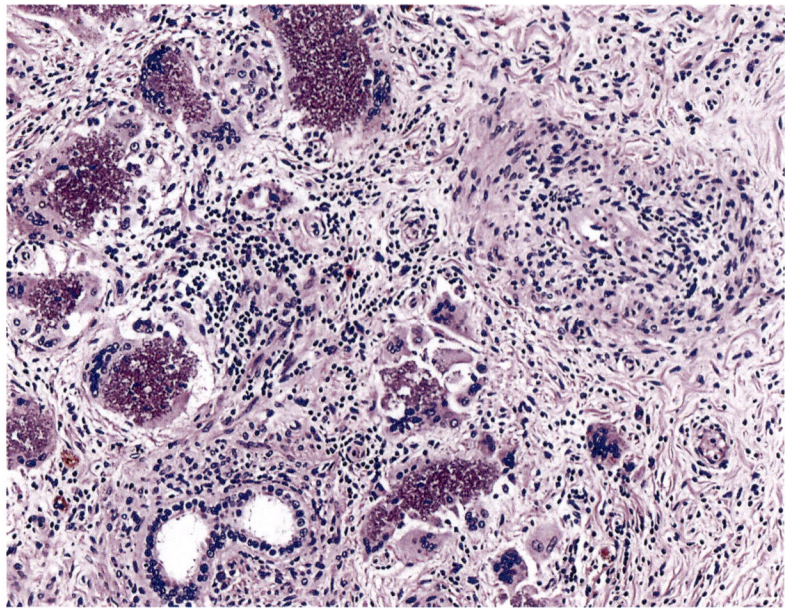

Fig. 8.16 Ischemic epididymitis. All the ductules show necrosis of the epithelium. Necrotic material, eosinophilic and granular in appearance, occupies the former lumen, surrounding and delimiting it are several multinucleated giant cells with nuclei arranged in a horseshoe pattern

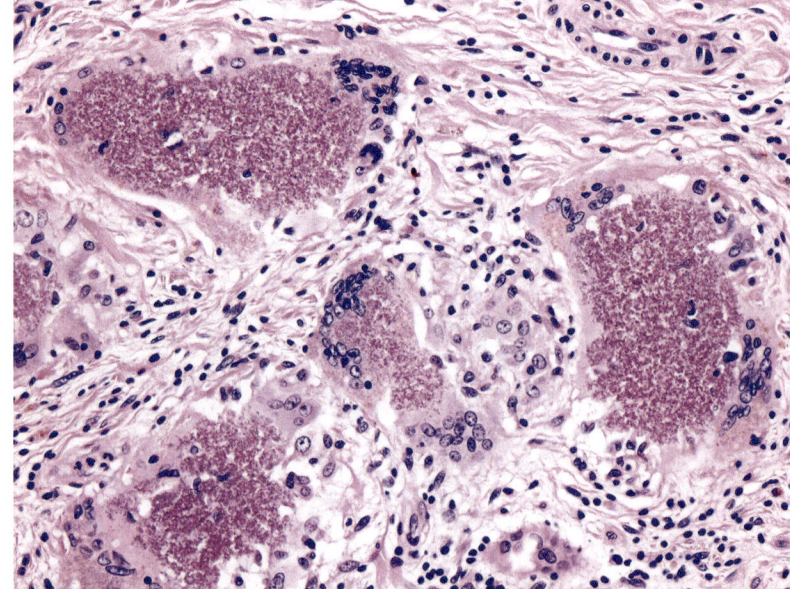

Fig. 8.17 Ischemic epididymitis. Presence of cholesterol crystals and abundant macrophages with lipofuscin (ceroid granuloma) in an old necrotic area of the epididymis

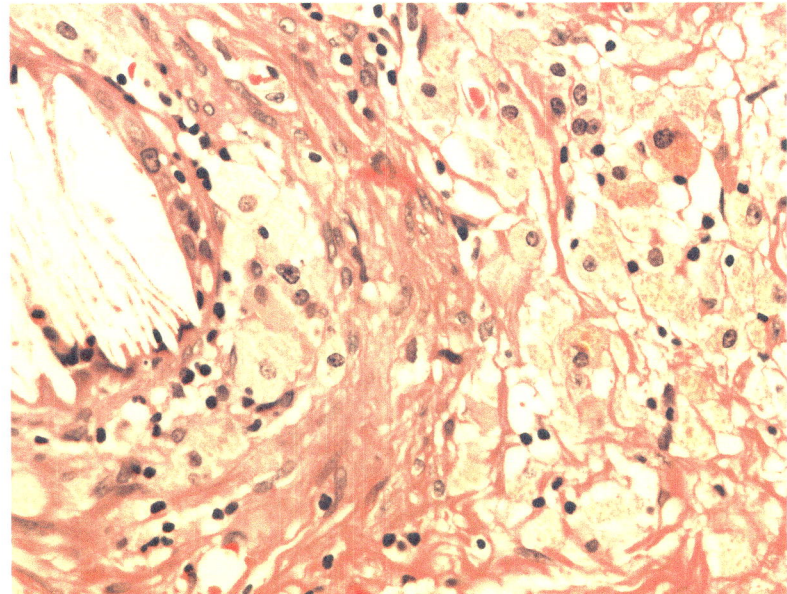

Fig. 8.18 Ischemic epididymitis. Numerous lumina of epithelial structures taking the form of glands or small ducts in a highly collagenized stroma. The picture is like that of vasitis and epididymitis nodosa

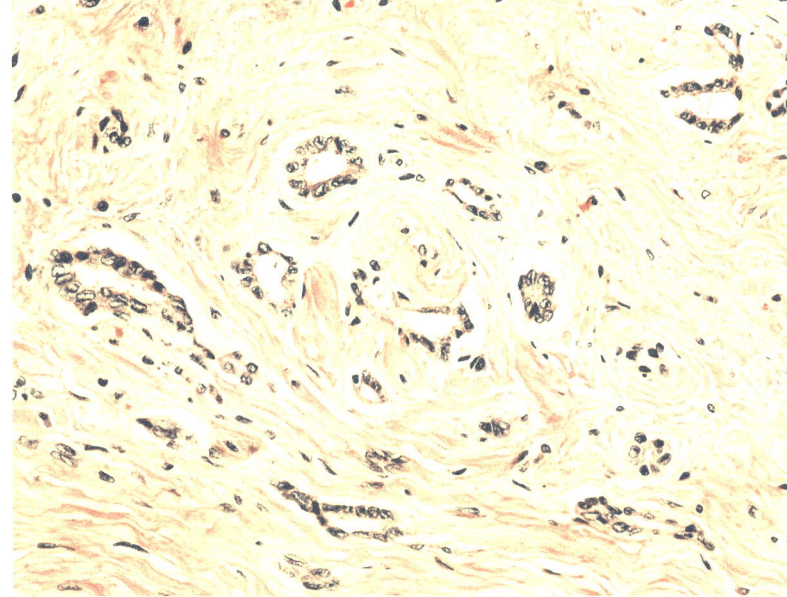

8.4   Hematoma of Paratesticular Structures

Hematomas of the epididymis and spermatic cord can be idiopathic, or secondary to well-known processes, such as trauma to the inguinal region, hernia repair [20, 21], or scrotum (ruptured epididymis) [22], rupture of a varicocele with or without previ-

ous trauma [23, 24], a complication of anticoagulant therapy [25, 26], or spread of intra-abdominal haemorrhage and vasculitis [27]. The age of presentation is very variable and is related to the pathology of the patient or the treatment used.

There is another group of patients who have no history of any kind and who present a hematoma in paratesticular structures [28]. Some are clinically diagnosed with epididymitis and treated with antibiotics without result. In others, a paratesticular tumour has been suspected. Most of the lesions are well-demarcated nodular formations varying in size from 1 cm to more than 5 cm. A small group of these hematomas are observed in elderly patients, who also show marked arteriosclerosis, both in the vessels located near the hematoma and in the testicle, which also usually presents ischemic lesions. These observations suggest a rupture of an arterial vessel with lesions of atherosclerosis either spontaneously or favoured by a trauma that went unnoticed (Figs. 8.19 and 8.20).

Histologically, the hematomas show different aspects that are consistent with the age of the hematoma itself and the attempted resorp-

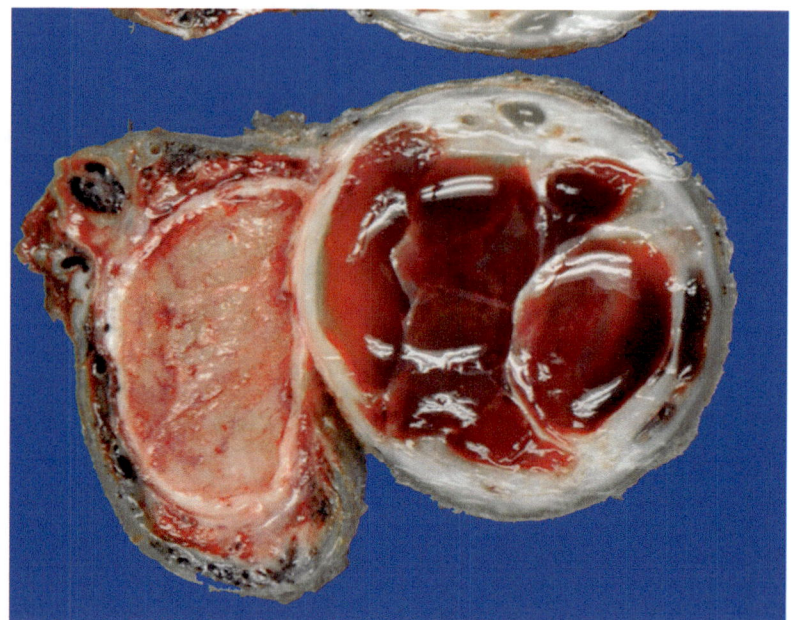

Fig. 8.19 Paratesticular hematoma. Slowly evolving paratesticular nodular formation in an 89-year-old patient. It has a fibrous capsule that is multi-cameral. The testicle is small

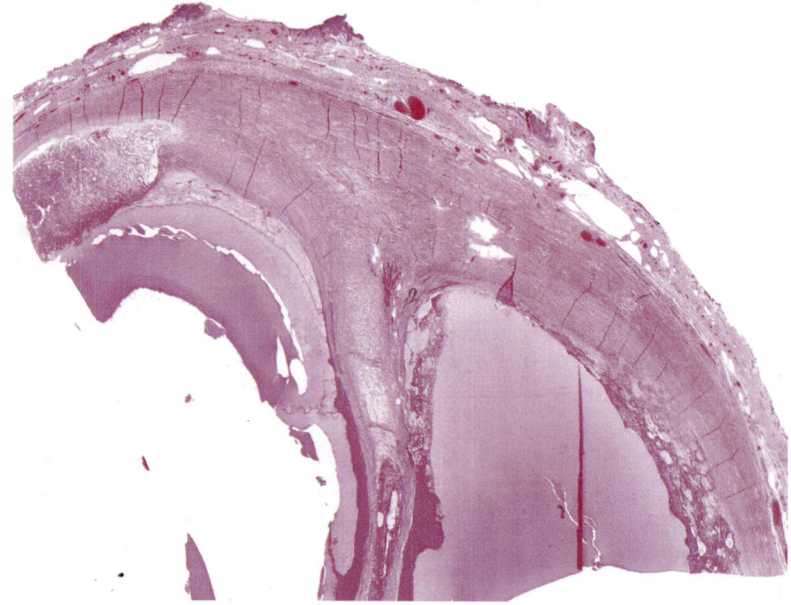

Fig. 8.20 Paratesticular hematoma. Fibrous tissue septum delimits cavities containing eosinophilic fluid in the central part and fibrin networks in the periphery

tion of the haematic material. In recent cases, there is a poorly-demarcated haemorrhagic area with even Zahn lines and macrophages with abundant hemosiderin. In other cases, the larger hematomas generally have multiple cavities with haematic material surrounded by a fibrous capsule. Inside the cavities, there may be coexisting areas of haemorrhage, fibrin networks, and clusters of cholesterol crystals (Figs. 8.21, 8.22, 8.23, and 8.24).

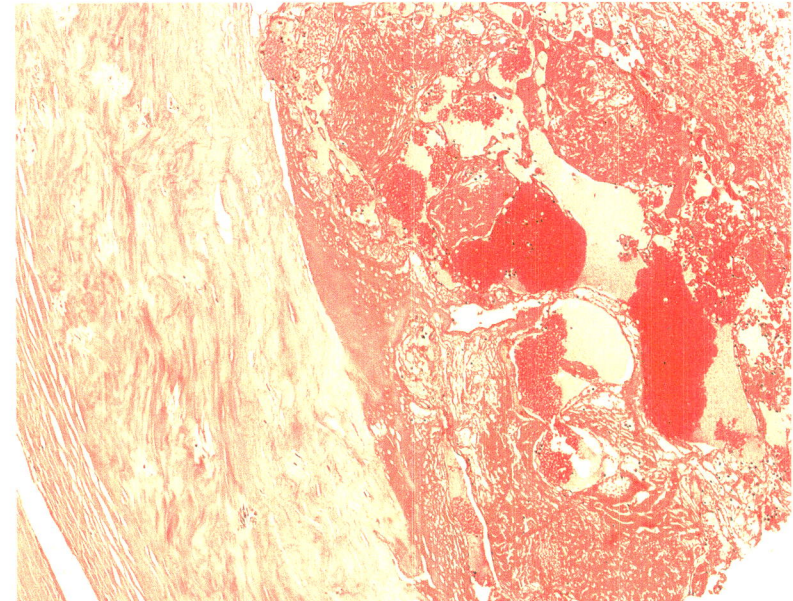

Fig. 8.21 Paratesticular hematoma. The wall is formed by a highly collagenized tissue. In the interior of one of the cavities, haematic material, and abundant fibrin networks still stand out

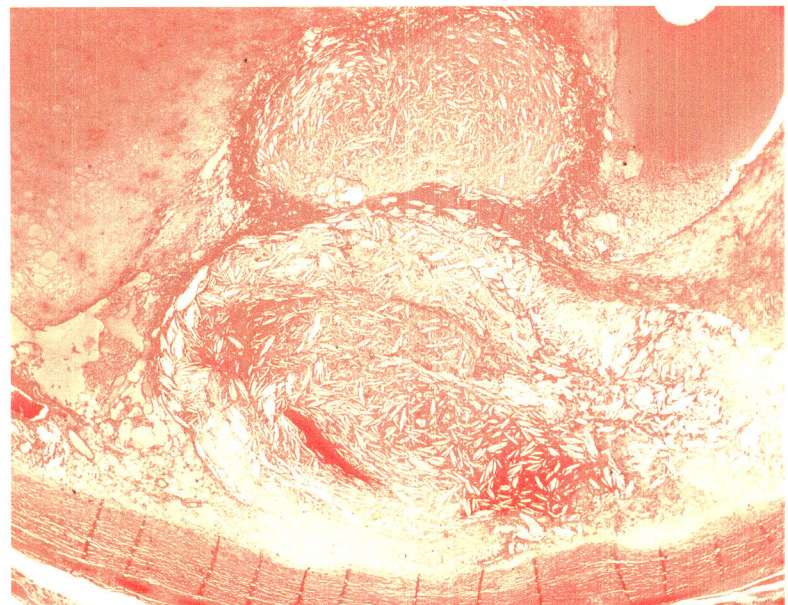

Fig. 8.22 Paratesticular hematoma. Two nodular formations inside a cavity. They consist of clusters of cholesterol needles

Fig. 8.23 Paratesticular hematoma. A 78-year-old patient with a small retroepididymal hematoma near the inferior pole of the testicle. The testicle is completely sclerosed (autopsy finding)

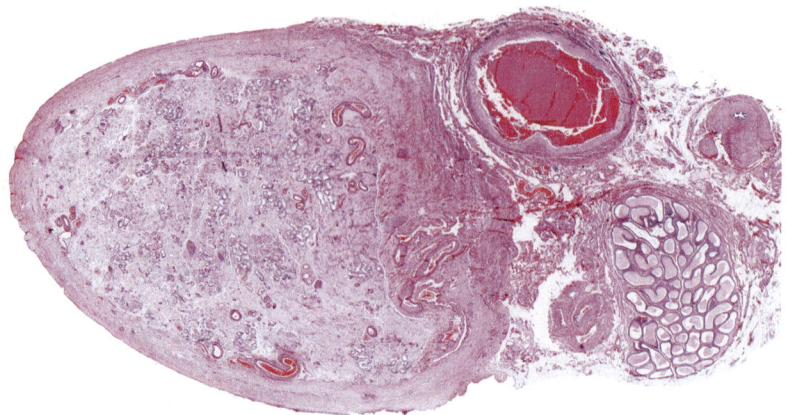

Fig. 8.24 Paratesticular hematoma. The wall of the large hematoma is in contact with the albuginea of the epididymis. Abundant cholesterol crystals and macrophages with hemosiderin are visible in the thickness of the hematoma

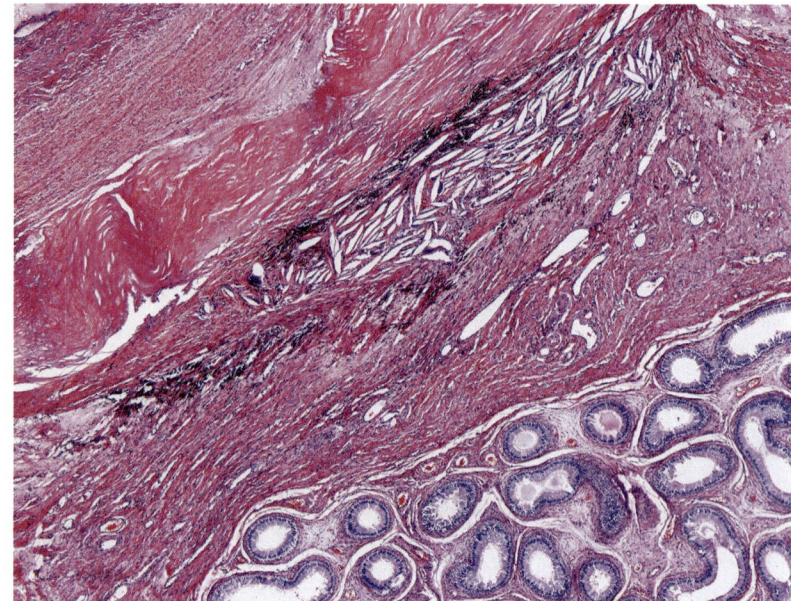

References

1. Adachi S, Tsutahara K, Kinoshita T, Hatano K, Kinouchi T, Kobayashi M, Inoue H, Takada T, Hara T, Yamaguchi S. Segmental testicular infarction due to cholesterol embolism: not the first case, but the first report. Pathol Int. 2008;58:745–8.
2. Thomas E, Parra BL, Patel S. Post-endovascular aneurysm repair (EVAR) testicular ischemia: a rare complication. Urol Case Rep. 2017;14:35–7.
3. Pathmarajah T, Abdelhamid M, Tenna AS, Paton DJW, Hockley JA, Jansen S. Acute global testicular infarction Post-EVAR from cholesterol embolisation can be mistaken for torsion. EJVES Short Rep. 2017;35:11–5.
4. McKenna AJ, Gambardella I, Collins A, Harkin DW. Testicular infarction: a rare complication of endovascular aneurysm repair treatment for aortoiliac aneurysm. J Vasc Surg. 2009;50:1487–9.
5. Finnerty N, Rancour S, King A. Acute testicular ischemia following endovascular abdominal aortic aneurysm repair identified in the emergency department. Case Rep Emerg Med. 2014;2014:591820.
6. Nistal M, Paniagua R. Nodular proliferation of calcifying connective tissue in the rete testis: a study of three cases. Hum Pathol. 1989;20:58–61.
7. Bustos-Obregón E, Holstein AF. The rete testis in man: ultrastructural aspects. Cell Tissue Res. 1976;175:1–15.
8. Kormano M, Suoranta H. Microvascular organization of the adult human testis. Anat Rec. 1971;170:31–9.

9. Suzuki F, Nagano T. Microvasculature of the human testis and excurrent duct system. Resin-casting and scanning electron-microscopic studies. Cell Tissue Res. 1986;243:79–89.

10. Nistal M, García-Cabezas MA, Regadera J, Castillo MC. Microlithiasis of the epididymis and the rete testis. Am J Surg Pathol. 2004;28:514–22.

11. Nistal M, Jiménez-Heffernan JA, García-Viera M, Paniagua R. Cystic transformation and calcium oxalate deposits in rete testis and efferent ducts in dialysis patients. Hum Pathol. 1996;27:336–41.

12. Ramachandran A, Das CJ, Razik A. Male genital tract tuberculosis: a comprehensive review of imaging findings and differential diagnosis. Abdom Radiol. 2021;46:1677–86.

13. Angulo JC, González J, Rodríguez N, Hernández E, Núñez C, Rodríguez-Barbero JM, Santana A, López JI. Clinicopathological study of regressed testicular tumors (apparent extragonadal germ cell neoplasms). J Urol. 2009;182:2303–10.

14. Al-Obaidy KI, Idrees MT, Abdulfatah E, Kunju LP, Wu A, Ulbright TM. Large cell calcifying sertoli cell tumor: a clinicopathologic study of 18 cases with comprehensive review of the literature and reappraisal of prognostic features. Am J Surg Pathol. 2022;46:688–700.

15. Kormano M, Reijonen K. Microvascular structure of the human epididymis. Am J Anat. 1976;145:23–7.

16. Nistal M, Mate A, Paniagua R. Granulomatous epididymal lesion of possible ischemic origin. Am J Surg Pathol. 1997;21:951–6.

17. Mitchinson MJ, Sherman KP, Stainer-Smith AM. Brown patches in the epididymis. J Pathol. 1975;115:57–62.

18. Peña Barreno C, Gonzalez-Peramato P, Nistal M. Vascular and inflammatory effects of estrogen and anti-androgen therapy in the testis and epididymis of male to female transgender adults. Reprod Toxicol. 2020;95:37–44.

19. Regadera J, Nistal M, Paniagua R. Testis, epididymis, and spermatic cord in elderly men. Correlation of angiographic and histologic studies with systemic arteriosclerosis. Arch Pathol Lab Med. 1985;109:663–7.

20. Maat S, Dreuning K, Nordkamp S, van Gemert W, Twisk J, Visschers R, van Heurn E, Derikx J. Comparison of intra- and extra-corporeal laparoscopic hernia repair in children: a systematic review and pooled data-analysis. J Pediatr Surg. 2021;56:1647–56.

21. Schulster ML, Cohn MR, Najari BB, Goldstein M. Microsurgically assisted inguinal hernia repair and simultaneous male fertility procedures: rationale, technique and outcomes. J Urol. 2017;198:1168–74.

22. Anastasiadis K, Godosis D, Kepertis C, Mouravas V, Lampropoulos V, Demiri C, Tsopozidi M, Spyridakis I. Partial epididymal rupture and spermatic cord haematoma with an associated secondary testicular torsion due to blunt scrotal injury, in a 12-year-old boy. Afr J Paediatr Surg. 2022;19:183–5.

23. Arif C, Kotoulas K, Georgellis C, Frigkas K, Bantis A, Patris E. Two case reports of varicocele rupture during sexual intercourse and review of the literature. Case Rep Urol. 2018;2018:4068174.

24. Gordon JN, Aldoroty RA, Stone NN. A spermatic cord hematoma secondary to varicocele rupture from blunt abdominal trauma: a case report and review. J Urol. 1993;149:602–3.

25. Handmaker H, Mehn WH. Hemorrhage into spermatic cord and testicle simulating incarcerated inguinal hernia. An unusual complication of anticoagulation therapy. IMJ Ill Med J. 1969;135:697–9.

26. McKenney MG, Fietsam R, Glover JL, Villalba M. Spermatic cord hematoma: case report and literature review. Am Surg. 1996;62:768–9.

27. Eyal I, Mizrachi S, Greif Z. Spermatic cord hematoma simulating torsion of testis in Henoch-Schönlein syndrome. Harefuah. 1989;116(5):260–1.

28. Nistal M, Martín-López PR. Idiopathic hematoma of the epididymis: presentation of three cases. Eur Urol. 1990;17:178–80.

9.1 Testicular Hemangioma

Hemangioma is a benign testicular tumour, generally occurring in childhood and adolescence, which can develop in any part of the body, but, in decreasing order of frequency, in the head and neck, trunk, and extremities. Only 2% of angiomas develop in the genitalia, with fewer than 60 cases having been reported [1]. The clinical presentation in prepubertal and adolescent patients is dominated by testicular asymmetry not usually associated with pain, which suggests in the first place a germinal tumour or a tumour of the sexual cords because of their greater frequency. In the adult, testicular angiomas are rare [2, 3], with described cases having presented either with tumour symptomatology [4] or with acute scrotal symptomatology (testicular infarction or torsion) [5], which broadens the differential diagnosis [6]. No angioma presents elevated tumour markers (AFP, b-HCG, and lactate dehydrogenase). Although multiparametric ultrasound can provide interesting data that is highly suggestive of an angioma, it is not sufficient, and surgical exploration, with intraoperative biopsy, is required to confirm the diagnosis, even more so if enucleation is to be performed [7].

Macroscopically, they are intraparenchymal tumours, well-circumscribed, tan-brown in colour and far from the albuginea. Histologically, there are four types of angiomas: cavernous, epithelioid, capillary, and anastomosing types [8].

They are generally small tumours (10–40 mm), well-circumscribed but poorly encapsulated. Regardless of the histological variety, the cells show no atypia, have low mitotic activity (<3–5%) and lack anaplasia. The immunohistochemical pattern, with positivity for CD31, CD34, and factor VIII, is typical of endothelial cells [9].

Most angiomas are capillary angiomas [10] that are formed by a proliferation of endothelial cells surrounded by pericytes, which form small vessels containing red blood cells, alternating with more solid areas which only occasionally contain vascular lumina. The tumour may adapt a lobular pattern. In its periphery the tumour frequently shows an infiltrative growth separating the seminiferous tubules [11] (Figs. 9.1, 9.2, 9.3, 9.4, 9.5, and 9.6).

Given the higher incidence of angiomas in the paediatric age group, many are considered congenital hemangiomas [12]. In this regard, to know their behaviour is of value the distinction made by the international Society for the Study of Vascular Anomalies [13]: (a) congenital hemangiomas, including non-involuting congenital hemangioma (NICH); (b) rapidly involuting congenital hemangioma (RICH) and (c) the GLUT-1 positive infantile hemangioma (IH). Endothelial cell positivity for GLUT-1 discriminates the evolutionary capacity of the tumours [14].

Cavernous angiomas of the testis are very rare, slow-growing, and can be seen at any age,

Fig. 9.1 Capillary angioma. A 13-year-old patient with enlargement of the left testicle. Negative tumour markers. After intraoperative biopsy, enucleation of the tumour was performed. The 1.5-cm nodule was reddish, had a lobular pattern, and was formed by small vessels

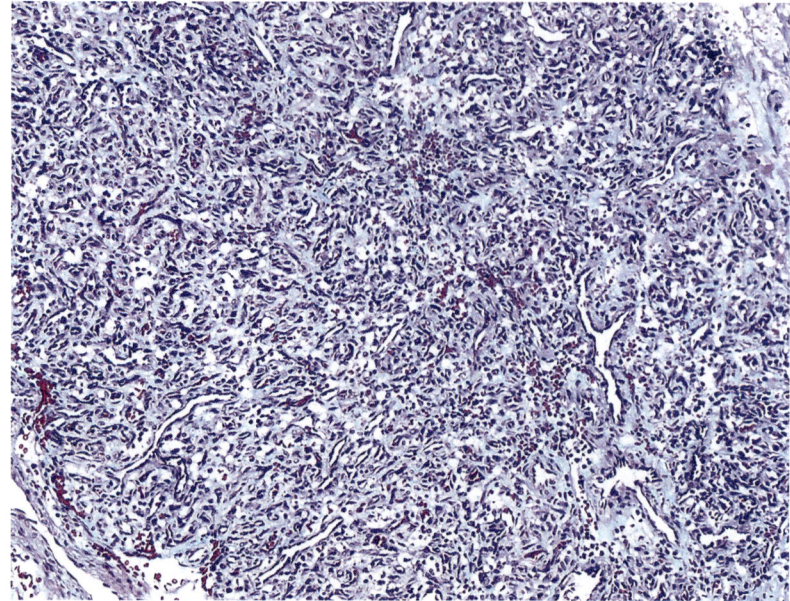

Fig. 9.2 Capillary angioma a. The tumour is constituted from solid cellular nests and ecstatic capillaries with prominent endothelia and thin wall. The larger vessels contain red blood cells

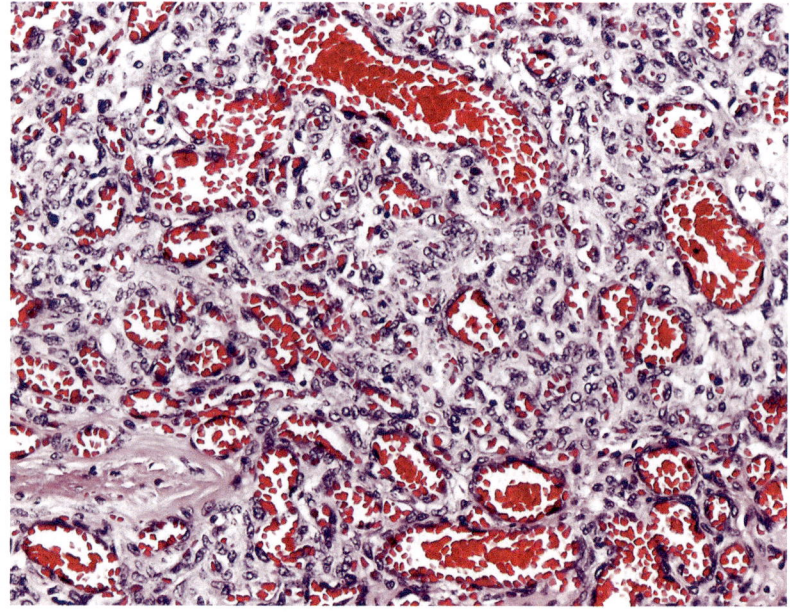

from 17-week-old foetuses to 77-year-old patients [15]. Clinically, they may mimic orchio-epididymitis or a tumour [16]. The case discussed in the figures debuted with an acute scrotum, and given the impossibility of ruling out a tumour, orchiectomy was performed. The subalbuginea tumour had three types of cavities. The most numerous had a relatively thick wall with connective tissue partitions inside. The deeper, intra-parenchymal cavities had a very thin wall. The third type of cavities was preferentially located in the most superficial area of the lesion. They consisted of flattened, or cystic, cisterns and were very thin-walled. The content of the first two types of cavities was blood, while the content of the third type was an acellular eosinophilic fluid. All endothelial cells of the three cavity types were CD31 positive. The endothelial cells of the

Fig. 9.3 Capillary
angioma. Intense CD31
positivity in a tumoural
area with larger vessels

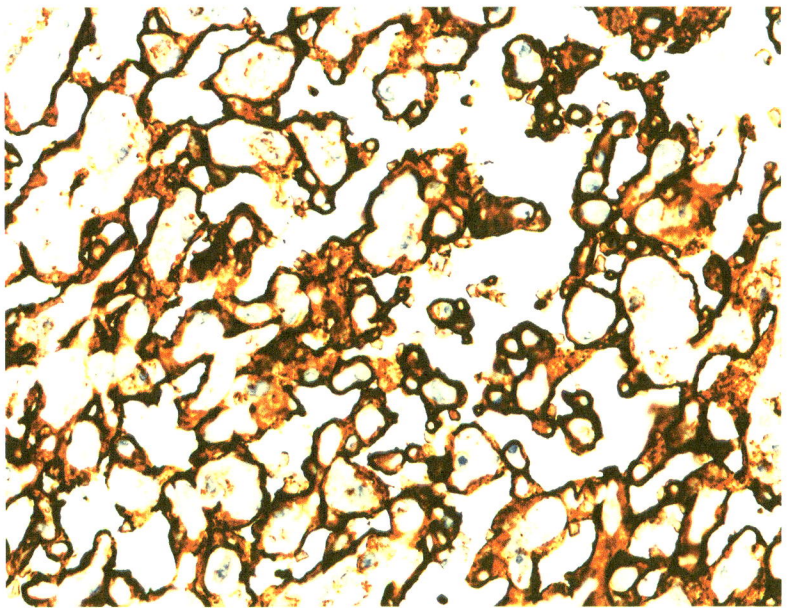

Fig. 9.4 Capillary
angioma. The tumour in
the peripheral part
extends between the
seminiferous tubules and
reaches an interlobular
septum

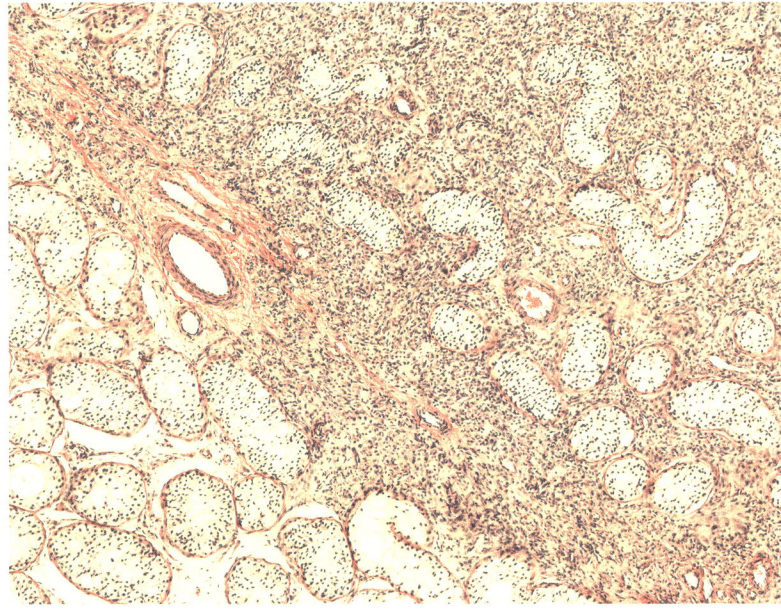

third type of cavity were also positive for D2-40, allowing them to be identified as lymphatic vessels. The neoformation, as is common in cavernous angiomas, had both thrombosis and small calcifications [17] (Figs. 9.7, 9.8, 9.9, and 9.10).

Given the presence of hematic and lymphatic vessels, the differential diagnosis between two processes, cavernous angioma and haemangiolymphangioma, was considered. The presence of lymphatic vessels only in the most superficial subalbuginea area of the tumour, and the existence of other lymphatic vessels also slightly dilated in the tunica vasculosa, separated from the tumour, led us to the diagnosis of cavernous angioma. The presence of ecstatic lymphatic vessels in the albuginea is common in a wide variety of situations which will be considered in detail in the chapters on lymphatic vessel pathology.

Fig. 9.5 Capillary angioma. Seminiferous tubules with initial pubertal development separated by an interstitium infiltrated by the tumour

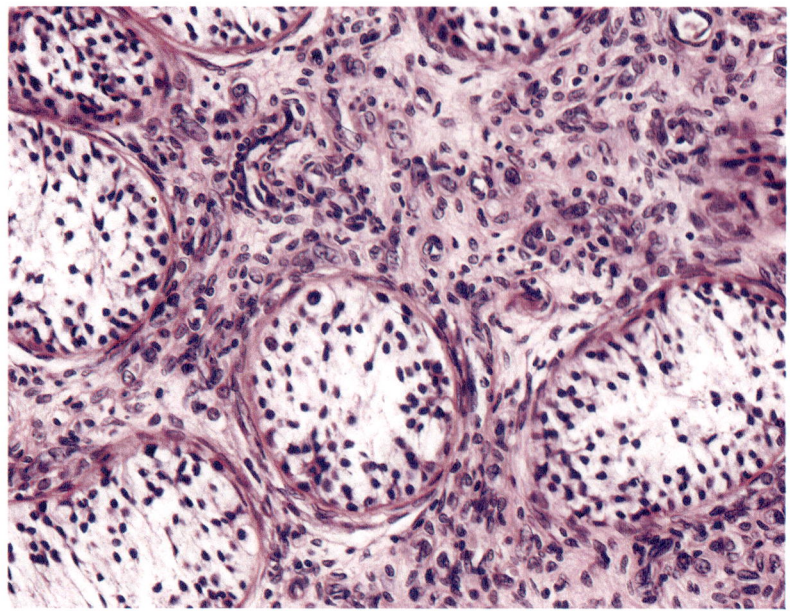

Fig. 9.6 Capillary angioma. Solid proliferation with abundant collapsed capillaries. Only occasionally small lumina are observed between the cells

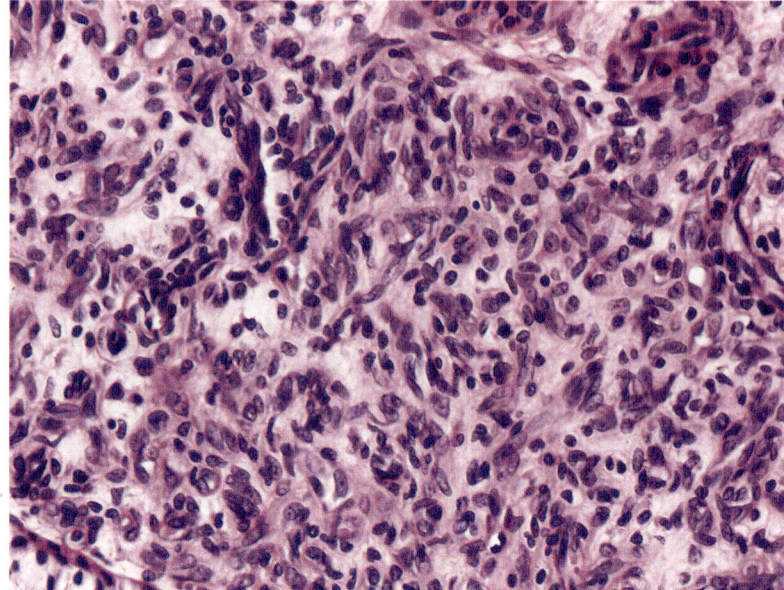

Fig. 9.7 Cavernous angioma. A 34-year-old patient consulted for acute pain in the left testicle. Imaging tests were unable to differentiate it from a testicular tumour. Orchiectomy was performed. The lesion was preferentially located in the tunica vasculosa of the albuginea

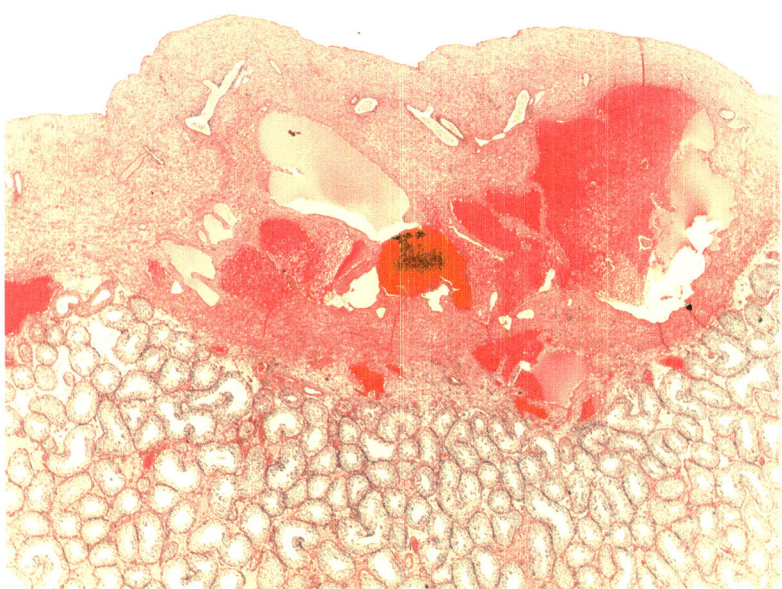

Fig. 9.8 Cavernous angioma. Irregularly shaped, blood-filled cavities in the testicular parenchyma beneath the albuginea. The lesion is partially surrounded by atrophic seminiferous tubules while in more distant tubules spermatogenesis is normal

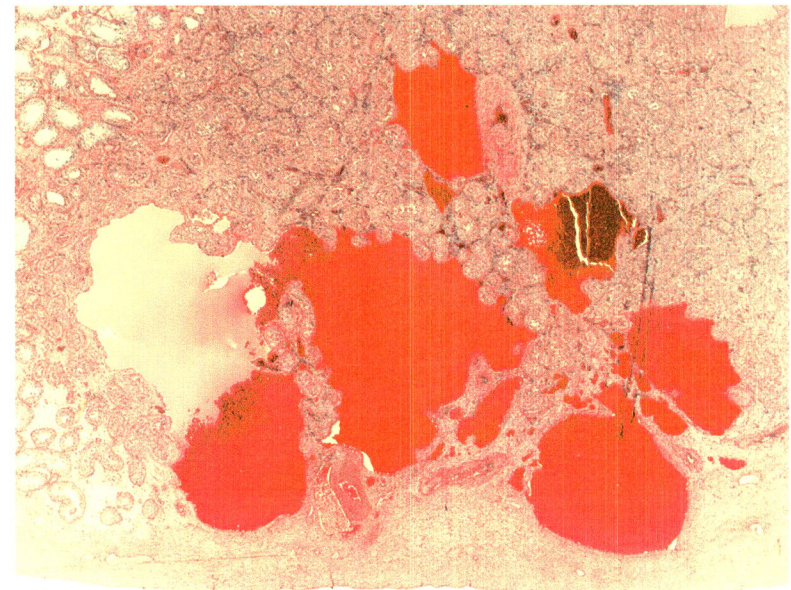

Fig. 9.9 Cavernous angioma. Connective tissue trabeculae partially separate the large cavities of the angioma located under the albuginea

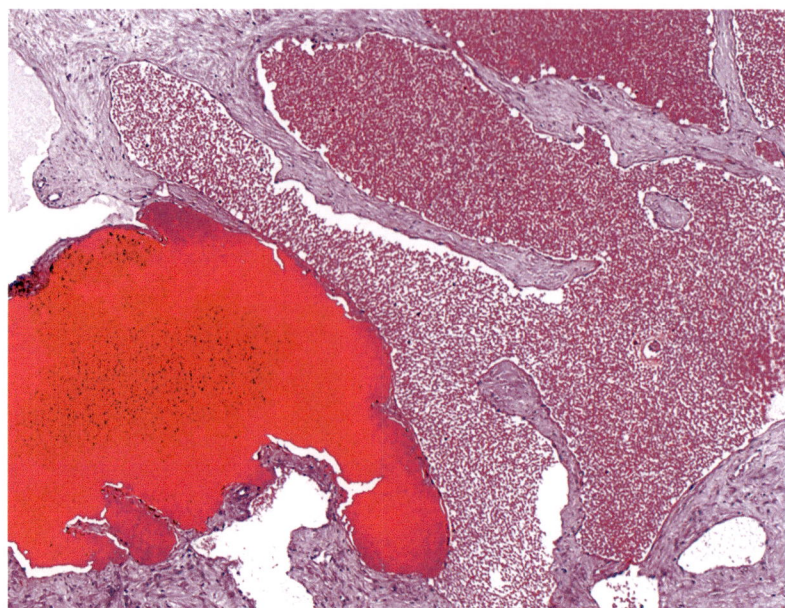

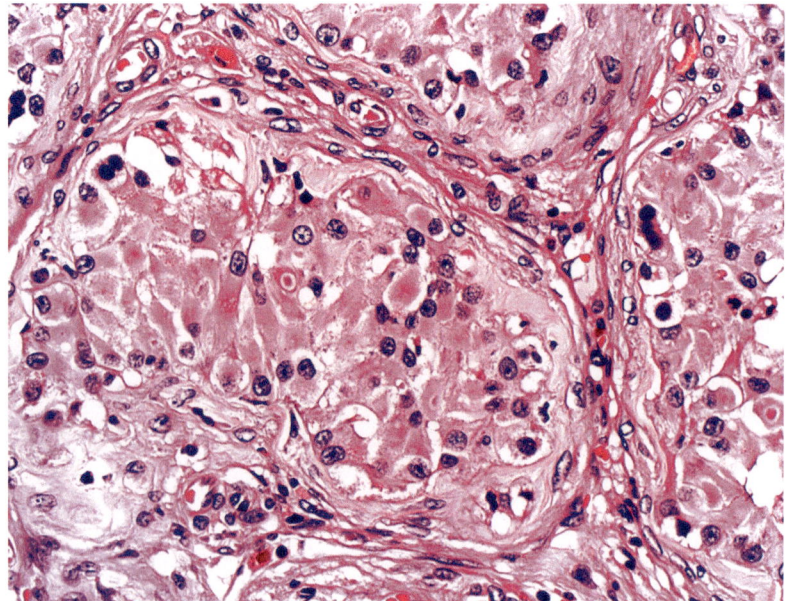

Fig. 9.10 Cavernous angioma. The seminiferous tubules show a peculiar atrophy. They lack lumina and even show isolated spermatogonia, some of which are binucleated. Sertoli cells have spherical nuclei instead of the classical triangular ones and two peculiar facts in the cytoplasm, the large eosinophilia which gives them an oncocytic appearance and the presence of eosinophilic inclusions surrounded by a clear halo whose size is like that of the nucleus of Sertoli cells. These inclusions bear a strong resemblance to spirolactone bodies

9.2   Testicular Hemangiomatosis

Capillary hemangiomatosis is a lesion that preferentially affects the lung [18] and, to a lesser extent, other organs such as the spleen, liver, skin, lymphatic vessels or bone marrow, in which case several organs are frequently affected [19, 20].

Testicular hemangiomatosis has been recently described [21] in a 12-year-old patient, who consulted for progressive enlargement of the right testicle in the previous 6 months. Serum FSH and LH levels remained at prepubertal levels, and no increase in testosterone was observed. AFP and HCG were negative. The ultrasound study was not definitive. The patient had no other pathology that would lead to suspicion of Carney or Peutz-Jegers syndrome. The contralateral testicle was normal. Orchiectomy was performed.

The testicle measured 4 × 3 × 4 cm. On section, the parenchyma had a reddish coloration but a tumor could not be identified. Histologically there was a diffuse proliferation of capillary vessels affecting most of the testicular sections. The vessels were grouped in clusters distributed between the seminiferous tubules. The endothelial cells of the neo-formed vessels had a morphology that varied from one cluster to another. In some clusters, the endothelial cells were cubic with a spherical, euchromatic nucleus with a prominent central nucleolus, and a minimal vascular lumen. Some cells had mitoses. In others, the endothelial cells were flat, the nuclei heterochromatic and the vascular lumen wide with numerous hematocytes. Focally, the endothelial cells expressed GLUT-1. The seminiferous tubules, widely separated by clusters of neo-formed capillaries, had delayed pubertal maturation. The mean diameter was 82 microns, the tubules lacked lumina, the Sertoli cells had elongated showing hyperchromatic nuclei with inhibin bodies in their cytoplasm. The population of spermatogonia varied from two to six per tubular section, some were binucleate. No first order spermatocytes were observed. No clusters of Leydig cells were observed in the interstitium (Figs. 9.11, 9.12, 9.13, 9.14, 9.15, and 9.16).

The clinical differential diagnosis, after ruling out the presence of a tumour, could consider, given that the patient was beginning puberty, two entities: compensatory hypertrophy of the testis and idiopathic benign enlargement of the testis. When compensatory hypertrophy occurs, most of the time, it happens when the contralateral testicle presents a pathology such as cryptorchidism, absence of testicle or varicocele and it develops very early (before the first 3 years of life) [22]. In this case the contralateral testis was considered normal. Idiopathic benign enlargement can be either bilateral or unilateral, and its presentation coincides with the onset of puberty or immediately after. The great disproportion in size between the two testes is a factor against. Idiopathic benign enlargement is considered the result of a peculiar sensitivity of the testicular parenchyma to the onset of hormonal stimulation [23].

Histologically, the vascular proliferation, which separates the seminiferous tubules, bears a

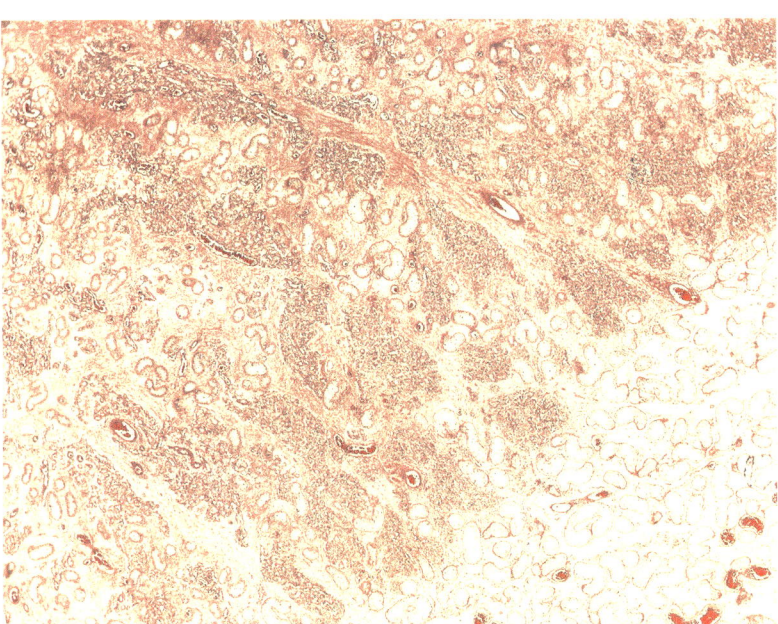

Fig. 9.11 Testicular hemangiomatosis. The testicular architecture is relatively well preserved, with partial recognition of the lobular organization of the parenchyma. There is an enlargement of the interstitium by a vascular proliferation that separates the seminiferous tubules

Fig. 9.12 Testicular hemangiomatosis. Cluster of dilated lumen capillaries and veins between the seminiferous tubules. These still show prepubertal development with absence of lumina and a pseudostratified arrangement of Sertoli cells

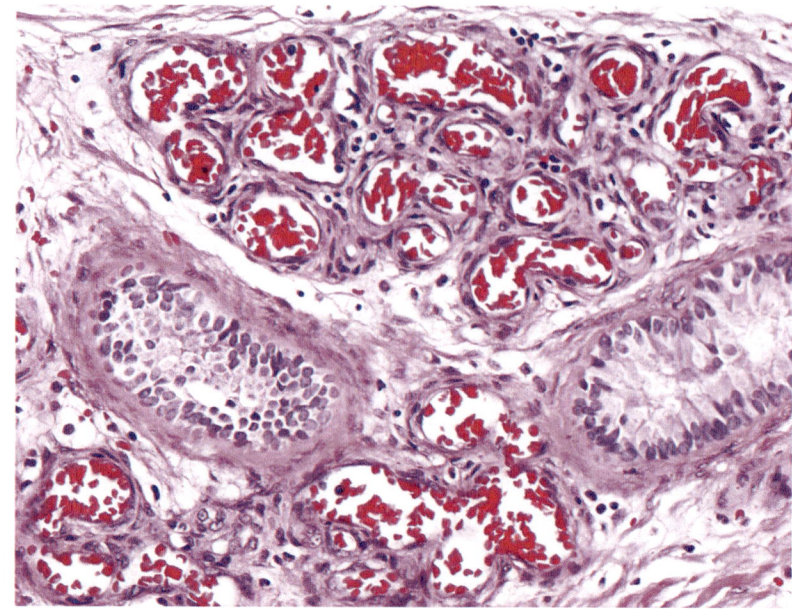

Fig. 9.13 Testicular hemangiomatosis. Area of vascular neoformation. The development varies from solid cords formed by cells of large nuclei with a prominent nucleolus to normal capillaries passing through others of tubular morphology lined by cubic cells

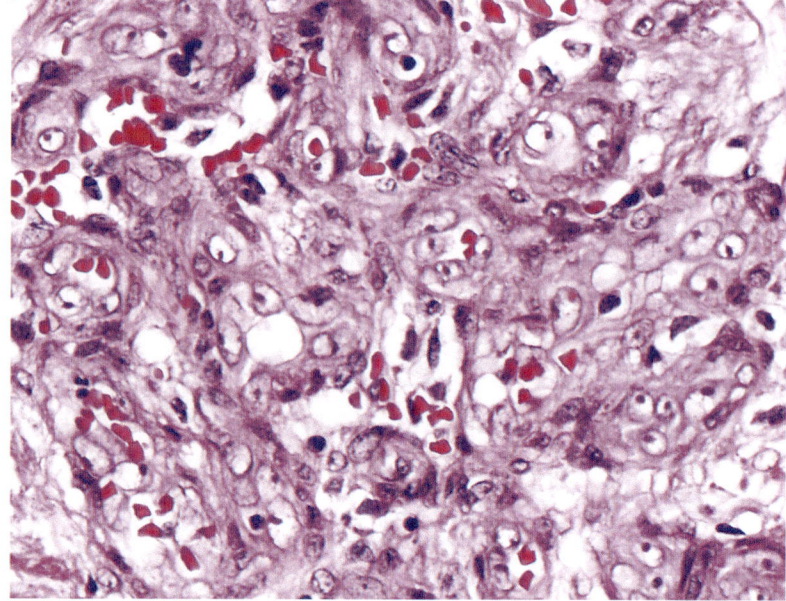

close resemblance to that seen in the periphery of capillary hemangiomas of the testis, which are also more frequent in the prepubertal age. However, the absence of a vascular tumour rules it out. On the other hand, the diffuse capillary proliferation with capillary clusters distributed irregularly throughout the parenchyma is like that described in capillary angiomatosis of other organs, making this diagnosis very attractive [3].

In this case, no pathology was observed in other organs.

Given the exceptional nature of this pathology, there are no adult cases in the literature to suggest the evolution of this angiomatosis. Recently, we have had the opportunity to study a peculiar case in our material. The patient was azoospermic and consulted for infertility. Testicular size was within normal limits. The hor-

Fig. 9.14 Testicular hemangiomatosis. Interrelationship between vascular proliferation and seminiferous tubules, highlighted by immunostaining with CD31

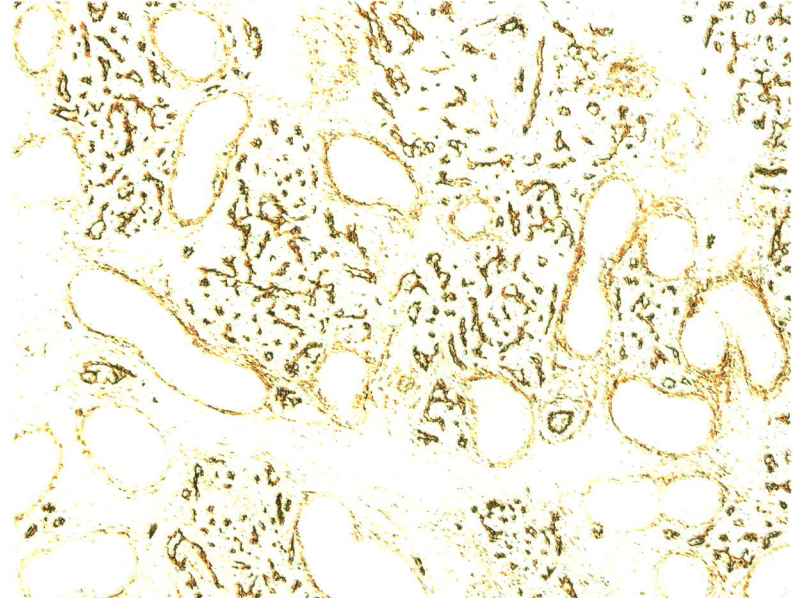

Fig. 9.15 Testicular hemangiomatosis. Marked proliferation of endothelial cells. Most vessels have some Ki67-positive cells, which contrasts with the minimal proliferative activity of some spermatogonia in the seminiferous tubule

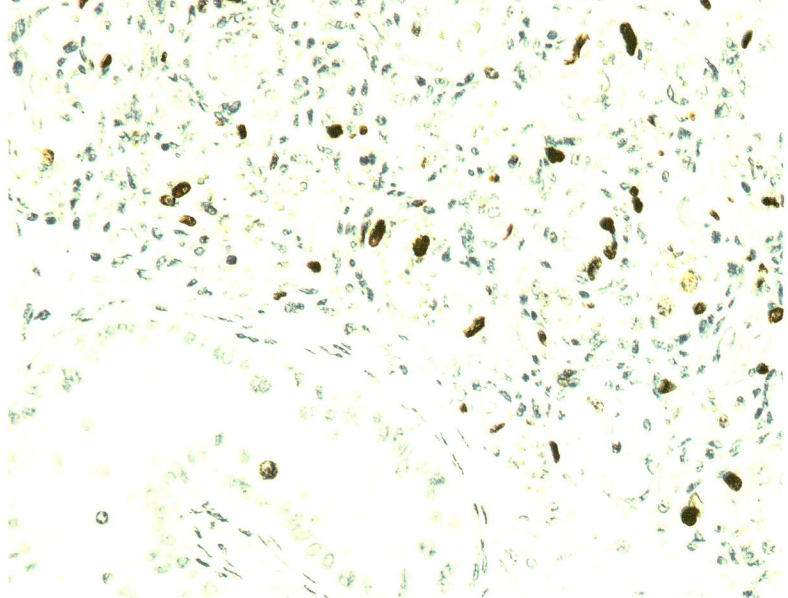

monal determinations of FSH, LH, testosterone, oestradiol, and prolactin were normal. He had no history of cryptorchidism, varicocele, chronic disease or groin surgery. The presence of the cystic fibrosis gene was excluded. The karyotype was normal and there were no microdeletions of the Y chromosome.

Histologically, the seminiferous tubules had a caliber at the lower limit of normal. Most seminif-

erous tubules showed slight thickening of their wall. Spermatogenesis was complete, although quantitatively abnormal with few tubules containing some spermatids that could be bi- and multinucleated. A small group of seminiferous tubules had complete hyalinisation of the wall. The most striking findings were in the interstitium. Multiple clusters of small vessels (capillaries and venules) were recognized between the sections of several

Fig. 9.16 Testicular hemangiomatosis. Intense WT1 positivity of both neo-formed vessels and Sertoli cell nuclei

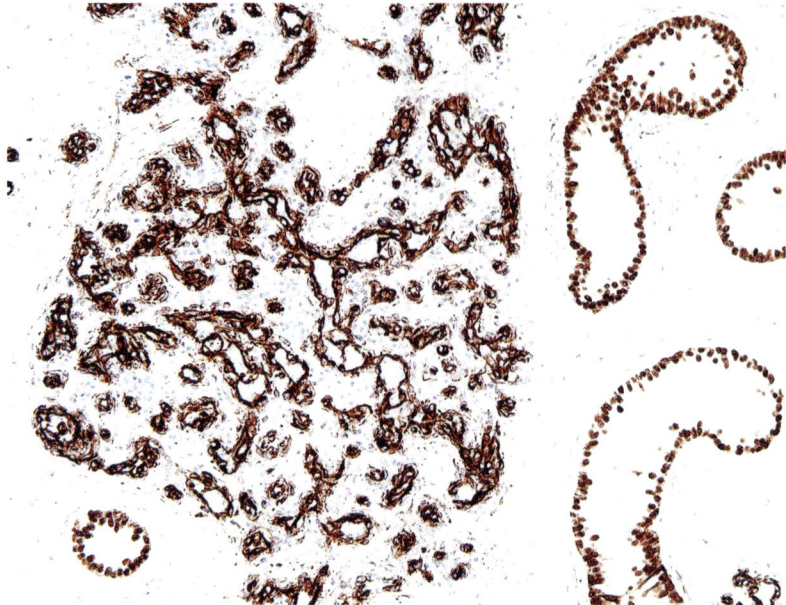

Fig. 9.17 Testicular haemangiomatosis. Adult testis of an infertile patient with azoospermia. Seminiferous tubules are separated by a wide interstitium in which small vessels, veins and ecstatic capillaries are prominent

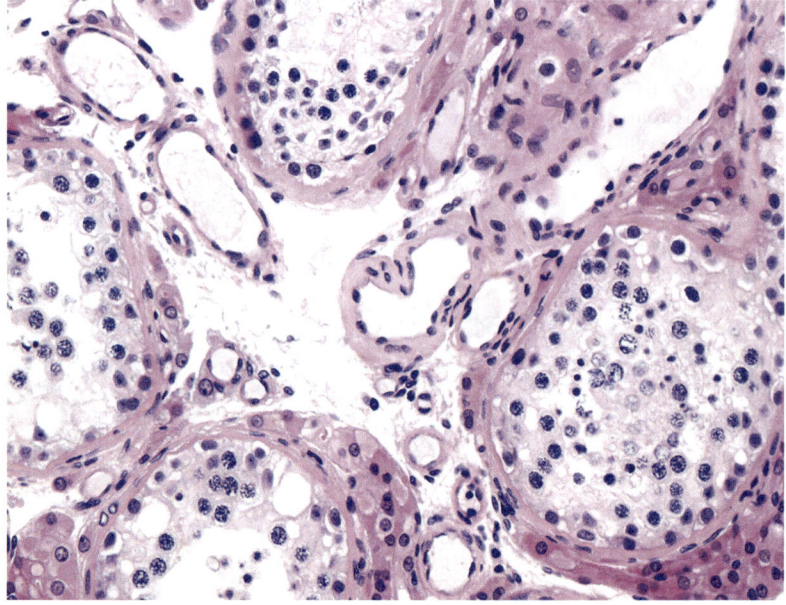

seminiferous tubules. Often these vessels extended radially dissecting the seminiferous tubules. No endothelia with atypia or mitosis figures or inflammatory infiltrates (tubulitis or vasculitis) were observed. Leydig cells were normal (Figs. 9.17, 9.18, 9.19, and 9.20).

Although the explanation for the patient's azoospermia is speculative, if we bear in mind, on the one hand, the absence of a history to justify it and, on the other hand, the sensitivity of the spermatogenesis process to the increase in temperature, it is suggestive that angiomatosis could have played an important role in the elevation of the temperature over a period of years. In this sense, among the causes of hypospermatogenesis and multinucleation of spermatids, which the patient presented, both experimentally and in the clinic, the harmful effects of hyperthermia are well-known [24, 25].

Fig. 9.18 Testicular haemangiomatosis. Seminiferous tubules of an adult testis with wall thickening and hypospermatogenesis with malformed spermatids. The tubules are surrounded by small vessels which are irregularly distributed and focally form a conglomerate

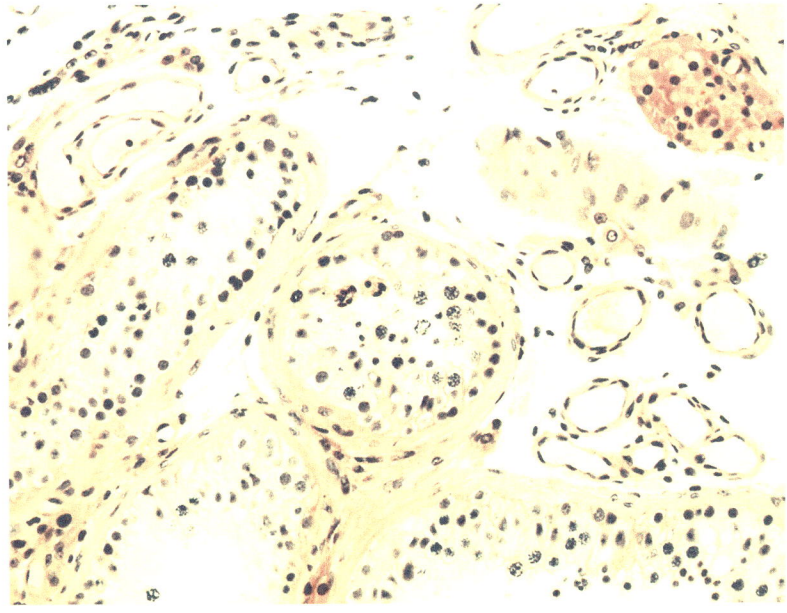

Fig. 9.19 Testicular haemangiomatosis. Cluster of small vessels between clusters of Leydig cells and part of several seminiferous tubules. The vessels are lined by one or two endothelial cells. The dilatation of the lumen is prominent

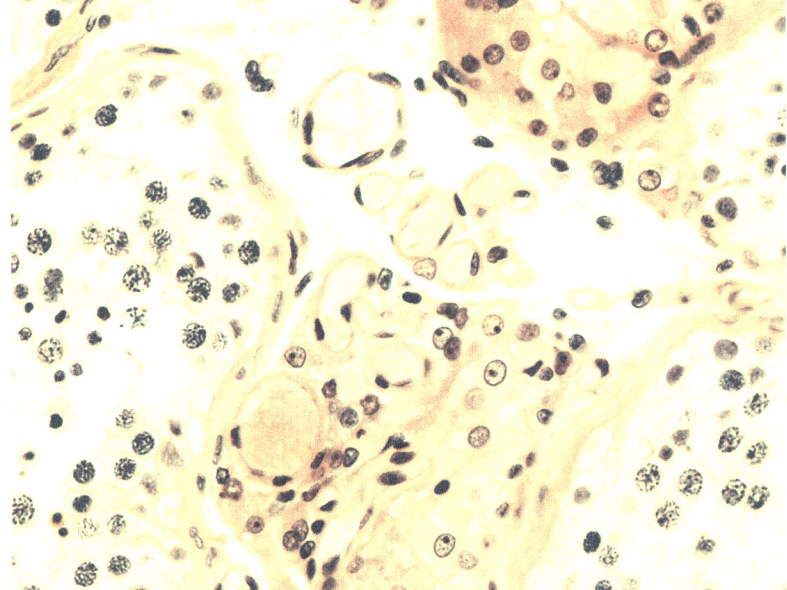

Fig. 9.20 Testicular haemangiomatosis. Cluster of veins and capillaries between sclerosed seminiferous tubules. Interstitial fibrosis and inflammatory infiltrates are absent

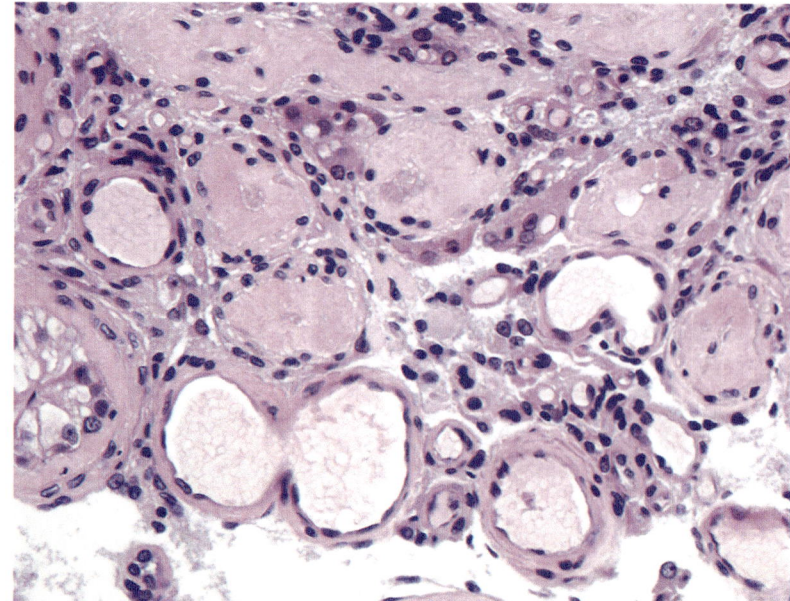

Fig. 9.21 Pseudoangioma. A 4-year-old patient with 46, XY female phenotype (CAIS). Inguinal testis. The central part is occupied by numerous sections of arterioles. Some have hyalinosis

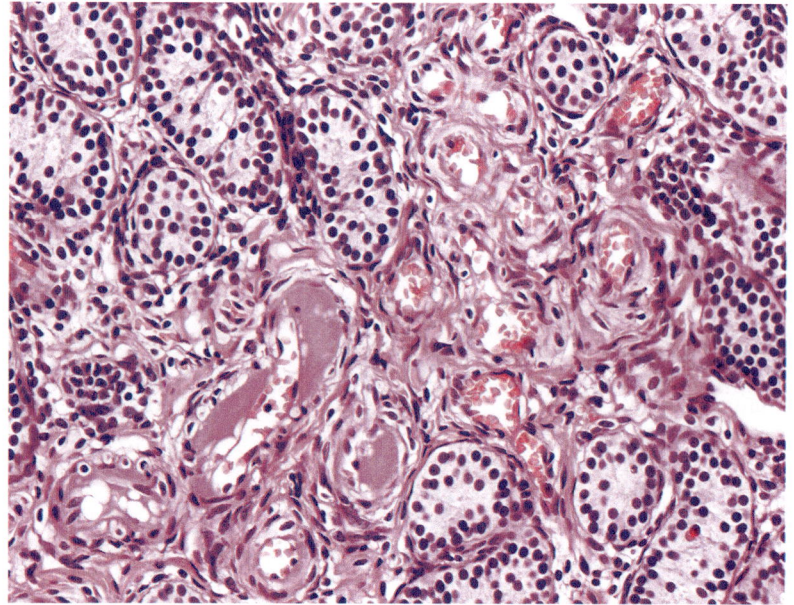

9.3   Testicular Pseudoangioma

Testicular pseudoangioma is a term we propose to describe a benign, multicentric lesion formed by small-caliber vessels that strongly resembles an angioma. They are well-demarcated lesions, without a capsule and in which the vessels are arranged back-to-back. Most of the vessels can be easily identified as arterioles, with a uniform caliber and thin wall (endothelium and a layer of smooth muscle cells). Arterioles may present hyalinosis with variable degrees of luminal stenosis (Figs. 9.21, 9.22, 9.23, and 9.24).

This lesion is most frequently observed in small testicles in childhood and puberty. Most cases are in patients with DSD, especially patients with androgen insensitivity. Although at first

Fig. 9.22 Pseudoangioma. Compact, rectangular formation of thin-walled arterioles, sharply separated from the seminiferous tubules

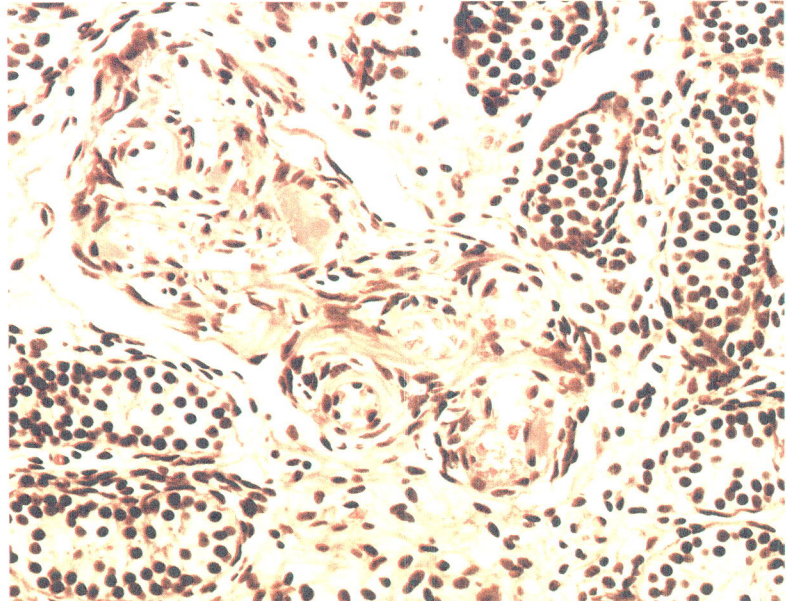

Fig. 9.23 Pseudoangioma. A glomeruloid formation of arterioles surrounded by seminiferous tubules containing only Sertoli cells

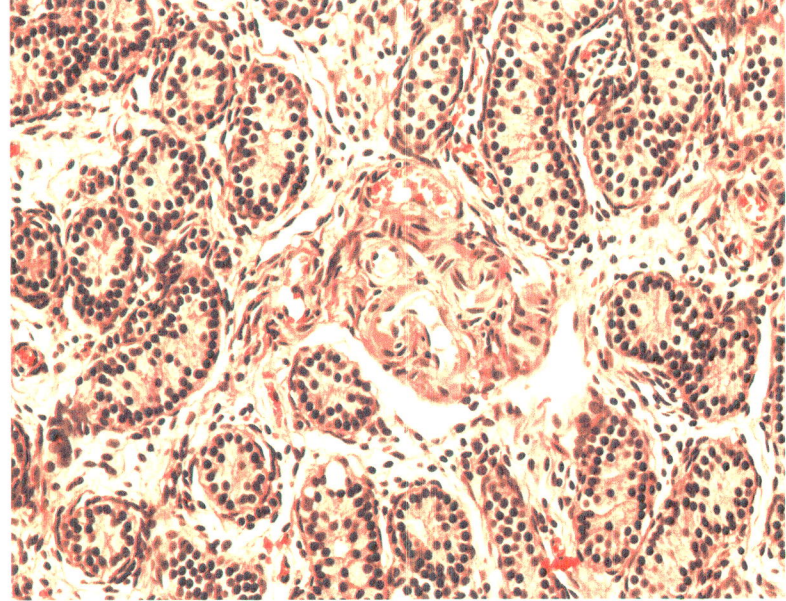

glance the lesion has a proliferative appearance, it is probably only an excessive folding of the spiral or corkscrew arteries of the testis.

The differential diagnosis could be posed with angiomas and hemangiomatosis. Angiomas are single tumour lesions and do not have a higher incidence in DSD patients. Angiomas share with hemangiomatosis the fact that they are multiple lesions, but they differ in that they are formed by capillaries instead of arterioles and they lack a clear delimitation between the vascular proliferation and the seminiferous tubules.

Fig. 9.24 Pseudoan-
gioma. The wall of the
arterioles consists only
of endothelium and
isolated smooth muscle
cells with almost no
interstitium between
them

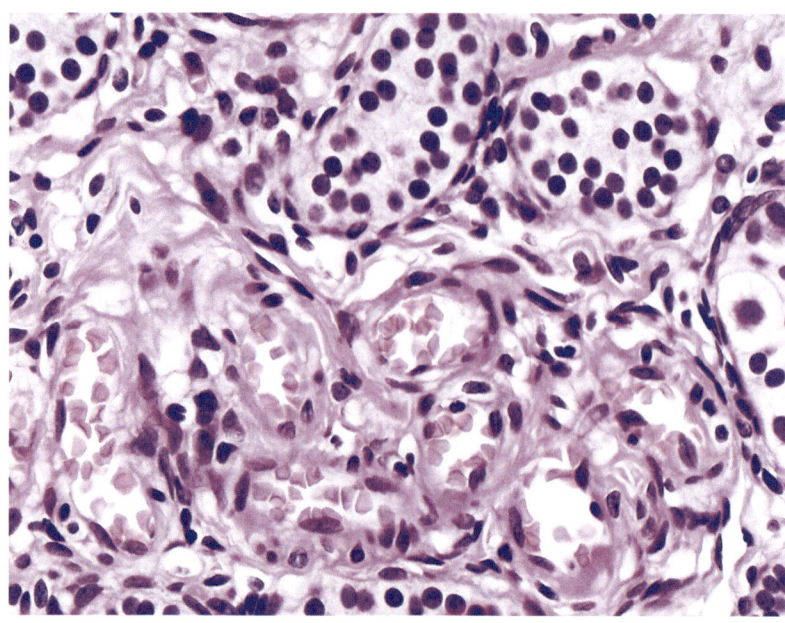

9.4   Aneurysm of the Testicular Artery

Testicular artery aneurysms are very rare. Most
aneurysms described are secondary to trauma, an
infectious process, vasculitis or arteriosclerosis
and the most common location is intratesticular.
The clinical presentation is limited to an increase
in scrotal size with or without pain [26–30]. True
aneurysms are exceptional [31–33]. They have
not been described in association with syndromes
related to the development of aneurysms, such as
Marfan syndrome. In many cases, given their rar-
ity, the diagnosis is histological. The clinical differential diagnosis is mainly with inguinal hernia
and varicocele. The gold standard diagnostic
technique is Doppler ultrasonography. Intratesticular aneurysms are often diagnosed histologically. A case of an association of testicular artery
aneurysm with a segmental infarction of the testis
has been reported [34].

9.5   Arteriovenous Malformation of the Spermatic Cord

Arteriovenous malformations of the male genital
tract have been described in all structures (testicle, epididymis, spermatic cord, scrotum, and

penis) [35]. The clinical presentation is very varied, asymptomatic, and it is usually an incidental
discovery during the evaluation of a testicular
tract [36], an infertility study [37, 38], an exploration for irreducible inguinal swelling [39], or of
recurrent acute testicular pain [40].

The ultrasound study is of particular importance in the diagnosis. Grey-scale ultrasound
images reveal a well-defined, hypoechoic lesion.
The colour Doppler reveals a lesion with tortuous
arterial and venous vessels, high peak systolic—
end diastolic velocities, and a low resistance
index.

Macroscopically they are small lesions (usually no larger than 1 cm) that are made up of arterial and venous vessels. The most typical
characteristics are observed in the veins, which
present dilated lumen and wall thickening.
Histologically at the level of the intima there is a
predominance of tissue poor in cells with abundant collagen and elastic fibres.

At the level of the media, in addition to smooth
muscle cells, there is a marked concentric
increase in elastic fibres. Among the venous sections, there are groups of capillary vessels with
dilated lumens. Arterialization of the vein wall
together with capillary neoformation constitutes
the two most important histological observations
(Figs. 9.25, 9.26, 9.27, 9.28, 9.29, and 9.30).

Fig. 9.25 Arteriovenous malformation of the spermatic cord. A 38-year-old patient consulted for recurrent pain in the left testicle. Clinical examination revealed a tumour of 0.9 cm in diameter separated from the testicle at the beginning of the spermatic cord. It could not be clearly identified as vascular on colour Doppler ultrasound examination. Cluster of thick-walled vessels

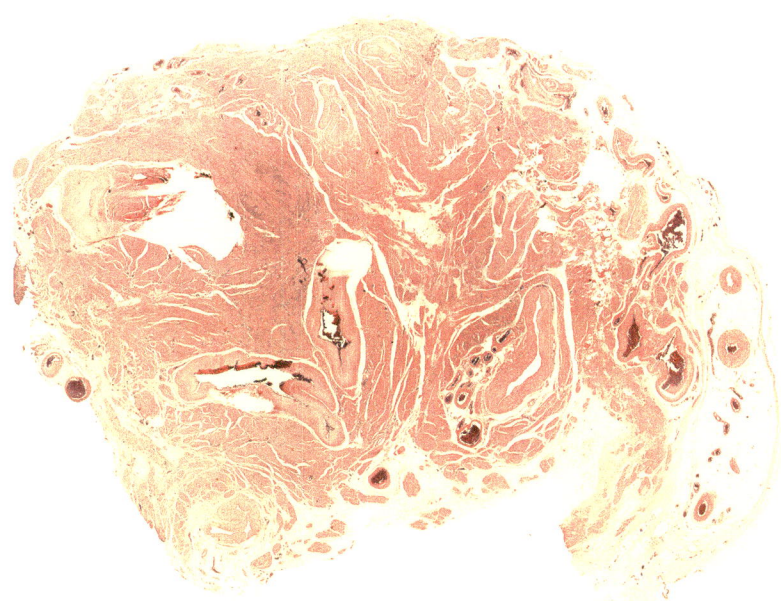

Fig. 9.26 Arteriovenous malformation. Cross section of a vessel folded on itself. It is surrounded by bundles of smooth muscle tissue

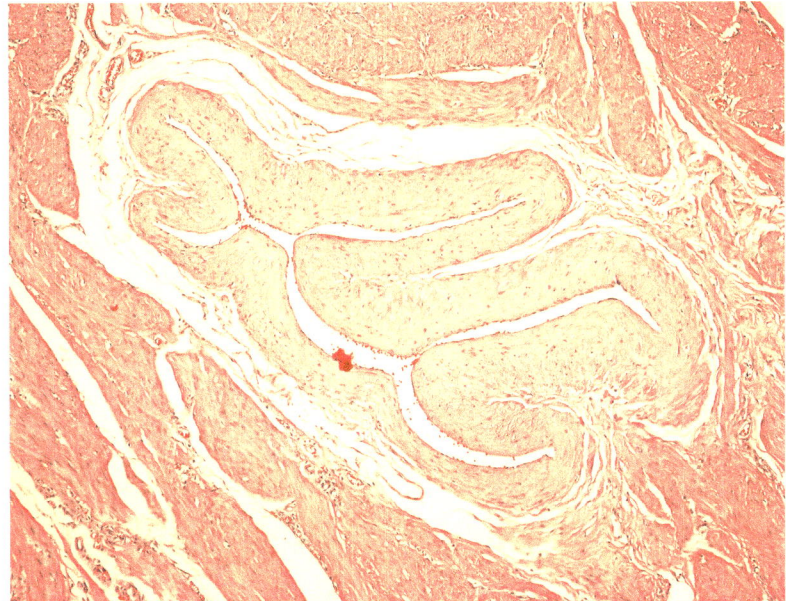

Both are probably reactive alterations in response to the high blood pressure to which the veins are exposed.

Intratesticular arteriovenous malformations, of which only half a dozen cases have been reported, deserve special mention because of their exceptionality. These anomalies pose a differential diagnosis with intratesticular varicocele, hemangiomas, and cystic transformation of the rete testis [41]. Ultrasonographic studies can exclude intratesticular varicocele and ectasia of the rete testis. Hemangiomas on grey-scale sonography are described as well-demarcated lesions, sometimes hypoechoic, sometimes hyperechoic, homogeneous or not, depending on whether they present fibrosis or calcifications. In most cases Doppler imaging allows a correct diagnosis. In one case, the malformations were associated with microlithiasis, and that testis was cryptorchid [42].

Fig. 9.27 Arteriovenous malformation. Thick-walled vessels are completely collapsed or have a minimal lumen

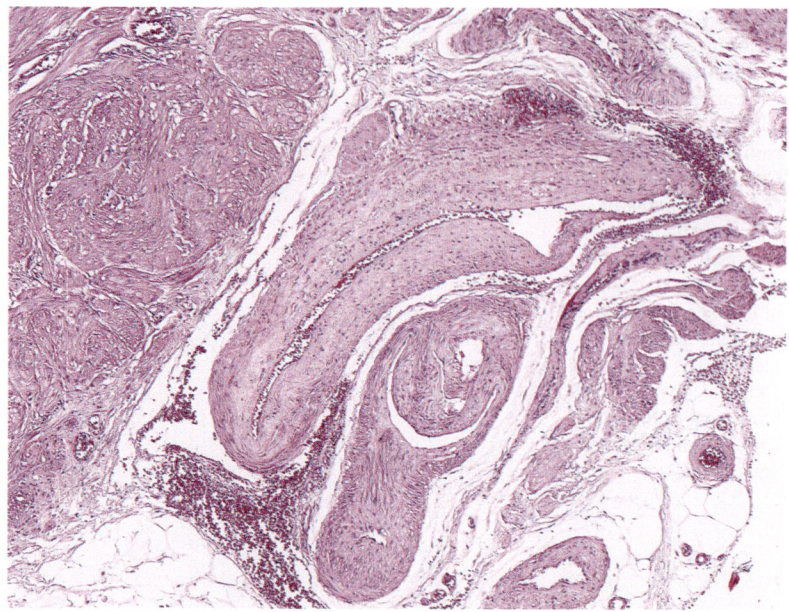

Fig. 9.28 Arteriovenous malformation. The wall of most vessels, apart from notable thickening lacks a clear layered organization. Of note is the marked fibrosis in all layers

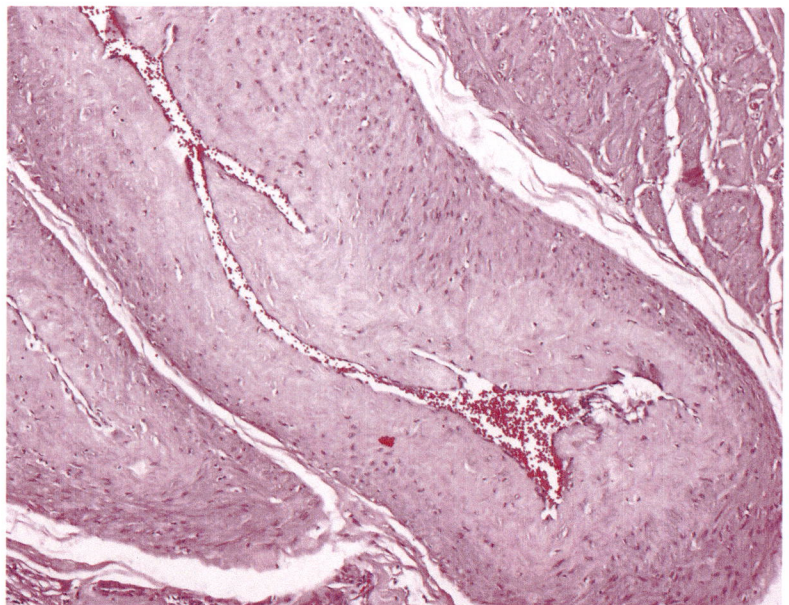

The treatment of arteriovenous malformation varies according to the clinical effects, and ranges from conservative, in asymptomatic cases, to microembolization, excision of the lesion, or even orchiectomy when the pain is intractable.

Fig. 9.29 Arteriovenous malformation. Marked proliferation of elastic fibres preferentially affecting inner- and outermost part of the vessel wall (orcein)

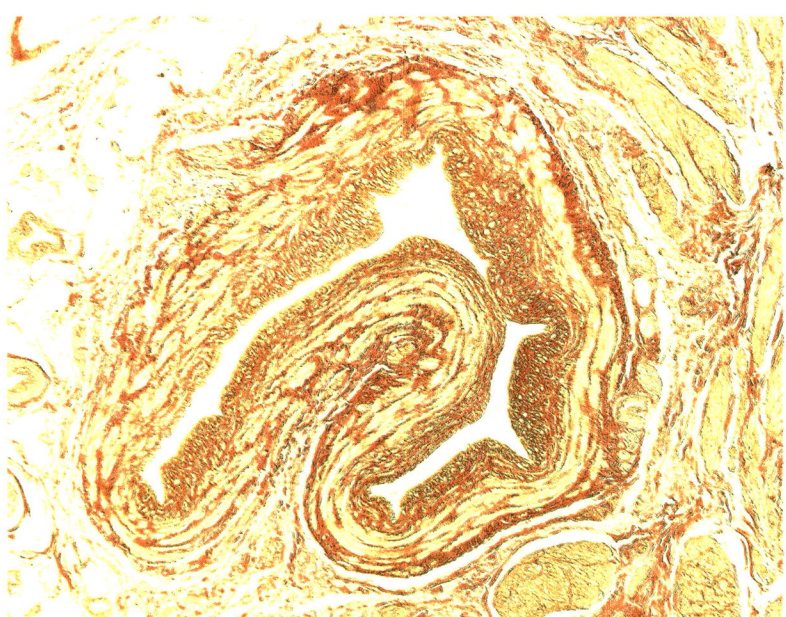

Fig. 9.30 Arteriovenous malformation. Cumulus of capillary vessels and venules in the vicinity of the arteriovenous malformation. Peripheral smooth muscle cell bundles are observable

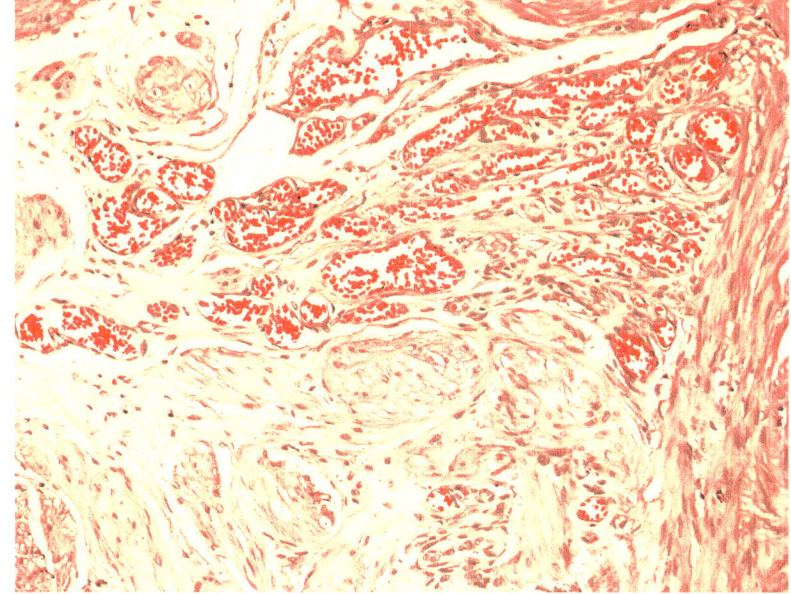

References

1. Kutsal C, Baloğlu İH, Albayrak AT. Hydrocele accompanying testicular cavernous hemangioma: a infant case report. Int J Surg Case Rep. 2021;82:105844.
2. Nistal M, Paniagua R, Regadera J, Abaurrea MA. Testicular capillary haemangioma. Br J Urol. 1982;54:433.
3. Nistal M, García-Cardoso JV, Paniagua R. Testicular juvenile capillary hemangioma. J Urol. 1996;156:1771.
4. Liu B, Chen J, Luo J, Zhou F, Wang C, Xie L. Cavernous hemangioma of the testis mimicking a testicular teratoma. Exp Ther Med. 2013;6:91–2.
5. Escolino M, Cerulo M, Insabato L, Puccio F, Borgogni R, Chiodi A, Lepore B, Califano G, Esposito C. Pediatric testicular cavernous hemangioma with acute onset mimicking testicular torsion: case report and review of the literature. J Pediatr Hematol Oncol. 2023;45:216–9.
6. Wong NC, Dason S, Pozdnyakov S, Alexopoulou I, Greenspan M. Capillary hemangioma of the testis: a rare benign tumour. Can Urol Assoc J. 2015;9:133–5.

7. He Y, Liao H, Xiang X, Cai D, Qiu L. High-frequency ultrasonography and contrast-enhanced ultrasound for the evaluation of testicular capillary hemangioma: a case report. Medicine. 2019;98(11):e14779.

8. Kryvenko ON, Epstein JI. Testicular hemangioma: a series of 8 cases. Am J Surg Pathol. 2013;37:860–6.

9. Talmon GA, Stanley SM, Lager DJ. Capillary hemangioma of the testis. Int J Surg Pathol. 2011;19:398–400.

10. Nistal M, Paniagua R, González-Peramato P, Reyes-Múgica M. Testicular and paratesticular tumors in the pediatric age group. Pediatr Dev Pathol. 2016;19:471–92.

11. Uchida K, Takahashi A, Miyao N, Takeda K, Tsutsumi H, Satoh M, Tsukamoto T. Juvenile hemangioma of the testis: analysis of expression of angiogenic factors. Urology. 1997;49:285–6.

12. Laarif S, Trabelsi F, Daïb A, Ben Abdallah R, Hellal Y, Kaabar N. Inguinoscrotal hernia revealing a testicular hemangioma: report of a neonatal case. Urol Case Rep. 2023;50:102491.

13. Idrees MT, Ulbright TM, Oliva E, Young RH, Montironi R, Egevad L, Berney D, Srigley JR, Epstein JI, Tickoo SK, Members of the International Society of Urological Pathology Testicular Tumour Panel. The World Health Organization 2016 classification of testicular non-germ cell tumours: a review and update from the International Society of Urological Pathology Testis Consultation Panel. Histopathology. 2017;70:513–21.

14. Hugar SB, Kadow BT, Davis A, Ranganathan S, Reyes-Múgica M, Schneck FX, Picarsic J. Pediatric testicular hemangioma in a 10-year-old: a rare entity that may mimic malignancy with appraisal of the literature. Urology. 2018;114:175–80.

15. Suriawinata A, Talerman A, Vapnek JM, Unger P. Hemangioma of the testis: report of unusual occurrences of cavernous hemangioma in a fetus and capillary hemangioma in an older man. Ann Diagn Pathol. 2001;5:80–3.

16. Isharwal S, Khot R, Gupta S, Tandon YK. Testicular cavernous hemangioma masquerading as testicular malignancy. J Clin Ultrasound. 2023;51:898–900.

17. Li F, Han S, Liu L, Xu S, Cai D, Liang Z, Wang H, Guo K. Benign testicular cavernous hemangioma presenting with acute onset: a case report. Mol Clin Oncol. 2020;13:19–22.

18. Kimmig LM, Stutz MR, Husain AN, Bag R. Identification of a novel EIF2AK variant and genetics-assisted approach to diagnosis of pulmonary capillary hemangiomatosis. Lung. 2022;200(2):217–9. https://doi.org/10.1007/s00408-022-00517-2.

19. Kapatia G, Mitra S, Gupta K, Menon P, Rao KLN. Splenic hemangiomatosis: an uncommon vascular lesion in an infant. Fetal Pediatr Pathol. 2018;37:372–6.

20. Mirali H, Kamaoui I, Aichouni N, Nasri S, Skiker I. Diffuse capillary spleen hemangiomatosis: a rare cause of hepatic dysmorphia. Cureus. 2021;13(5):e15320.

21. Nistal M, Gonzalez-Peramato P. Testicular hemangiomatosis with capillary hemangioma pattern. In: Atlas of peculiar and common testicular and paratesticular tumors. Cham: Springer; 2020.

22. Lee PA, Marshall FF, Greco JM, Jeffs RD. Unilateral testicular hypertrophy: an apparently benign occurrence without cryptorchidism. J Urol. 1982;127:329–31.

23. Laron Z, Dickerman Z, Ritterman I, Kaufman H. Follow-up of boys with unilateral compensatory testicular hypertrophy. Fertil Steril. 1980;33:297–301.

24. Liu YX. Temperature control of spermatogenesis and prospect of male contraception. Front Biosci. 2010;2:730–55.

25. Abdelhamid MHM, Walschaerts M, Ahmad G, Mieusset R, Bujan L, Hamdi S. Mild experimental increase in testis and epididymis temperature in men: effects on sperm morphology according to spermatogenesis stages. Transl Androl Urol. 2019;8:651–65.

26. Ohmor K, Isokawa Y. Aneurysm of the testicular artery. J Urol. 1994;151:1646–7.

27. Deck KE, Deck A, Waitches GM. Intratesticular pseudoaneurysm after blunt trauma. Rev Am J Roentgenol. 2000;174:1136.

28. Zicherman JM, Mistry KD, Sarokhan CT, DeCarvalho VS. CT angiography, sonography, and MRI of aneurysm of the testicular artery. AJR Am J Roentgenol. 2004;182:1088–9.

29. Mujoomdar A, Maheshwari S, Zand F, Sircar K, Mesurolle B. Sonographic diagnosis of a ruptured intratesticular pseudoaneurysm secondary to orchitis. AJR Am J Roentgenol. 2007;189:20–2.

30. Parker WP, Nangia AK. Testicular artery pseudoaneurysm: a case report. F1000Res. 2014;3:2.

31. Reddy YP, Murphy JK, Sheridan WG. Spontaneous aneurysm of the testicular artery. Br J Urol. 1998;82:599–600.

32. Valle-Leal JG. Testicular artery aneurysm: case report and review of the literature. Bol Med Hosp Infant Mex. 2018;75:373–6.

33. Verma M, Ojha V, Chandrashekhara SH, Kumar S. 'Spontaneous aneurysm of left testicular artery with an anomalous origin': detection of a rare entity on CT. BMJ Case Rep. 2021;14(1):e240456.

34. Rao K, Aswani Y, Priya S, Kemp S, Rajput M. Segmental testicular infarct with an associated testicular artery aneurysm: case report of a rare clinical entity. Radiol Case Rep. 2022;17:2150–4.

35. Bapir R, Kakamad FH, Aghaways I, Abdullah AM, Hassan MN, Abid AAM, Hasan SJ, Salih KM, Hamasalih HM. Para testicular arteriovenous malformation: a case report and mini review of the literature. Med Int. 2023;3:28.

36. Jafarpishefard MS, Momeni M, Baradaran Mahdavi MM, Momeni F, Kamal S. An intratesticular arteriovenous malformation identified incidentally during ultrasound evaluation of scrotal trauma. Adv Biomed Res. 2016;5:202.

37. Skiadas V, Antoniou A, Primetis H, Moulopoulos L, Vlahos L. Intratesticular arteriovenous malformation. Clinical course, ultrasound and MRI findings of an extremely rare lesion on a 7 year follow-up basis. Int Urol Nephrol. 2006;38:119–22.

38. Monoski MA, Gonzalez RR, Thomas AJ, Goldstein M. Arteriovenous malformation of scrotum causing virtual azoospermia. Urology. 2006;68:203.

39. Joshi MA, Gadhire M, Dhake A, Patil M. A diagnostic dilemma: arteriovenous malformation of spermatic cord presenting as irreducible inguinal swelling. J Postgrad Med. 2011;57:339–40.

40. Sountoulides P, Bantis A, Asouhidou I, Aggelonidou H. Arteriovenous malformation of the spermatic cord as the cause of acute scrotal pain: a case report. J Med Case Rep. 2007;1:110.

41. Kutlu R, Alkan A, Soylu A, Sigirci A, Dusak A. Intratesticular arteriovenous malformation: color Doppler sonographic findings. J Ultrasound Med. 2003;22:295–8.

42. McDaniels JQ, Morganstern BA. Intratesticular arteriovenous malformation: a rare benign testicular lesion in an adolescent male. Urol Case Rep. 2023;48:102406.

10.1 Amyloidosis

Amyloidosis refers to the extracellular deposition of a proteinaceous, eosinophilic, insoluble material that stains with Congo red [1]. At least 36 different proteins have been identified as amyloid fibril proteins. Classically, amyloidoses can be grouped as follows: a) AL amyloidosis or primary amyloidosis, with localized forms in different organs including the testis and the acquired forms of primary amyloidosis, which are generally due to deposits of Ig light-chain fragments produced by clonal plasma cells in the bone marrow, b) AA amyloidosis or secondary amyloidosis, characteristic of chronic granulomatous diseases (tuberculosis, Crohn's, leprosy, arthritis, arthritis), pyogenic diseases, vasculitis, familial Mediterranean fever and neoplasms, and c) Hereditary amyloidosis, of which many subtypes are known, in which amyloid fibrils derive from mutations in genes encoding any of the following proteins: transthyretin, apolipoprotein A-I, apolipoprotein A-II, apolipoprotein CII, apolipoprotein CIII, lysozyme, beta2-microglobulin, fibrinogen Alpha-chain, cystatin C, and gelsolin among others [2–4].

Although infrequently the clinical picture may be highly suggestive of amyloidosis, definitive diagnosis requires the identification of amyloid deposits in tissues. Tissue selection has classically been based on tissue accessibility. The most common method for amyloid detection is rectal biopsy, its sensitivity depending on whether it includes submucosa. Skin biopsy including subcutaneous cellular tissue, or aspiration of subcutaneous fat is also a frequently used method, but it should be noted that in some AA type amyloidoses such as those associated with familial Mediterranean fever, no deposits are observed [5]. Renal or liver biopsies have a high risk of haemorrhagic complications [6]. Other tissues that have allowed diagnosis in the past are gingival biopsy, but it has a high incidence of false negatives, and in individual cases, biopsy of the labial salivary glands, bone marrow, peripheral nerves, endocardium, or thyroid in patients with amyloid goitre [7].

Testicular biopsy is more sensitive for diagnosing systemic amyloidosis than rectal biopsy. Data from a large series yield the following results. Testicular biopsy was diagnostic in 91.7% of patients with primary amyloidosis, 85% in patients with systemic amyloidosis, and 87.5% of patients with familial Mediterranean fever, compared to 75%, 51.7%, and 40.6% of the respective different groups in whom a rectal biopsy was positive [8].

The testicle can be affected in all three types of amyloidosis; however, although AA type amyloidosis is five times more frequent than AL type, testicular involvement in hereditary amyloidosis varies greatly depending on the subtype. The first striking feature is testicular size, especially if we bear in mind that more than 50% of patients are

© The Author(s), under exclusive license to Springer Nature Switzerland AG 2024

M. Nistal, P. González-Peramato, *Testicular Vascular Lesions*,

https://doi.org/10.1007/978-3-031-57847-2_10

infertile and frequently show azoospermia. The testicles are of normal or increased size and macro-orchidism is not uncommon. Lesions are seen in both the seminiferous tubules and the interstitium. In the seminiferous tubules, there is thickening of the basement membrane due to amyloid deposits and impaired spermatogenesis in 84% of cases. In the interstitium, there are fibrillar deposits and a decrease in Leydig cells.

Amyloid deposits can be seen in arterioles, venules, and capillaries (Fig. 10.1, 10.2, 10.3 and 10.4). Lymphatic vessels may also be affected. Amyloid, in addition to having an appetite for Congo Red stain (Fig. 10.5), shows apple green birefringence when polarized and it stains with cresyl violet [9] (Fig. 10.6). Under the electron microscope, it consists of 7–10 nm diameter fibrils [10].

Fig. 10.1 Secondary amyloidosis. Patient with long-standing rheumatoid arthritis. All vessels of the testis show deposited eosinophilic material in their walls. The seminiferous tubules show variable degrees of atrophy of the seminiferous epithelium and wall thickening

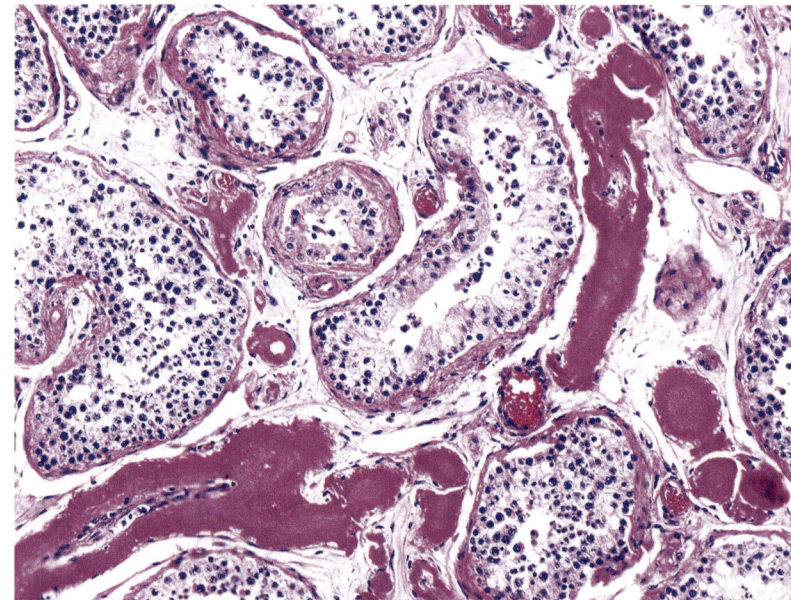

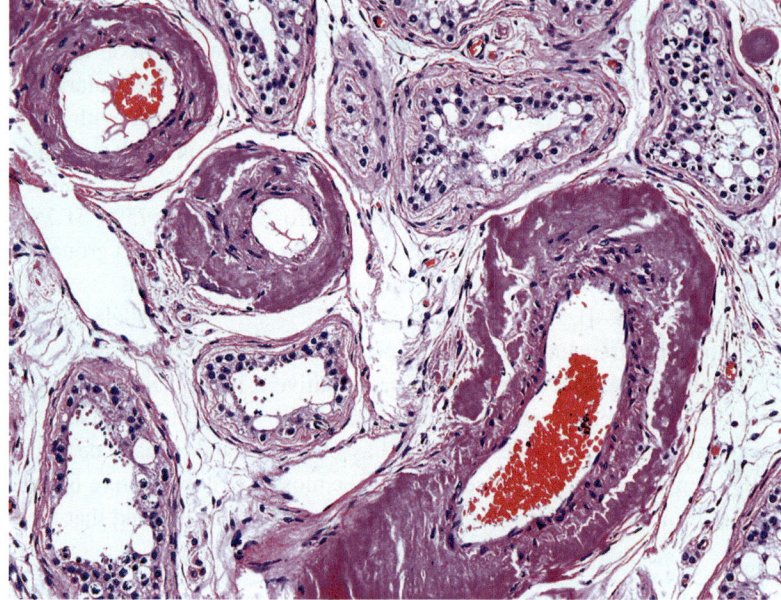

Fig. 10.2 Secondary amyloidosis. Cross sections of several vessels with circumferential deposits in all layers. Note the rigidity of the wall allowing the lumen not to appear collapsed and the deposits in the adventitia. Other findings are dilatation of the lymphatic vessels and vacuolization of the Sertoli cells

Fig. 10.3 Secondary amyloidosis. Circumferential deposits in the media of two arterioles causing luminal stenosis in one of them. One of the seminiferous tubules has a complete but quantitatively abnormal spermatogenesis

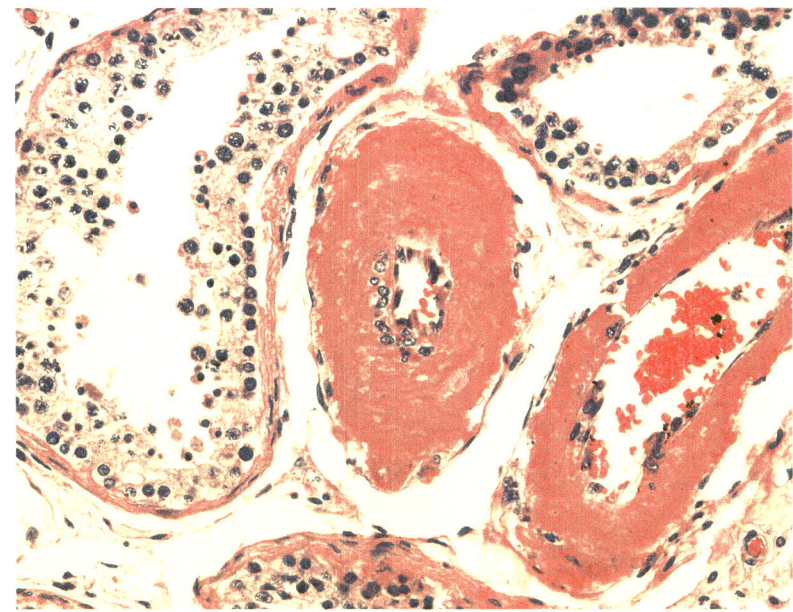

Fig. 10.4 Secondary amyloidosis. Amyloid deposits in four small veins in the vicinity of the vas deferens

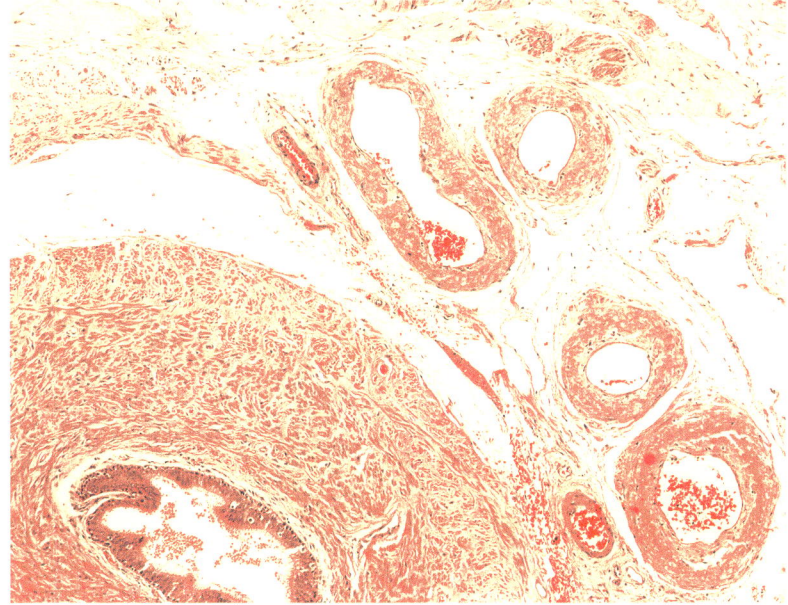

The impact of testicular amyloidosis on testicular function is related to the type of clinical entity. While testicular localization of the amyloid in AL diseases rarely results in azoospermia and hypogonadism, in AA amyloidoses, and especially in familial Mediterranean fever [11], testicular amyloidosis may actually be the first sign of systemic amyloidosis. This amyloidosis can manifest itself by hypergonadotropic hypo-gonadism, sterility or macro-orchidism [12], or even simulate a tumour [13, 14]. The same occurs in hereditary apolipoprotein A-I amyloidosis in which testicular involvement (macro-orchidism and hypergonadotropic hypogonadism) also occurs earlier than in other systemic forms of amyloidosis [15–18]. Testicular enlargement may be associated with giant hepatomegaly [19].

Fig. 10.5 Secondary amyloidosis. Deposits of Congo red-positive material of very irregular shape and size in the media and adventitia of lymphatic vessels. Absence of deposits in the wall of the arteries

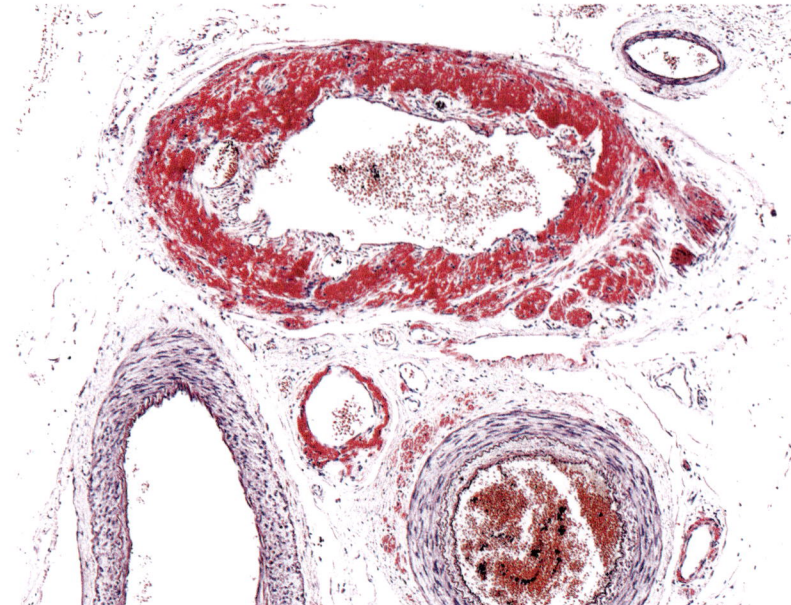

Fig. 10.6 Secondary amyloidosis. Patient with chronic renal failure, hemodialyzed for several years. Beta2-microglobulin deposits in the adventitia of veins and lymphatic vessels of the pampiniform plexus (Cresyl violet) (same patient as in the previous figure)

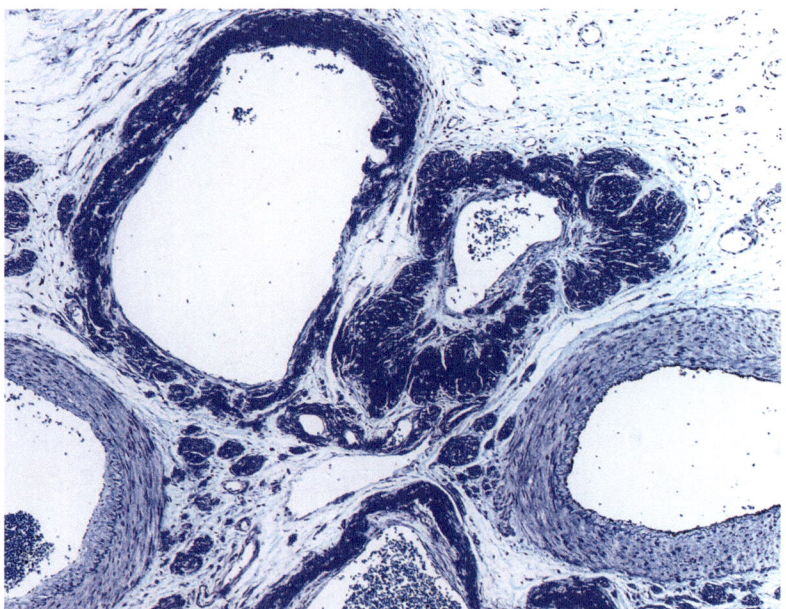

The amyloid deposits must be detected early so as to institute appropriate therapy and preserve fertility. Therapy is effective in all types of amyloidosis except hereditary amyloidosis or patients with poorly preserved renal function [20].

The pathogenetic mechanism is related to the amount of amyloid deposited in the vessels and interstitium. The amyloid deposited in the vascular walls not only causes a thickening of the wall, but also stenosis of the vascular lumen. In this situation, on the one hand, there is ischaemia of the parenchyma, and on the other, as vascular permeability is altered, a change in the interstitial microenvironment, leading to an eventually impairing both spermatogenesis and Leydig cell function [8].

References

1. Puchtler H, Sweat F. Congo red as a stain for fluorescence microscopy of amyloid. J Histochem Cytochem. 1965 Nov-Dec;13(8):693–4.

2. Westermark P, Benson MD, Buxbaum JN, Cohen AS, Frangione B, Ikeda S, Masters CL, Merlini G, Saraiva MJ, Sipe JD. Amyloid fibril protein nomenclature—2002. Amyloid. 2002;9:197–200.

3. Sipe JD, Benson MD, Buxbaum JN, Ikeda SI, Merlini G, Saraiva MJ, Westermark P. Amyloid fibril proteins and amyloidosis: chemical identification and clinical classification International Society of Amyloidosis 2016 nomenclature guidelines. Amyloid. 2016;23:209–13.

4. Moutafi M, Ziogas DC, Michopoulos S, Bagratuni T, Vasileiou V, Verga L, Merlini G, Palladini G, Matsouka C, Dimopoulos MA, Kastritis E. A new genetic variant of hereditary apolipoprotein A-I amyloidosis: a case-report followed by discussion of diagnostic challenges and therapeutic options. BMC Med Genet. 2019;20:23.

5. Orfila C, Giraud P, Modesto A, Suc JM. Abdominal fat tissue aspirate in human amyloidosis: light, electron, and immunofluorescence microscopic studies. Hum Pathol. 1986;17:366–9.

6. Yood RA, Skinner M, Rubinow A, Talarico L, Cohen AS. Bleeding manifestations in 100 patients with amyloidosis. JAMA. 1983;249:1322–4.

7. Ozdemir BH, Akman B, Ozdemir FN. Amyloid goiter in familial Mediterranean fever (FMF): a clinicopathologic study of 10 cases. Ren Fail. 2001;23:659–67.

8. Ozdemir BH, Ozdemir OG, Ozdemir FN, Ozdemir AI. Value of testis biopsy in the diagnosis of systemic amyloidosis. Urology. 2002;59:201–5.

9. Puchtler H, Waldrop FS, Meloan SN. A review of light, polarization and fluorescence microscopic methods for amyloid. Appl Pathol. 1985;3(1–2):5–17.

10. Nistal M, Santamaria L, Codesal J, Paniagua R. Secondary amyloidosis of the testis: an electron microscopic and histochemical study. Appl Pathol. 1989;7:2–7.

11. Haimov-Kochman R, Prus D, Ben-Chetrit E. Azoospermia due to testicular amyloidosis in a patient with familial Mediterranean fever. Hum Reprod. 2001;16:1218–20.

12. Handelsman DJ, Yue DK, Turtle JR. Hypogonadism and massive testicular infiltration due to amyloidosis. J Urol. 1983;129:610–2.

13. Casella R, Nudell D, Cozzolino D, Wang H, Lipshultz LI. Primary testicular amyloidosis mimicking tumor in a cryptorchid testis. Urology. 2002;59:445.

14. Corvino C, Balloni F, Meliani E, Giannini A, Serni S, Carini M. Testicular amyloidosis. Urol Int. 2002;69:162–3.

15. Schrepferman CG, Lester DR, Sandlow JI. Testicular amyloid deposition as a cause of secondary azoospermia. Urology. 2000;55:145.

16. Scalvini T, Martini PR, Obici L, Tardanico R, Biasi L, Gregorini G, Scolari F, Merlini G. Infertility and hypergonadotropic hypogonadism as first evidence of hereditary apolipoprotein A-I amyloidosis. J Urol. 2007;178:344–8.

17. Scalvini T, Martini PR, Gambera A, Tardanico R, Biasi L, Scolari F, Gregorini G, Agabiti RE. Spermatogenic and steroidogenic impairment of the testicle characterizes the hereditary leucine-75-proline apolipoprotein a-I amyloidosis. J Clin Endocrinol Metab. 2008;93:1850–3.

18. Facondo P, Delbarba A, Pezzaioli LC, Ferlin A, Cappelli C. Osteoporosis in men with hypogonadism because of ApoA-I Leu75Pro amyloidosis under long-term testosterone therapy. Andrology. 2023;11:1077–85.

19. Yoshinaga T, Katoh N, Yazaki M, Sato M, Kametani F, Yasuda H, Watanabe K, Kawata K, Nakagawa M, Sekijima Y. Giant hepatomegaly with Splenotesticular enlargement in a patient with apolipoprotein A-I amyloidosis: an uncommon type of amyloidosis in Japan. Intern Med. 2021;60:575–81.

20. Livneh A, Zemer D, Langevitz P, Laor A, Sohar E, Pras M. Colchicine treatment of AA amyloidosis of familial Mediterranean fever. An analysis of factors affecting outcome. Arthritis Rheum. 1994;37:1804–11.

The return of blood to the testicular veins begins when the interstitial and peritubular capillaries join to form veins that converge in the intralobular veins that drain into veins located in the interlobular septa. Most of the blood collected in the deep 2/3 of the parenchyma drains through centripetal veins that run into the mediastinum, traverse it, exit the testis and join the pampini-form plexus [1] (Fig. 1). The peripheral third of the parenchyma is drained by veins that also follow the interlobular septa but are directed toward the albu-ginea (centrifugal veins) (Fig. 2). They follow the tunica vasculosa and, at the level of the inferior pole of the testis, perforate the albuginea to join the pampiniform plexus of the spermatic cord [2] (Fig. 3).

The marginal vein of the epididymis is also involved in the formation of the pampiniform plexus. As a whole, it is made up of 10–12 veins which are

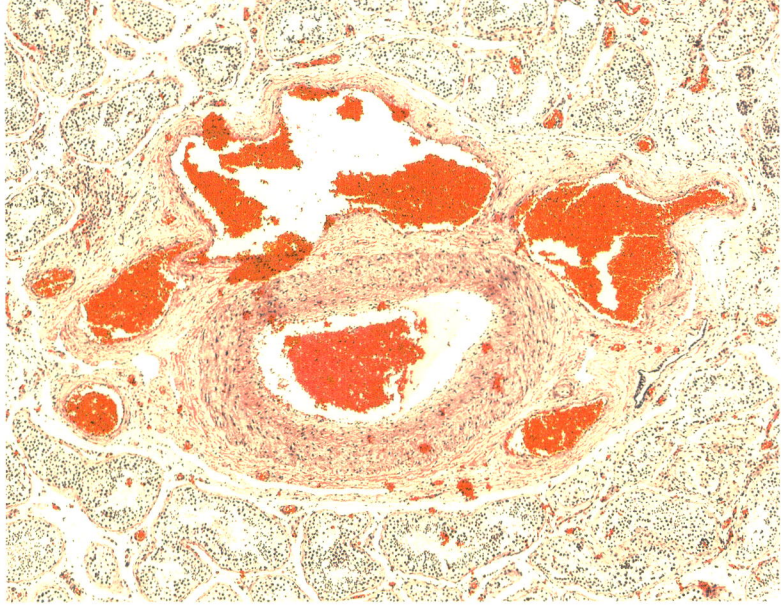

Fig. 1 Sections of veins obliquely crossing the testicular parenchyma following a thin interlobular septum. Note the thin wall of the veins and the moderate congestion

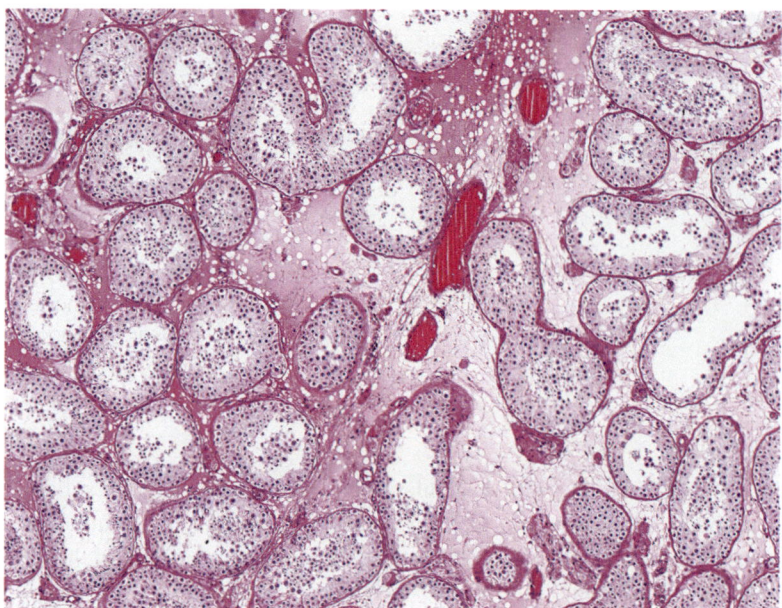

Fig. 2 Several centripetal veins surrounding the hilar artery in the vicinity of the rete testis. Despite their calibre, the wall consists only of an endothelium and one or two layers of smooth muscle cells with a ring of connective tissue in the adventitia

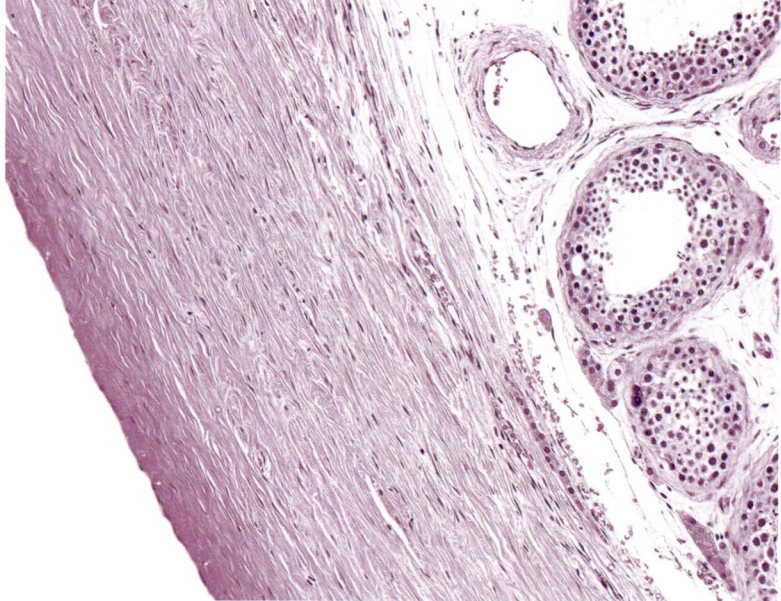

Fig. 3 Cross section of a vein and several seminiferous tubules located close to the tunica vasculosa of the albuginea

divided into anterior and posterior groups according to their topography. The venous return of the testis also includes the deferential vein, which accompanies the vas deferens, and the cremasteric vein, which is located between the internal and external spermatic fascia and drains into the inferior epigastric vein. At the level of the inferior pole of the testis, there are numerous connections between the three vascular systems [3] (Fig. 4).

At the level of the deep inguinal ring, the pampiniform plexus is continued by the spermatic vein which has numerous valves. On the right side, the spermatic vein drains directly into the inferior vena cava at an oblique angle four centimetres from the renal vein. The left spermatic vein is located ventral to the iliopsoas muscle and drains into the renal vein at a right angle (Fig. 5).

Studies in cadavers [4–6], with phlebography [7, 8], or multidetector computed tomography [9], have shown that the presence of multiple testicular veins is frequent, as well as is their atypical drainages. A single testicular vein is identified on the right side in 85% of cases and two testicular veins in 5%. In 25% of cases there are communicating veins with the colon. On the left side, there is a testicular vein in 82% of the cases, two veins in 15%, three veins in 2%, and four veins in 1% of the cases. Some 31% of men show communications with the veins of the colon. The most frequent testicular vein drainages are: to the vena cava on the right side in 83% of cases, to the junction of the renal vein with the cava in 12% and to the renal vein in 4.2%. On the left side, regardless of the number of veins, they all flow into the renal vein [10].

The venous drainage of the vessels of the deferential compartment is to the pelvic plexus, while the cremasteric vessels drain into the inferior epigastric veins.

In the following chapters, reference is made to the classic entities produced by altered venous return such as torsion of the spermatic cord and varicocele. Two chapters are dedicated to recently-described vascular lesions, some of known aetiology and others of uncertain significance. The last one is

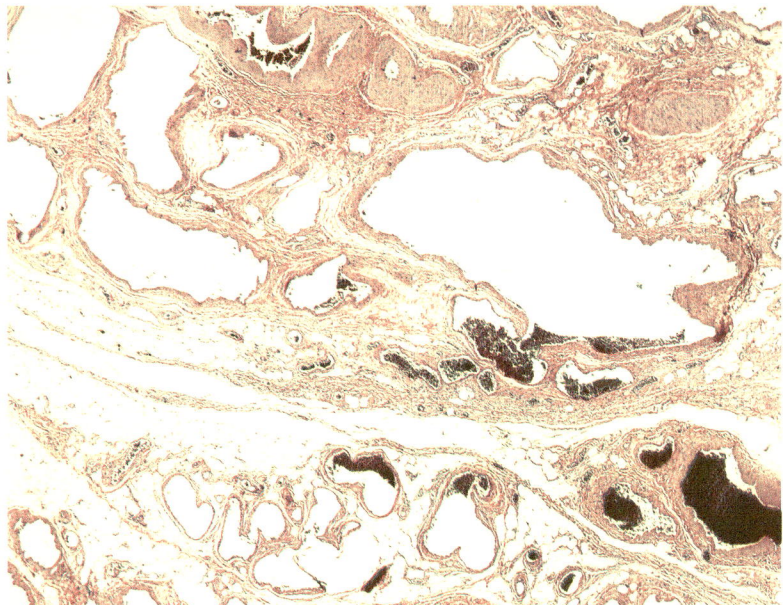

Fig. 4 Partial section of the pampiniform plexus. Some sections show blood in their interior, others, the majority, are optically empty. The vein walls are quite thin

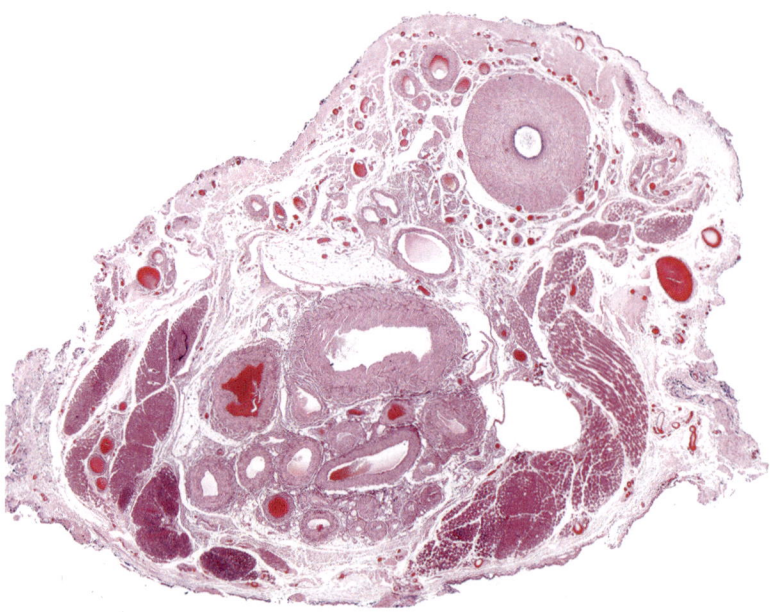

Fig. 5 Cross section of the spermatic cord. In the central part, there are two thick-walled veins and an artery surrounded by several small veins. Peripherally, lie the cremaster muscle and the vas deferens

dedicated, on the one hand, to thrombosis of the testicular vein, pampiniform plexus, and intraparenchymatous veins and small vessels, and on the other, to two other entities, segmental infarction of the testicle and polypoid granulomatous endophlebitis of the spermatic cord.

References
1. Suzuki F, Nagano T. Microvasculature of the human testis and excurrent duct system. Resin-casting and scanning electron-microscopic studies. Cell Tissue Res. 1986;243:79–89.
2. Kormano M, Suoranta H. Microvascular organization of the adult human testis. Anat Rec. 1971;170:31–9.
3. Gaudin J, Lefèvre C, Person H, N'Guyen-Huu, Senecail B. The venous hilum of the testis and epididymis: anatomic aspect. Surg Radiol Anat. 1988;10:233–42.
4. Shafik A, Moftah A, Olfat S, Mohi-el-Din M, el-Sayed A. Testicular veins: anatomy and role in varicocelogenesis and other pathologic conditions. Urology. 1990;35:175–82
5. Wishahi MM. Anatomy of the venous drainage of the human testis: testicular vein cast, microdissection and radiographic demonstration. A new anatomical concept. Eur Urol. 1991;20:154–60.
6. Asala S, Chaudhary SC, Masumbuko-Kahamba N, Bidmos M. Anatomical variations in the human testicular blood vessels. Ann Anat. 2001;183:545–9.
7. Coolsaet BL. The varicocele syndrome: venography determining the optimal level for surgical management. J Urol. 1980;124:833–9.

8. Bensussan D, Huguet JF. Radiological anatomy of the testicular vein. Anat Clin. 1984;6:143–54.

9. Kara T, Younes M, Erol B, Karcaaltincaba M. Evaluation of testicular vein anatomy with multidetector computed tomography. Surg Radiol Anat. 2012;34:341–5.

10. Favorito LA, Costa WS, Sampaio FJ. Applied anatomic study of testicular veins in adult cadavers and in human fetuses. Int Braz J Urol. 2007;33:176–80.

Impact of Spermatic Cord Torsion on Testicular Structure and Function

11.1 Introduction

Testicular torsion occurs when the spermatic cord is twisted. This disrupts blood circulation and leads to testicular ischaemia with parenchymal necrosis if it is not corrected. Two types of torsion are distinguished: extravaginal and intravaginal torsion. Extravaginal torsion is characteristic of the perinatal period when the attachments of the tunica vaginalis to the scrotal wall are incompletely developed. Intravaginal torsion is more common in puberty and young adults and is favoured by anatomical abnormalities of the tunica vaginalis that allow the testis to be suspended within the tunica vaginalis, resulting in bell-clapper deformity [1, 2].

The incidence of testicular torsion is estimated to be 1 in 4000 men under the age of 25 years [3]. Sixty-six percent of torsions occur between the ages of 12 and 18 years old, with the peak incidence at 14 years of age [4]. Neonatal torsion accounts for 5% of torsions and has an estimated incidence of 1 in 7500 newborns [5, 6]. Seventy two percent are intrautero torsions and 28% occur within the first month of life [7, 8]. In rare cases, familial presentation is observed [9]. The association of testicular torsion and an undescended testicle is rare [10].

Torsion can be uni- or bilateral. Torsion is more frequent in the left testicle than the right one [11]. Bilateral torsion mainly affects neonates and is observed in less than 2% of testicular torsions [12]. Pubertal cases of bilateral testicular torsion are rare [13, 14] and cases of bilateral testicular torsion in adults are exceptional [15].

The future of the testicle is related to two factors: the duration of symptoms before detorsion and the degree of torsion. The viability of the testicle worsens rapidly with a "golden window" for saving testicular function being estimated at between 4 and 8 h from the onset of symptoms [16]. If the degree of torsion is greater than 360 degrees for 24 h, the testicles are irreversibly damaged. There are always exceptions—either because arterial flow is not completely interrupted or because the torsion may be intermittent [17].

11.2 Parenchymal Injuries in Children and Adults

In perinatal torsions, the testicular lesions are always very severe, which is not surprising, as in a high percentage of cases they are congenital. They range from haemorrhagic infarction to necrosis of the entire parenchyma (Figs. 11.1, 11.2, 11.3, 11.4, 11.5 and 11.6). Haemorrhage is very extensive, starting under the albuginea, interlobular septa, and testicular mediastinum. In the seminiferous tubules, vacuolisation of the cytoplasm of the spermatogonia is initially prominent. In the testicles with very advanced lesions, subalbuginea and testicular mediastinum haem-

M. Nistal, P. González-Peramato, *Testicular Vascular Lesions*, https://doi.org/10.1007/978-3-031-57847-2_11

Fig. 11.1 Perinatal spermatic cord torsion. Haemorrhagic infarction affecting both testis and epididymis. Despite haemorrhage, tubular structures are still recognizable in both the testis and the epididymis

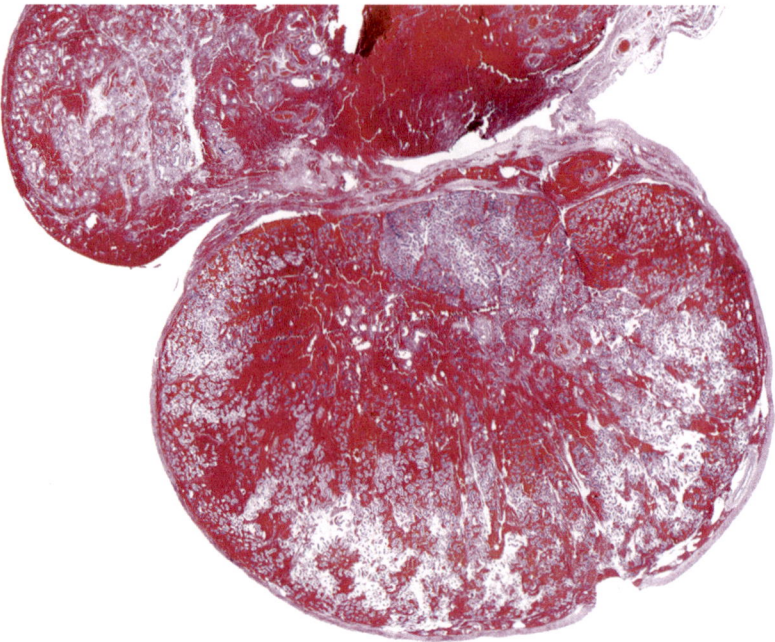

Fig. 11.2 Perinatal spermatic cord torsion. The haemorrhagic areas are preferentially distributed under the albuginea and in the interlobular septa

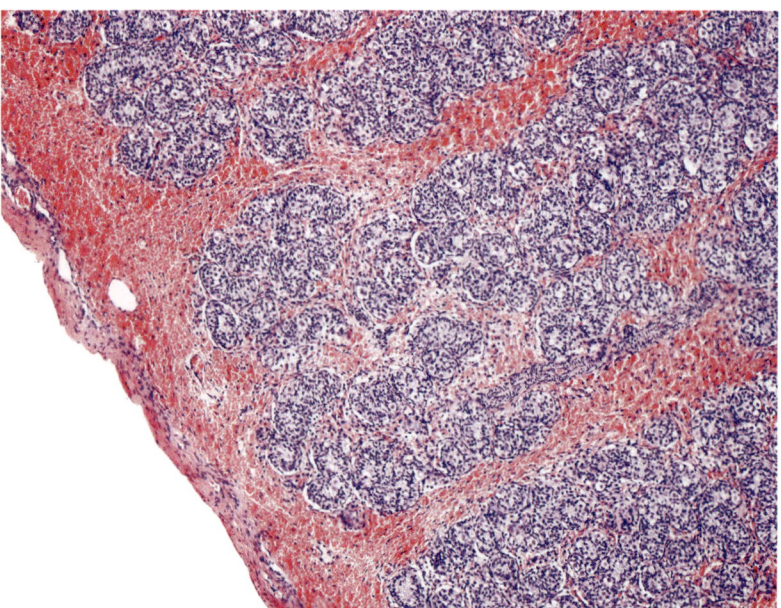

orrhages are preserved while the outline of the seminiferous tubules is barely visible in the necrotic parenchyma. The epididymis shows haemorrhagic infarct lesions like those of the testis. The testicle is finally fibrosed. The section on the evanescent testis will discuss the possible findings seen in an old torsioned testis.

In the pubertal and adult testis (Fig. 11.7), lesions secondary to torsion have been classified into three grades [18]. Grade I is characterized by testicular enlargement due to marked oedema, vascular congestion, dilatation of the lymphatic vessels, and focal haemorrhage. The seminiferous tubules show enlargement of the lumen and

Fig. 11.3 Perinatal spermatic cord torsion. Relatively well-preserved group of seminiferous tubules. Haemorrhagic area and lymphoid infiltrates on the side

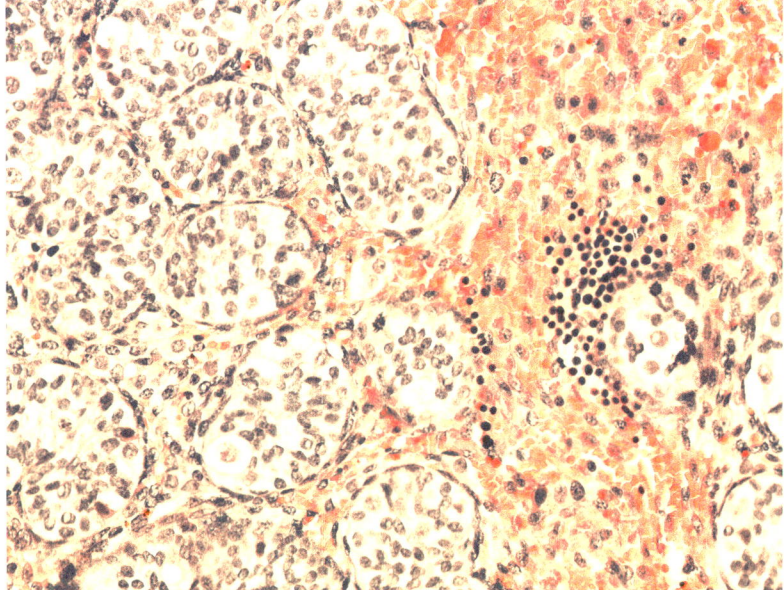

Fig. 11.4 Perinatal spermatic cord torsion. Longitudinal section of a testis showing parenchymal necrosis, congestion, and haemorrhage at the level of the mediastinum, neighbouring seminiferous tubules and under the albuginea

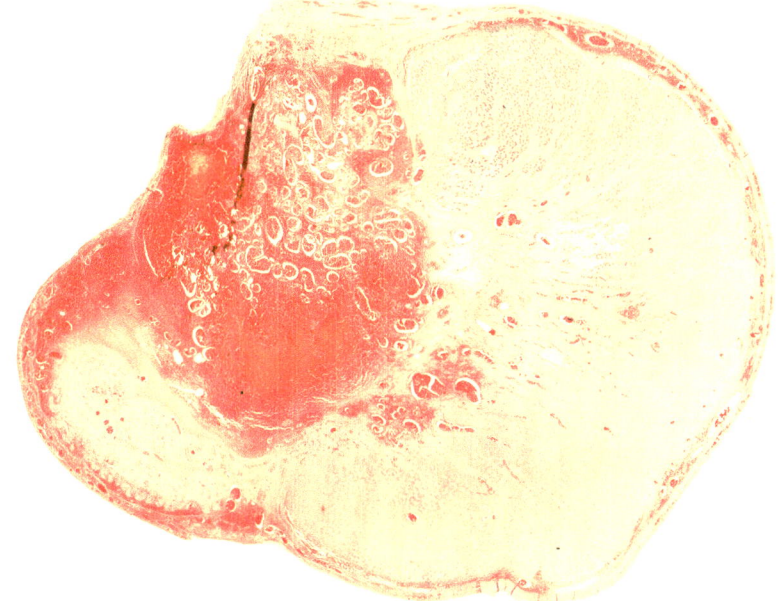

increased diameter. The seminiferous epithelium is altered in the Sertoli cells, which show marked cytoplasmic vacuolisation, as well as in the germ cells, which undergo early spermiation (Fig. 11.8). In our series, grade I was observed in 28.5% of the torsioned adult testes. Most came from patients with less than 4 h since symptom onset. These lesions are considered reversible after detorsion.

Grade II. Interstitial haemorrhage is more extensive and separates the seminiferous tubules. In many cases, it is even more extensive in the vicinity of the testicular mediastinum than in the periphery of the testis, which can underestimate the severity of the injuries as the information that can be provided by biopsy material usually only includes a peripheral part of the parenchyma.

Fig. 11.5 Perinatal spermatic cord torsion. Testicular parenchyma with extensive subalbuginea haemorrhage in the interlobular and intertubular septa, characteristic of advanced ischaemic lesions

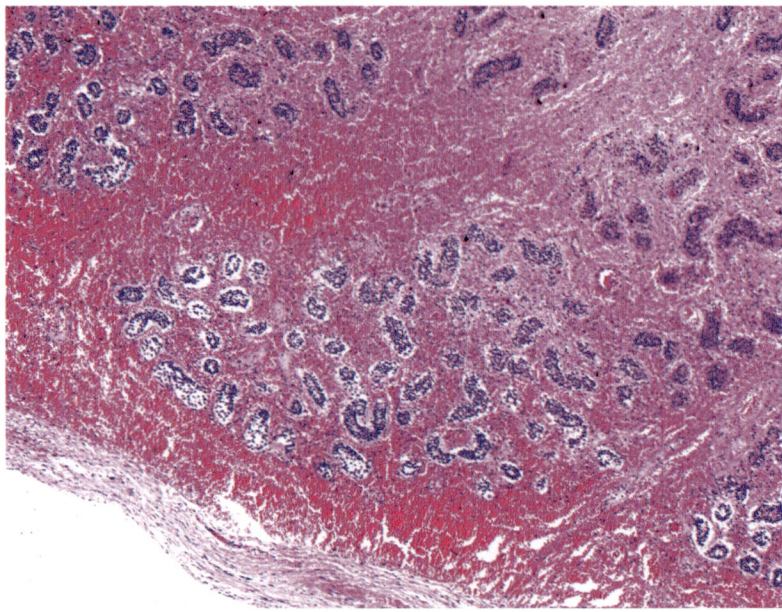

Fig. 11.6 Perinatal spermatic cord torsion. Parenchymal necrosis. The outline of the seminiferous tubules can still be seen in a haemorrhagic interstitium

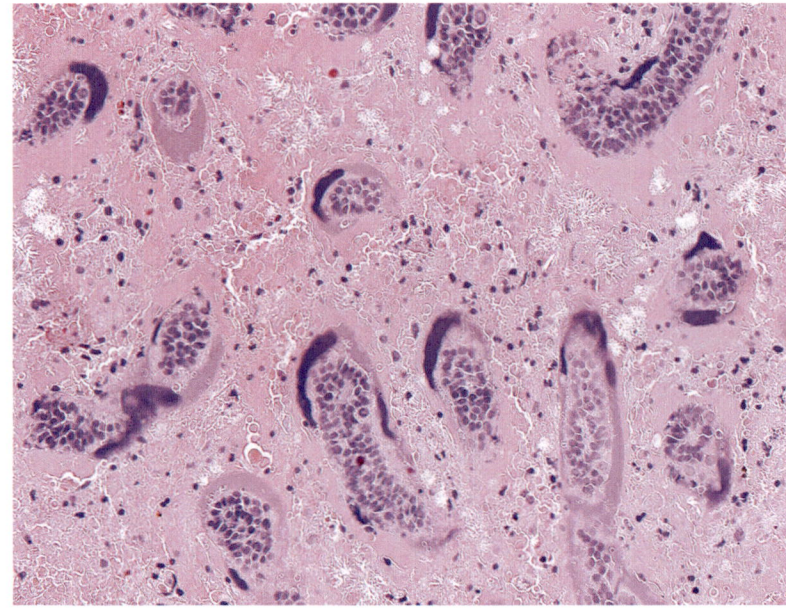

This fact is probably related to the distribution pattern of intraparenchymal veins. Most of the parenchyma drains via centripetal veins into the testicular mediastinum while only a small part of the peripheral parenchyma drains via centrifugal veins. Congestion first, followed by rupture of the wall of the large centripetal veins later may explain the topographical distribution of the lesions. The seminiferous tubules show marked dilatation of the lumen while the seminiferous epithelium is detached from the basement membrane in large areas and all cell types in these areas are desquamated (Figs. 11.8 and 11.9). Tubular ectasia is probably also related to the compression that the veins may exert against the spermatic pathways including the intratesticular ones [19]. The lesion is observed in 26.5% of torsioned testes. Most of them correspond to patients with a torsion of 4–8 h' duration (Fig. 11.10).

Fig. 11.7 Pubertal
testicular torsion.
Blackish discolouration
of both the testis and the
epididymis. Torsion is
seen at the level of the
cord

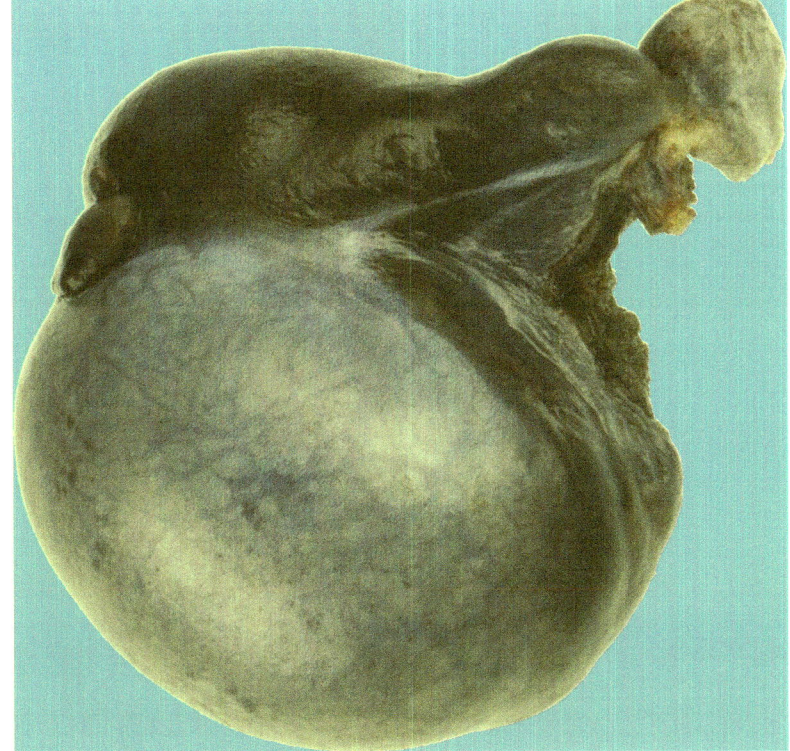

Fig. 11.8 Pubertal
testicular torsion. Type I
lesions. The tubules
have a slightly enlarged
lumen. The seminiferous
epithelium is well
preserved.
Spermatogenesis is
complete

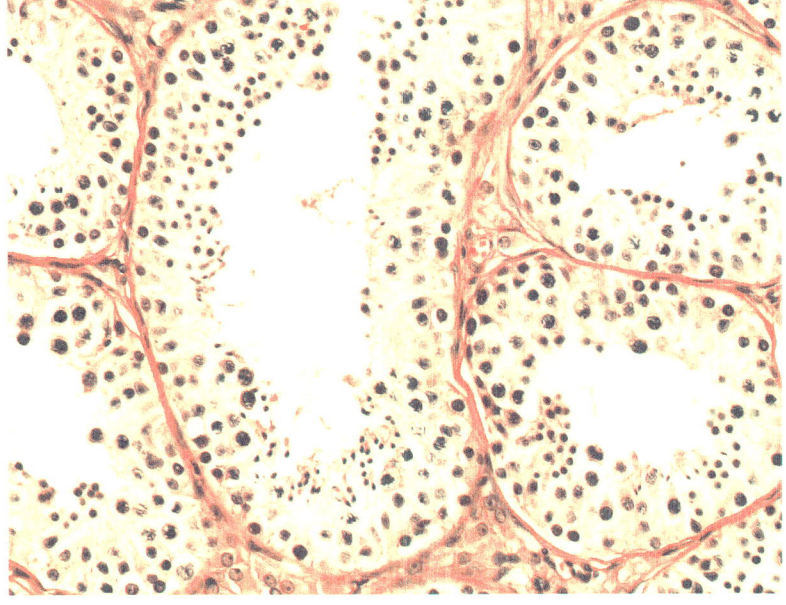

Grade III. The interstitium is diffusely haemorrhagic. The seminiferous epithelium shows diffuse necrosis (Fig. 11.11). These lesions are
observed in 45.7% of torsions in patients with
more than 12 h of evolution. Although the type of
torsion in most cases correlates well with the
time from symptom onset to detorsion, there are
approximately 6.5% of cases in which this is not

Fig. 11.9 Pubertal testicular torsion. Type II lesions. The interstitium shows focal haemorrhages and the seminiferous tubules have moderate ectasia. The seminiferous epithelium shows a decrease in height

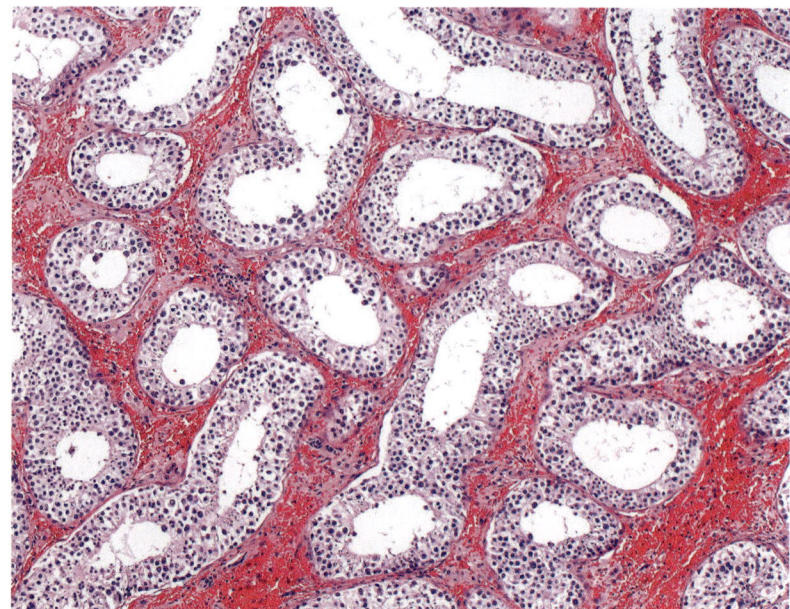

Fig. 11.10 Pubertal testicular torsion. Type II lesions. Extensive interstitial haemorrhage. In each tubule, different lesions are observed ranging from lumen enlargement to germ cell desquamation and necrosis of the seminiferous epithelium in contiguous tubules

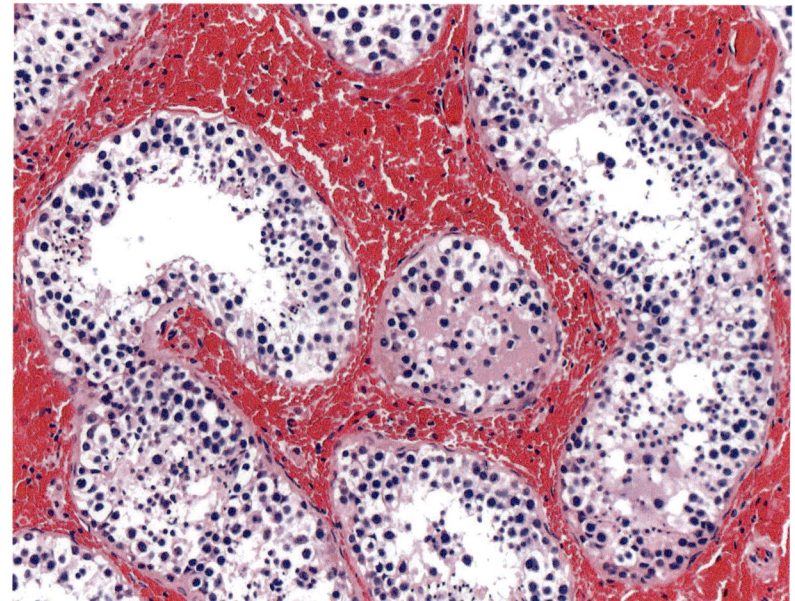

true. In these cases, the cause probably lies either in the degree of twisting of the spermatic cord or in the intermittency of the twisting.

An observation that, in our opinion has not received the necessary attention, probably because in some cases the biopsy only provides partial information and in others because testicular lesions are very advanced in the orchiectomy specimens, is the presence of primary alterations

in the torsioned testis that go beyond the abnormalities of vaginal implantation. At least one of the following lesions has been observed in 15% of torsioned testes: hypospermatogenesis, mixed atrophy, Sertoli cell nodules, and microlithiasis (Figs. 11.12, 11.13, 11.14 and 11.15). None of these lesions can be explained by the elapsed ischaemia time. Although it is possible that the testes with hypospermatogenesis are related to

Fig. 11.11 Pubertal testicular torsion. Type III lesions. Necrosis of the testicular parenchyma. Only the outline of the seminiferous tubules is visible in an area close to the albuginea

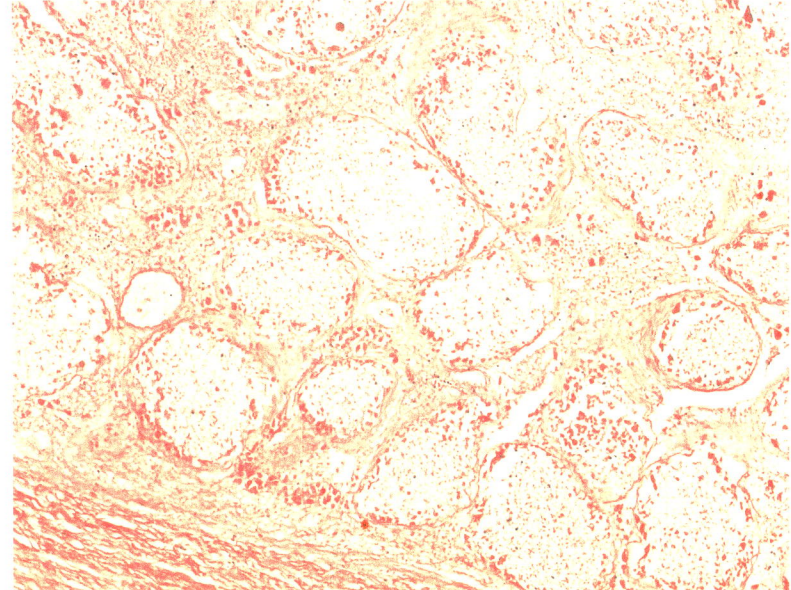

Fig. 11.12 Torsion of an adult testis with primary lesions. Intense hypospermatogenesis. The tubular lumen is slightly dilated. The Sertoli cells have abundant cytoplasmic vacuoles and the seminiferous epithelium only forms spermatozoa in some tubules. Marked interstitial oedema

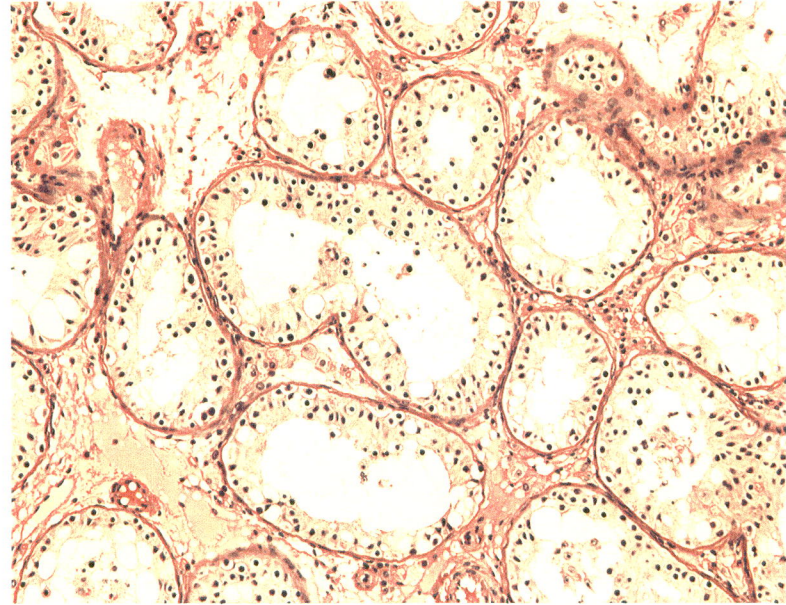

the age of the patient and reflect incomplete puberty, in the remaining cases, these lesions cannot be attributed to another pathology, such as cryptorchidism, in which their presence has been reported in only 2% of the cases. Although in most cases the lesions are focal and given that the contralateral testicle also carries the same vaginal reflection anomaly, the bilateral presence of these lesions may be the cause of the cases of subfertility that have been reported [20, 21].

Fig. 11.13 Torsion of an adult testis with primary lesions. Seminiferous tubules with hypospermatogenesis associated with involuted Sertoli cells (elongated hyperchromatic nuclei with abundant folds)

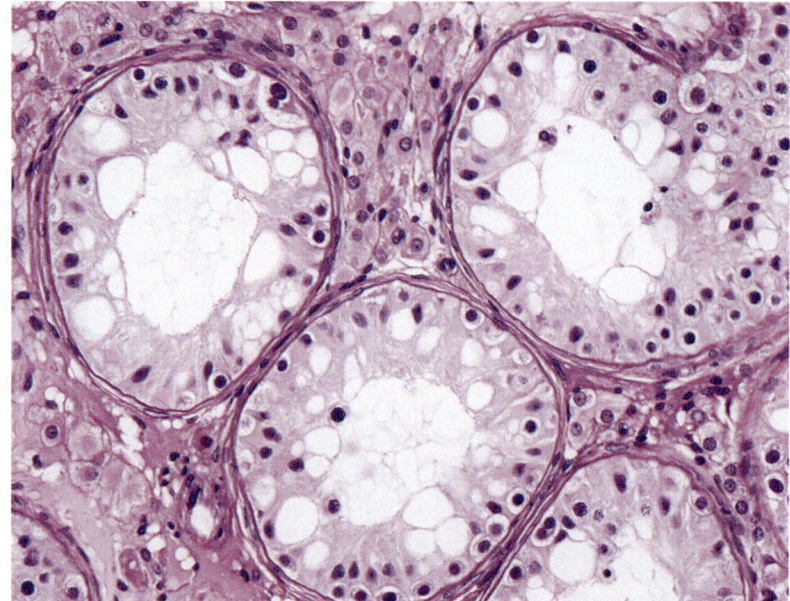

Fig. 11.14 Torsion of an adult testis with primary lesions. Apart from minimal interstitial haemorrhages, more than half of the tubules have decreased size, tubular wall thickening and the seminiferous epithelium consists only of Sertoli cells

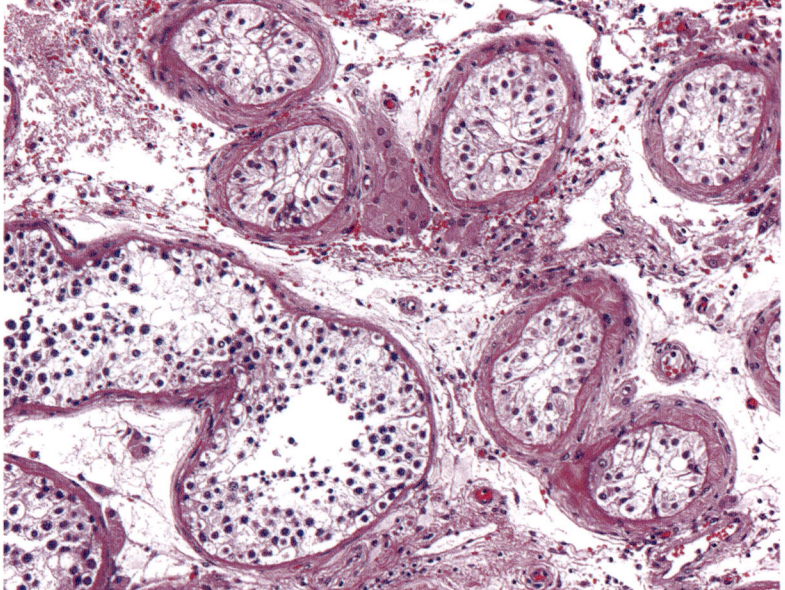

Fig. 11.15 Torsion of an adult testis with primary lesions. Mixed atrophy, seminiferous tubular ectasia with only Sertoli cells, focal haemorrhages, and presence of a microlith

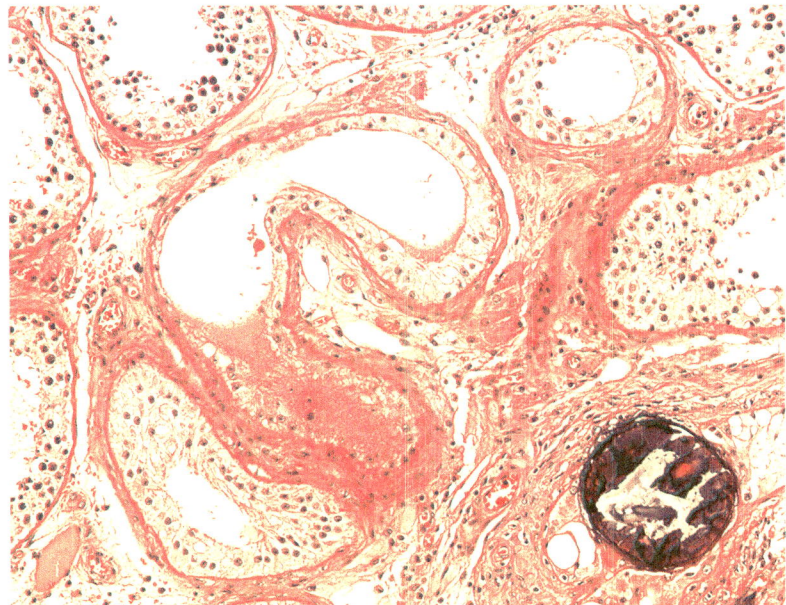

11.3   Injuries to Veins, Arteries, and Nerves of the Cord After Torsion

11.3.1   Intraparenchymal Vein Thrombosis

Even after the first few days following an uncorrected torsion, the veins of the spermatic cord still show marked congestion, which contrasts with the necrotic appearance of the testis. Some intraparenchymal veins can be distinguished between the necrotic seminiferous tubules. They seem well-demarcated, of good size, and most are notable for the presence of recent thrombosis. In some of them, clusters of red blood cells are still visible in the lumen. The thrombus shows signs of recanalization (Figs. 11.16, 11.17 and 11.18). There is, as evidenced by CD31 (Fig. 11.19) and Ki67, an intense proliferation of endothelial cells, which is very evident 1 week after torsion.

In the testes studied more than 1 month after a torsion, only fibrous tissue with a few macrophages with haemosiderin is recognizable and it is difficult to identify organized and recanalized venous thrombi.

11.3.2   Obliteration of Spermatic Cord Arteries

During a spermatic cord torsion, the venous flow is strangulated due to the weakness of the structure of the vein wall, while arterial flow is maintained for a certain time, resulting in a haemorrhagic infarction of the testicle. After the first few hours, arterial flow is also interrupted, and the vessels develop significant lesions (Figs. 11.20 and 11.21). After the first 24 h, the diameter of the testicular arteries and their branches decreases. The vascular lumen is reduced to a slit. The intima shows an apparent thickening. With the orcein technique, the internal elastic lamina appears reduplicated, and the media has an apparent increase in thickness (Fig. 11.22). The adventitia shows no alterations. With CD31 staining there are very few vasa vasorum in the media. The vascular lesion is not associated with inflammatory infiltrates. These changes give the arteries the appearance of solid cords rather than tubular formations (Fig. 11.23). These same atrophic changes are seen in some arteries of the tunica vasculosa. As time passes and probably due to ischaemia, the vessels become unrecognizable or fibrotic.

Fig. 11.16 Eight-day testicular torsion in an 18-year-old patient. Longitudinal section of the testicle. The haemorrhagic infarction is very advanced. No bleeding was observed at the albuginea incision

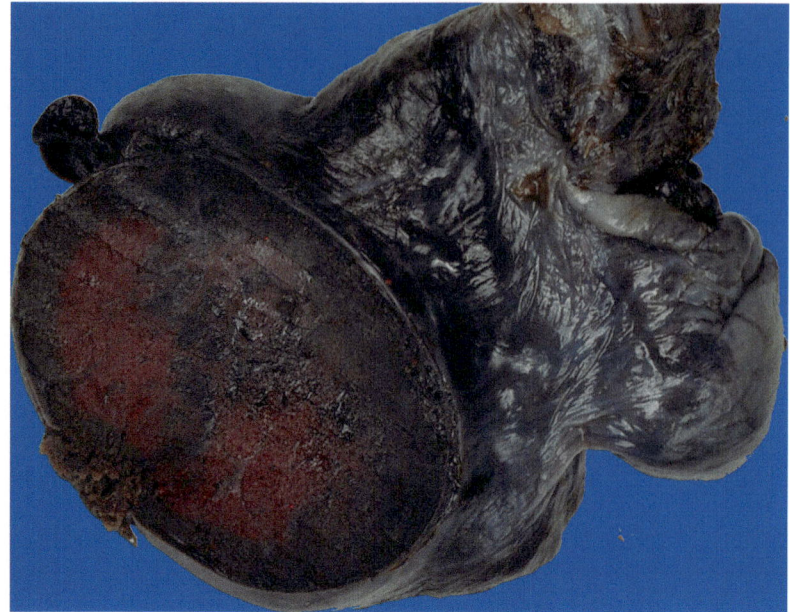

Fig. 11.17 Testicular torsion. Intraparenchymal vein with thrombosis. The testicular parenchyma shows necrotic tubules (type III lesions)

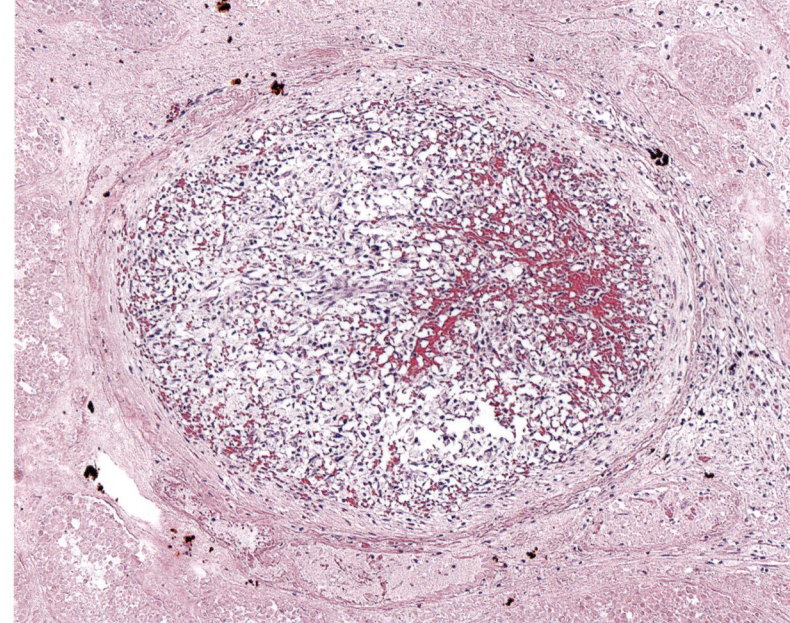

11.3.3 Morton-Like Neuroma in the Spermatic Cord

The first reference to an apparent hyperplasia of the spermatic cord nerves was described in the 1980s [22]. It was a finding in histological studies of the spermatic cord and testicular debris of patients who presumably had a history of torsion (fibrosis, calcifications, small clusters of seminiferous tubules). This curious lesion can be observed in both testes with a history of neonatal torsion and torsion during puberty.

The testicle is a nerve-rich organ. The testicle is innervated by the superior spermatic nerves, the

Fig. 11.18 Testicular torsion. Thrombal in organization. The lumen is occupied by numerous capillary vessels

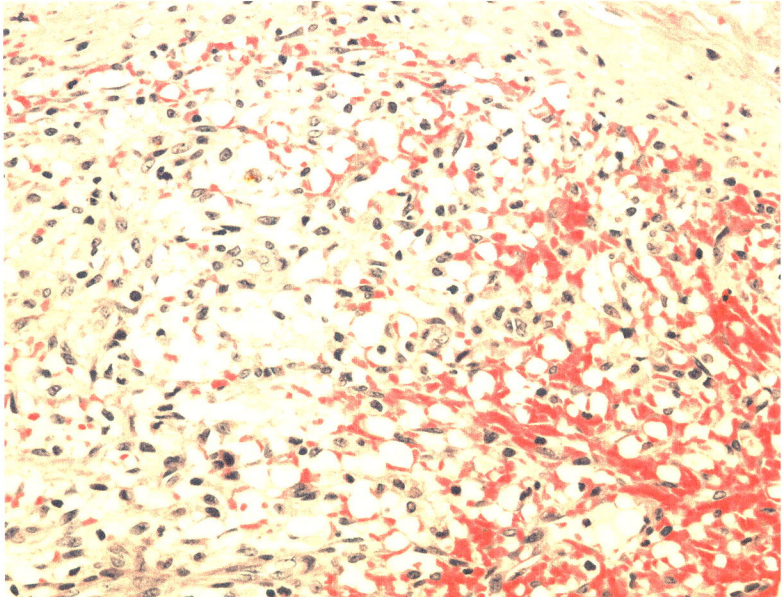

Fig. 11.19 Testicular torsion. Intense CD31 positivity in the vascular endothelium of the neoformed vessels of the thrombus

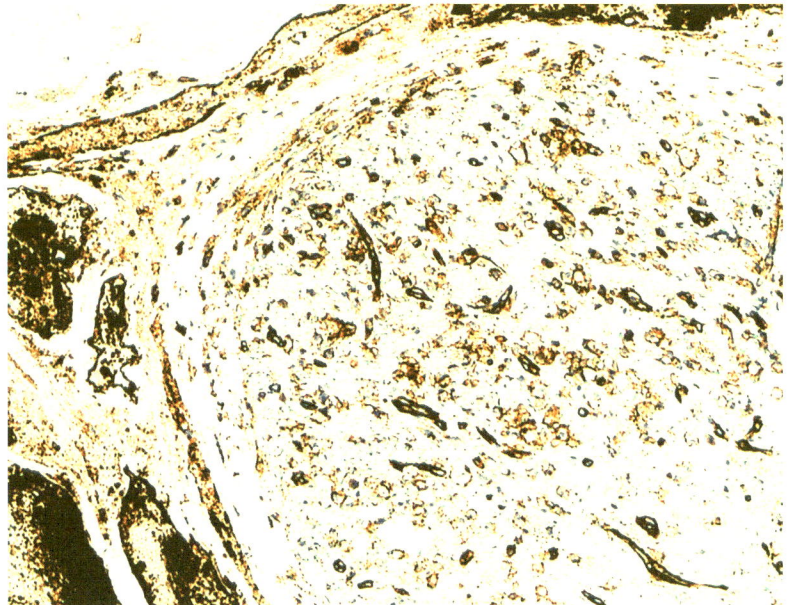

intermediate spermatic nerve, and the inferior spermatic nerve. The superior spermatic nerves originate from the intermesenteric nerves and the renal plexus, follow the testicular artery down its length and terminate in the testis. The intermediate spermatic nerve originates in the upper portion of the hypogastric plexus, crosses the internal inguinal canal, and joins the spermatic cord. Its terminal branches innervate the epididymis and the initial part of the deferens. The inferior spermatic nerve is supplied by fibres of dual origin. Most come from the pelvic plexus and the remainder from the inferior mesenteric plexus, which innervates the vas deferens, the epididymis, and only partially the testicle. Within the testicle, fine nerves are found both in the interlobular septa and

Fig. 11.20 Testicular torsion. At the level of the spermatic cord, the deferens, several congestive veins and two solid spherical formations stand out

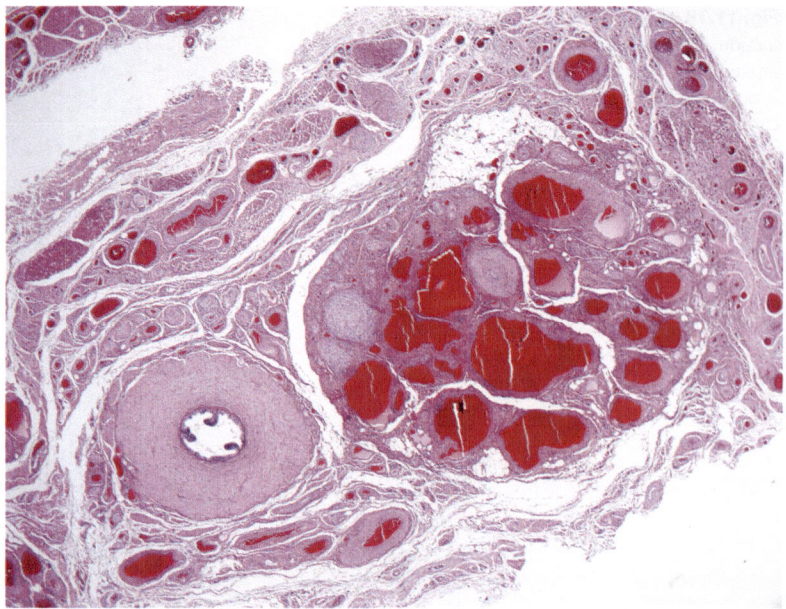

Fig. 11.21 Chordal formation close to the wall of a vein. The circumferential distribution of its constituent cells can be seen

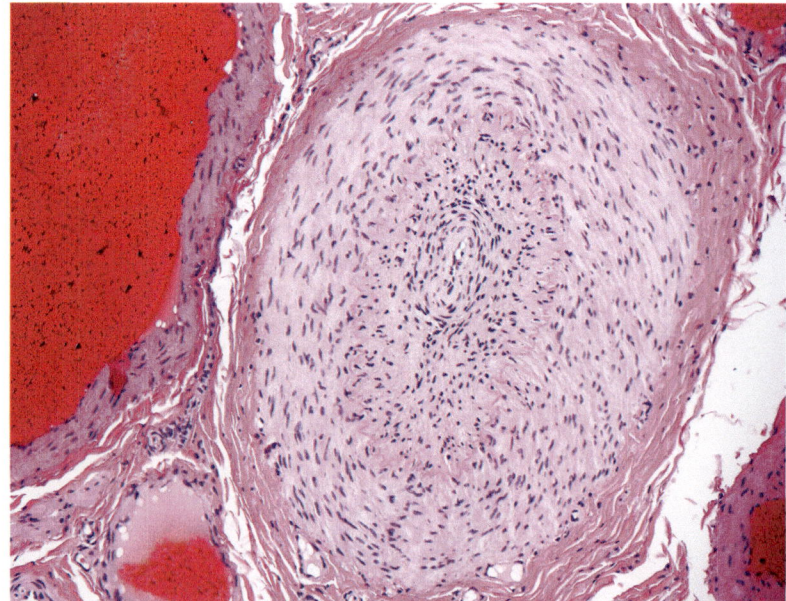

in the testicular mediastinum. Many nerve fibres innervate the vessels while others end up in the vicinity of the Leydig cells [23, 24] or even between the myoid cells of the tubular wall [25]. In the adult, peptidergic innervation is considered to be the most important in mediating the testicular functions of the cells involved [26]. The albuginea, especially at the level of the tunica vasculosa, shows abundant nerves and a plexus of fine catecholaminergic fibres.

The nerves observed in patients with a history of spermatic cord torsion are remarkable at this level not only for their thickening due to oedema, but also for the marked fibrosis that particularly affects the perineurium. The nerves more closely resemble a Morton's neuroma than a traumatic

Fig. 11.22 Orcein staining shows that the chordal formation corresponds to an artery. Note the reduplication of the internal elastic lamina, the thickness of the media, and the stenosis of the lumen

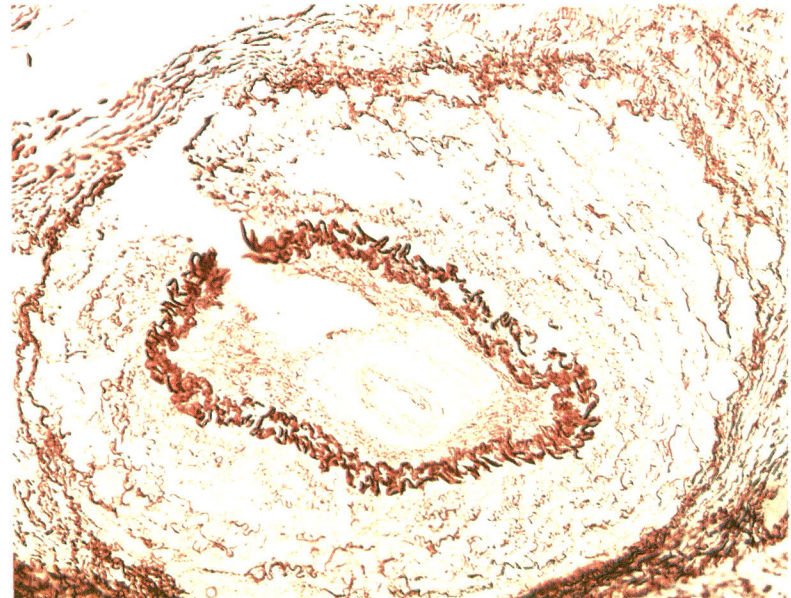

Fig. 11.23 The stenosed artery has thickening of the intima and apparent hyperplasia of the smooth muscle cells of the medial layer with immunostaining for smooth muscle actin

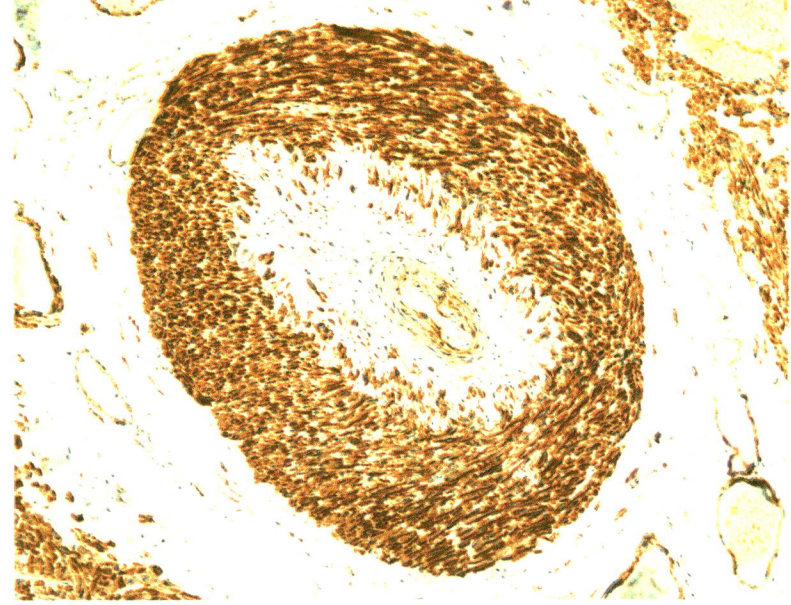

neuroma (Figs. 11.24 and 11.25). They differ histologically from Morton's neuroma in that their vicinity often holds traces of inflammation such as haemosiderin-containing macrophages or fibrosis of the structures through which they pass.

The aetiology of this appearance "neuroma" is probably due to inflammatory irritation following testicular torsion rather than compression by the torsioned structures of the spermatic cord, or loss of the testicle.

Fig. 11.24 Twisting of the spermatic cord. Transverse sections of several nerves with fibrosis of the perineurium. Surrounding them is connective tissue with small vessels and abundant haemosiderin-containing macrophages

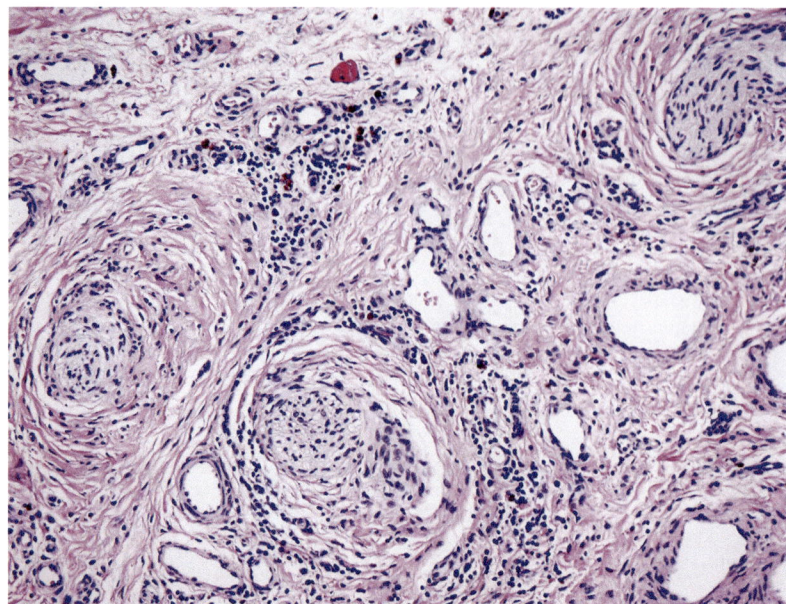

Fig. 11.25 Twisting of the spermatic cord. Section of two nerves with marked fibrosis of the perineurium

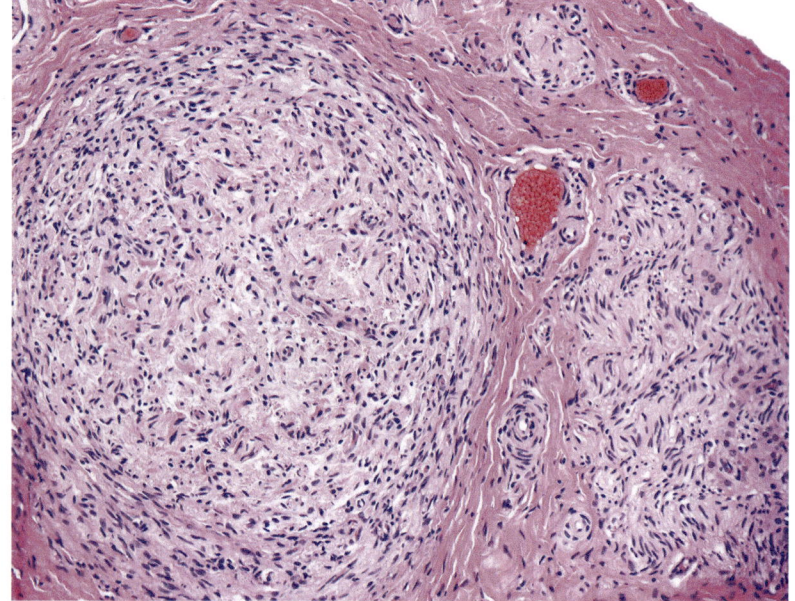

11.4   Management of Vanishing Testis Secondary to Testicular Torsion

About 20% of undescended testicles in the paediatric age group are clinically impalpable [27]. In 21% of surgical examinations performed to descend the testis, the testicle is unrecognizable (Fig. 11.26). In most cases, only testicular remnants are observed. In these anorchias, also known as evanescent testis, only blind-ended cord structures are discovered in the inguinal canal (59%), abdomen (21%), superficial inguinal ring (18%), or scrotum (2%) [28]. The aetiology is related to untreated perinatal torsion.

Macroscopic changes occur after an unresolved perinatal torsion in all distal structures of

Fig. 11.26 Perinatal testicular torsion. Cross section with an atrophic epididymis, arterial and venous vessels and necrotic testis

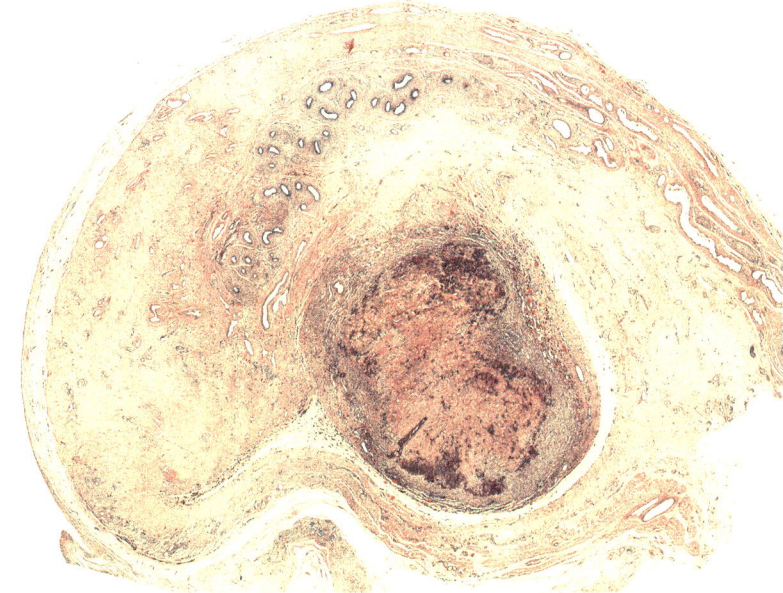

Fig. 11.27 Perinatal testicular torsion. The nubbin shows vas deferens, arteries, and veins and an atrophic testis with a small number of seminiferous tubules

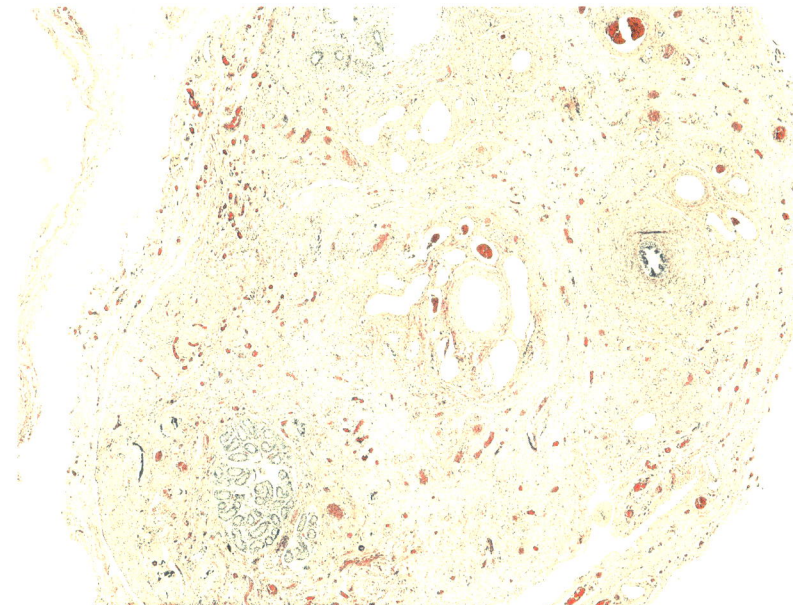

the spermatic cord. The spermatic cord is notable for being transformed into a thin cord with a slight thickening of fibrous tissue at the distal end. Histologically, in 69–83% of cases, structures of the cord, epididymis or remnants of seminiferous tubules are recognizable [29]. The most frequent finding is in the vas deferens (79%), followed by the epididymis (36%) and clusters of seminiferous tubules whose incidence varies from 0 to 20% of cases. Abundant veins that may correspond to spermatic and cremasteric veins or thickening of nerve trunks are recognizable in only 24% of cases (Fig. 11.27).

Dystrophic calcification (35.5–60% of cases), (Fig. 11.28) macrophages with haemosiderin or multinucleated giant cell reaction (44%) (Fig. 11.29) are observed in the fibrous thickening, which is likely to correspond to the twisted

Fig. 11.28 Perinatal testicular torsion. Dystrophic calcifications in the fibrous tissue of the testicular remnants

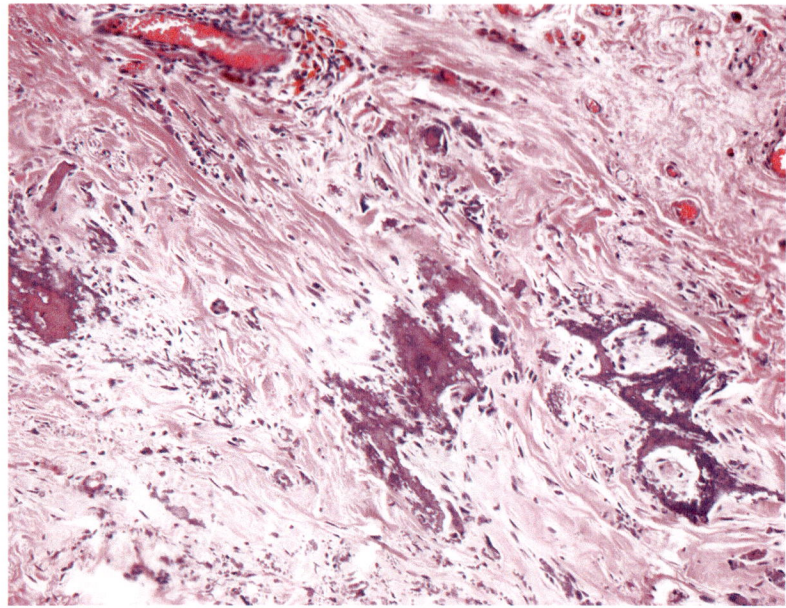

Fig. 11.29 Perinatal testicular torsion. Macrophages and giant cells in the fibrous tissue of the testis

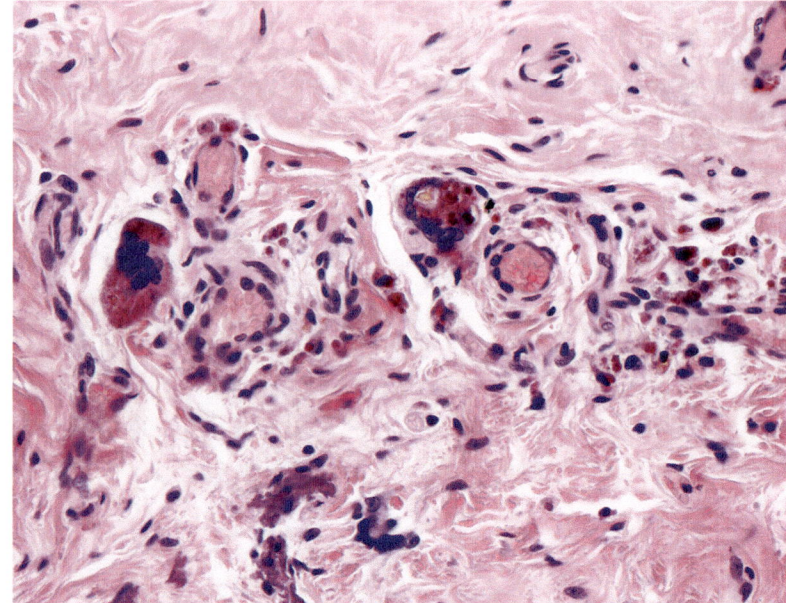

testis. In cases in which seminiferous tubules are identified, these usually do not contain germ cells (Fig. 11.30).

The controversy in the literature regarding the management of vanishing testis secondary to torsion is mediated by the possibility of developing a germ cell tumour. Some advocate surgical exploration and removal of any remains found. Others, based on the low number of cases in which seminiferous tubules are identified, and the fact that germ cells are identified in only 1–16% of these cases [30, 31], consider surgery unnecessary [32, 33]. Differentiating the cases according to the location of the testicular remnants does not seem to provide sufficient justification for the removal of remnants found in a scrotal or inguinal position, and only some doubt persists as to whether those located intra-

Fig. 11.30 Perinatal testicular torsion. Cluster of seminiferous tubules with only Sertoli cells surrounded by scar tissue

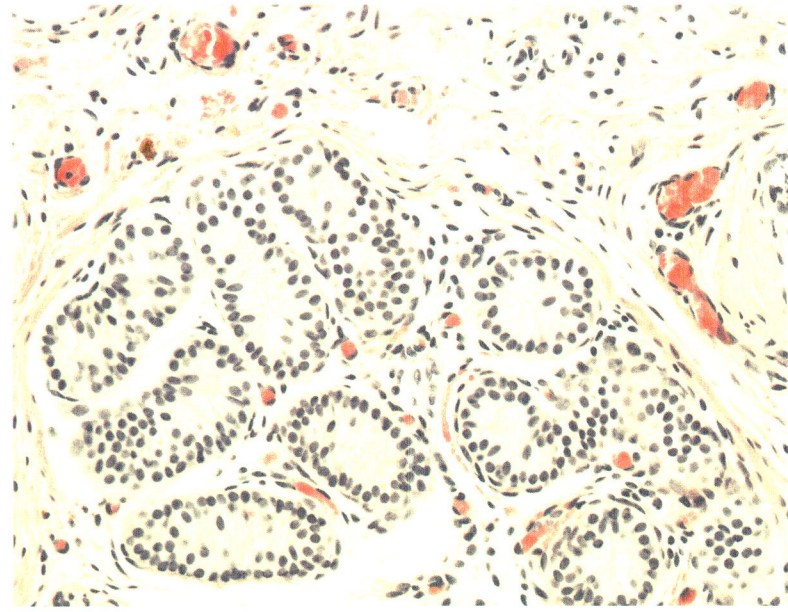

abdominally should be removed. Only one case of germ cell neoplasia in situ (GCNIS) is known [34].

Another, not less important question is what attitude to take towards the contralateral testicle. Loss of a solitary testicle by torsion leads to the catastrophic situation of anorchia. Even though there is no scientific evidence on the need for orchidopexy, most surgeons favour fixation of the contralateral solitary testicle [35].

11.5   Impact of Spermatic Cord Torsion on Testicular Function

Although in the past it was considered that patients with a history of testicular torsion who underwent detorsion or orchiectomy presented alterations, such as low sperm count, in their semen analysis and the number of sperm abnormalities was higher in patients who underwent detorsion [36], more recent studies show no statistical differences with the control population. Hormone function (FSH, LH, Testosterone, and inhibin B) is not affected in the majority of patients after testicular torsion [37]. However, patients with a history of preterm birth do show

subtle alterations such as slightly elevated FSH, low inhibin B, and low inhibin B/FSH ratio [38].

Variations in paternity rates are more closely related to age at torsion. The partner's pregnancy rates are higher in patients with torsion in childhood and slightly lower in patients with torsion in puberty. Adult patients have the worst outcomes [39, 40]. No differences in paternity rates have been observed between the partners of patients who underwent orchiectomy and those whose partners underwent surgical detorsion and orchiopexy [41].

The fact that paternity is preserved does not contradict the fact that torsion has deleterious effects on both the viable detorsioned testis and the contralateral testis. Damage to the torsioned testis is the result of both the ischaemia and the oxidative stress to which it is subjected after detorsion. At detorsion the oxygen-rich blood causes the formation of reactive oxygen species (ROS) in the parenchyma. ROS damages DNA and causes germ cell apoptosis. Three hypotheses have been proposed for the damage to the contralateral testis [42]: (a) reperfusion damage produces contralateral reflectory sympathetic mediated vasoconstriction and consequent hypoxia; (b) twisting of the spermatic cord produces an alteration of the blood-testicular barrier, triggering an immunological process leading to the production of anti-sperm antibodies that would be responsible for the decrease in sperm concentrations and decreased motility; and c) the contralateral testis is a carrier of congenital lesions.

References

1. Ringdahl E, Teague L. Testicular torsion. Am Fam Physician. 2006;74:1739–43.
2. Bokhari A, Aldarwish H, Alharbi T, Alrashidi Y, Alharbi A, Alsulami L. Bilateral testicular torsion: a systematic review of case reports. Cureus. 2023;15(5):e38861.
3. Burgher SW. Acute scrotal pain. Emerg Med Clin North Am. 1998;16:781–809.
4. Sharp VJ, Kieran K, Arlen AM. Testicular torsion: diagnosis, evaluation, and management. Am Fam Physician. 2013;88:835–40.
5. Ahmed SJ, Kaplan GW, DeCambre ME. Perinatal testicular torsion: preoperative radiological findings and the argument for urgent surgical exploration. J Pediatr Surg. 2008;43:1563–5.
6. Fu T, Li Q, Zhai H, Pu S, Wang H, Liang Y, Qiu Z, Chen L. Testicular torsion in neonates. Minerva Pediatr (Torino). 2023;75:432–3.
7. Gerbo M, Crigger C, Samadi Y, Ost MC, Al-Omar O. Prenatally diagnosed testicular torsion: a rare condition that causes dilemma in management. Case Rep Pediatr. 2021;2021:8825763.
8. Erlich T, Ghazzaoui AE, Pokarowski M, O'Kelly F, Lorenzo AJ, Bagli DJ, Koyle MA. Perinatal testicular torsion: the clear cut, the controversial, and the "quiet" scenarios. J Pediatr Surg. 2021;S0022–3468(21):00683–7.
9. Zetawi M, Altawil W, Ashour M, Abughali M, Ghousheh A. Familial testicular torsion in siblings of different age groups: a case report. Urol Case Rep. 2023;48:102408.
10. Melani AL, Faruk M, Palinrungi MA. Torsion in a right undescended testis: a case report. Urol Case Rep. 2023;50:102480.
11. Castañeda-Sánchez I, Tully B, Shipman M, Hoeft A, Hamby T, Palmer BW. Testicular torsion: a retrospective investigation of predictors of surgical outcomes and of remaining controversies. J Pediatr Urol. 2017;13(5):516.e1–4.
12. Haynes BE, Bessen HA, Haynes VE. The diagnosis of testicular torsion. JAMA. 1983;249:2522–7.
13. Lorenzo L, Martínez-Cuenca E, Broseta E. Bilateral testicular torsion in an adolescent: a case with challenging diagnosis. Int Braz J Urol. 2018;44:393–6.
14. Taheem MK, Ziada M, Arumugam V, Lamond Z, Almpanis S. Bilateral synchronous intravaginal testicular torsion presenting with unilateral testicular pain. J Surg Case Rep. 2022;2022(1):rjab586.
15. Smith T, Gross CL, Ryan M, Hwang CW. A rare case of bilateral testicular torsion in a 57-year-old man. J Am Coll Emerg Physicians Open. 2021;2(5):e12545.
16. Michail A, Ioanna G, Euaggelia S, Ioannis T, Christina P, Ioannis P. New insights about prognosis of spermatic cord torsion. Urologia. 2023;90:559–62.
17. Howe AS, Vasudevan V, Kongnyuy M, Rychik K, Thomas LA, Matuskova M, Friedman SC, Gitlin JS, Reda EF, Palmer LS. Degree of twisting and duration of symptoms are prognostic factors of testis salvage during episodes of testicular torsion. Transl Androl Urol. 2017;6:1159–66.
18. Mikuz G. Testicular torsion: simple grading for histological evaluation of tissue damage. Appl Pathol. 1985;3:134–9.
19. Nistal M, Paniagua R, Regadera J, Santamaria L. Obstruction of the tubuli recti and ductuli efferentes by dilated veins in the testes of men with varicocele and its possible role in causing atrophy of the seminiferous tubules. Int J Androl. 1984;7:309–23.
20. Nistal M, Martínez C, Paniagua R. Primary testicular lesions in the twisted testis. Fertil Steril. 1992;57:381–6.
21. Nistal M, Paniagua R, González-Peramato P, Reyes-Múgica M. Perspectives in pediatric pathology, chapter 14. Natural history of undescended testes. Pediatr Dev Pathol. 2016;19:183–201.
22. Nistal M, Paniagua R, Regadera J, Queizan A. Hyperplasia of spermatic cord nerves: a sign of testicular absence. Urology. 1987;29:411–5.
23. Nistal M, Paniagua R. Leydig cell differentiation induced by stimulation with HCG and HMG in two patients affected with hypogonadotropic hypogonadism. Andrologia. 1979;11:211–22.
24. Prince FP. Ultrastructural evidence of indirect and direct autonomic innervation of human Leydig cells: comparison of neonatal, childhood and pubertal ages. Cell Tissue Res. 1992;269:383–90.
25. Nistal M, Paniagua R, Abaurrea MA. Varicose axons bearing "synaptic" vesicles on the basal lamina of the human seminiferous tubules. Cell Tissue Res. 1982;226:75–82.
26. Gong YG, Feng MM, Hu XN, Wang YQ, Gu M, Zhang W, Ge RS. Peptidergic not monoaminergic fibers profusely innervate the young adult human testis. J Anat. 2009;214:330–8.
27. Vikraman J, Hutson JM, Li R, Thorup J. The undescended testis: clinical management and scientific advances. Semin Pediatr Surg. 2016;25:241–8.
28. Merry C, Sweeney B, Puri P. The vanishing testis: anatomical and histological findings. Eur Urol. 1997;31:65–7.
29. Cendron M, Schned AR, Ellsworth PI. Histological evaluation of the testicular nubbin in the vanishing testis syndrome. J Urol. 1998;160(3 Pt 2):1161–2.
30. Hegarty PK, Mushtaq I, Sebire NJ. Natural history of testicular regression syndrome and consequences for clinical management. J Pediatr Urol. 2007;3:206–8.

31. Antic T, Hyjek EM, Taxy JB. The vanishing testis: a histomorphologic and clinical assessment. Am J Clin Pathol. 2011;136:872–80.

32. Woodford E, Eliezer D, Deshpande A, Kumar R. Is excision of testicular nubbin necessary in vanishing testis syndrome? J Pediatr Surg. 2018;53:2495–7.

33. Gao L, Tang D, Gu W. Histopathological features of vanishing testes in 332 boys: what is its significance? A retrospective study from a tertiary hospital. Front Pediatr. 2022;10:834083.

34. Nataraja RM, Yeap E, Healy CJ, Nandhra IS, Murphy FL, Hutson JM, Kimber C. Presence of viable germ cells in testicular regression syndrome remnants: is routine excision indicated? A systematic review. Pediatr Surg Int. 2018;34:353–61.

35. Babu R, Miglani HS, Shah RS. Is routine excision of dysplastic testicular remnants/nubbins associated with nonpalpable testis necessary? Is routine fixation of contralateral solitary testis indicated? A survey on the prevalent practice among Indian pediatric surgeons. J Indian Assoc Pediatr Surg. 2022;27:723–7.

36. Turner TT, Brown KJ. Spermatic cord torsion: loss of spermatogenesis despite return of blood flow. Biol Reprod. 1993;49:401–7.

37. Arap MA, Vicentini FC, Cocuzza M, Hallak J, Athayde K, Lucon AM, Arap S, Srougi M. Late hormonal levels, semen parameters, and presence of antisperm antibodies in patients treated for testicular torsion. J Androl. 2007;28:528–32.

38. Hansen AH, Priskorn L, Hansen LS, Carlsen E, Joensen UN, Jacobsen FM, Jensen CFS, Jørgensen N. Testicular torsion and subsequent testicular function in young men from the general population. Hum Reprod. 2023;38:216–24.

39. Zhang X, Zhang J, Cai Z, Wang X, Lu W, Li H. Effect of unilateral testicular torsion at different ages on male fertility. J Int Med Res. 2020;48(4):300060520918792.

40. Almekaty K, Zahran MH, Eid A, Ralph D, Rashed A. Azoospermia and sperm retrieval in post-pubertal testicular torsion: benefits and limitations. Urology. 2023;171:121–6.

41. Mäkelä EP, Roine RP, Taskinen S. Paternity, erectile function, and health-related quality of life in patients operated for pediatric testicular torsion. J Pediatr Urol. 2020;16:44.e1–4.

42. Jacobsen FM, Rudlang TM, Fode M, Østergren PB, Sønksen J, Ohl DA, Jensen CFS, CopMich Collaborative. The impact of testicular torsion on testicular function. World J Mens Health. 2020;38:298–307.

12.1 Spermatic Cord Lipomembranous Fat Necrosis

Lipomembranous fat necrosis is a form of fat necrosis characterized by the presence of eosinophilic, crenulated, and/or serpiginous membranes constituting cystic formations of different sizes. It has been described as affecting the bone marrow under different names such as membranous reticulin dysplasia of bones [1], lipomembranous dystrophy [2, 3], and lipomembranous polycystic osteodysplasia [4, 5], for which the name Jarvi-Hakola-Nasu disease has been proposed. It is an autosomal recessive disorder caused by loss-of-function variants in TYROBP/DAP12 or TREM2 [6, 7]. Lipomembranous fat necrosis was initially considered pathognomonic for this disease.

Similar images of lipomembranous fat necrosis have been described in a variety of tissues in patients without hereditary disease and have recently been reviewed by Matsukuma et al. [8]. *These images have been found in/In* lower limbs with impaired blood flow (arteriosclerotic obliterans, thromboangiitis obliterans, progressive systemic sclerosis); *and conditions of* venous insufficiency (varicose veins, thrombophlebitis, stasis dermatitis, panniculitis, lipogranulomas, erythema nodosum, erythema induratum, necrobiosis lipoidica, scleroderma, lupus, vasculitis, diabetes mellitus, and sarcoidosis). *This fat necrosis* has also been observed in some breast tumours, epiploic appendix, intra-articular free bodies, heart valves, and tumours (lipomas, mature cystic teratomas). Lipomembranous fat necrosis is associated with lesions related to ischaemic conditions, venous insufficiency, or malnourishment, although no history has been recognized in 16% of patients [9–12]. The clinical picture varies according to the associated pathology [13].

Lipomembranous fat necrosis of the spermatic cord has been described in pubertal patients with a history of testicular torsion [14]. Macroscopically, it is a hard, yellowish lesion located at the level of the epididymis and first part of the spermatic cord associated with an atrophic, necrotic or fibrotic testicle, which has retracted to the superficial inguinal orifice (Fig. 12.1).

The histological appearance varies according to the age of the torsion. In the first few weeks, there is predominantly peripherally poorly demarcated fat necrosis with numerous cavities. The interior of the cavities is occupied by a honeycomb structure. The walls of this honeycomb are corrugated, hyaline, refringent membranes with a crenulated inner surface. The interior of the cavities is optically empty. Some have yellowish colouration, probably due to some deposition of non-ferric haemoglobin pigments. Peripherally there is an infiltrate between the cavities with abundant macrophages, some lymphocytes, and thrombosed venous vessels. In

Fig. 12.1 Lipomembranous fat necrosis of the spermatic cord. Cross section of a 39-year-old patient with a history of untreated left testicular torsion. Cross section of the testicle with grade III lesions. Thickening of the paratesticular tissues in which only the deferens is recognizable

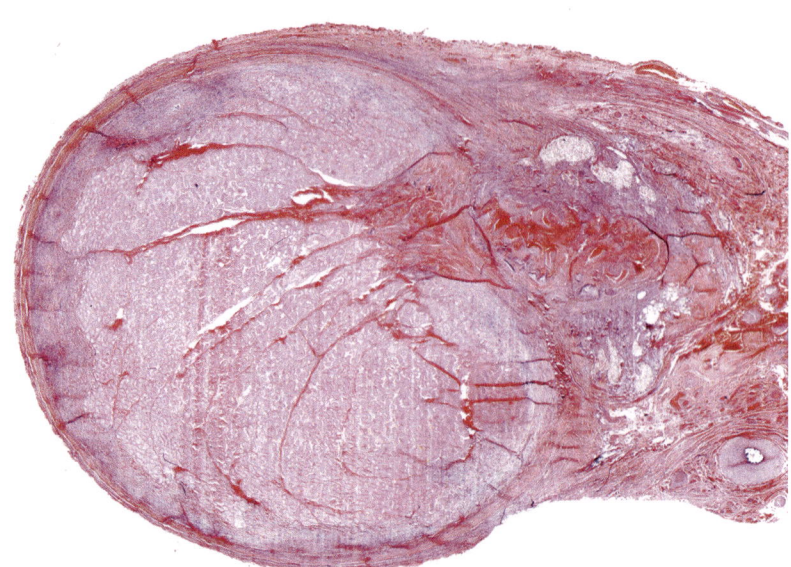

Fig. 12.2 Lipomembranous fat necrosis of the spermatic cord. Two groups of membranes separated by dense connective tissue. The membranes are arranged parallel to each other delimiting optically empty spaces

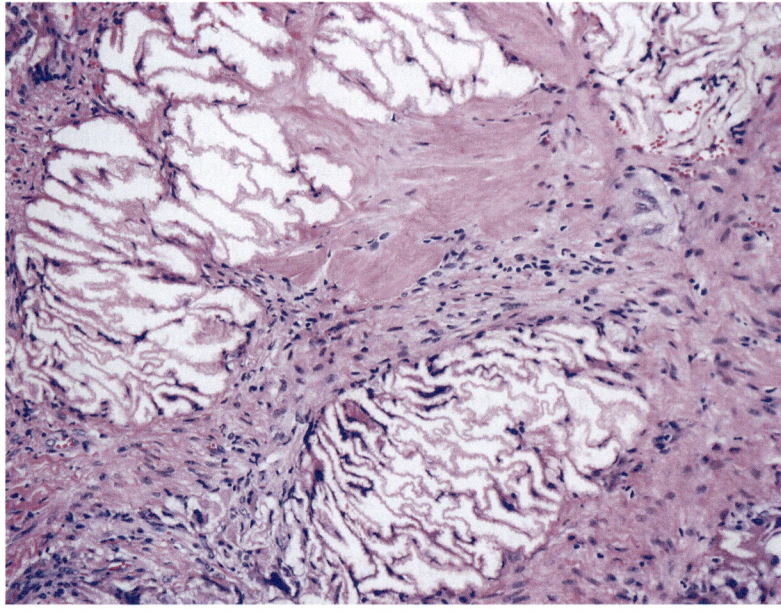

older lesions, there is fracturing of the membranes and intense phagocytosis by multinucleated giant cells (Figs. 12.2, 12.3 and 12.4).

Histochemically, the membranes are strongly PAS positive (before and after digestion with diastase) and stain red with Masson's trichrome. They also stain with orcein, sudan black, oil red O, acid phosphotungstic haematoxylin, and luxol fast blue [15–17] (Figs. 12.5 and 12.6). Unstained samples show yellowish green autofluorescence when observed with fluorescence microscopy [18]. These observations suggest that they are mainly composed of ceroid materials [19]. Immunohistochemically, they are positive for CD68 and lysozyme and negative for S100, CD34 protein, and factor XIIIa [20]. Ultrastructurally, they are composed of minute tubule-like and vesicle-like structures [21].

Fig. 12.3 Lipomembranous fat necrosis of the spermatic cord. The membranes are acellular. The profiles often show a crenellated appearance

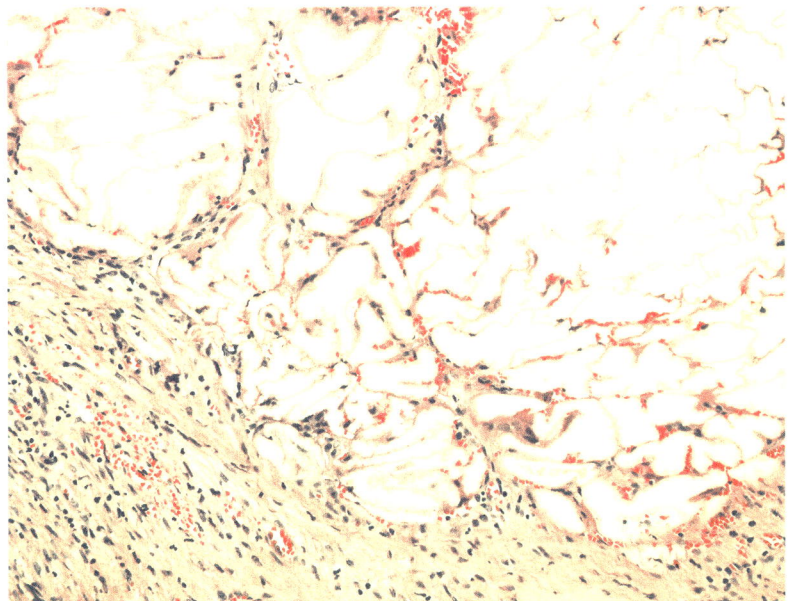

Fig. 12.4 Lipomembranous fat necrosis of the spermatic cord. Macrophages and multinucleated giant cells are phagocytosing refringent membrane debris

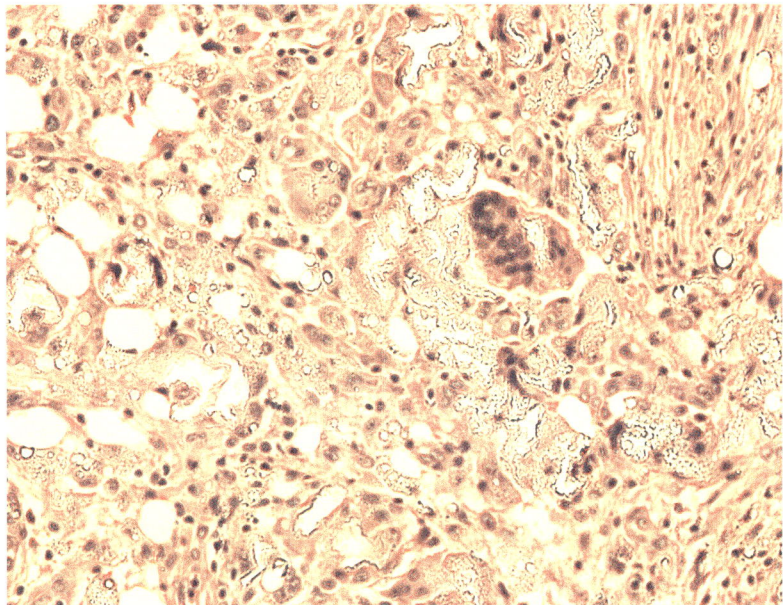

The lesion generally does not lend itself to differential diagnosis with other forms of fat necrosis (enzymatic fat necrosis, coagulation-like necrosis, lipogranuloma type fat necrosis). In late lesions of spermatic cord lipomembranous fat necrosis, the membranes may be suggestive of parasite cuticles, a granulomatous reaction to a ruptured testicular prosthesis or a sclerosing lipogranuloma. The parasites most frequently affect-

ing the urogenital tract are filariae and schistosomes. Both provoke an inflammatory reaction with numerous giant cells that surround the eggs or material derived from dead worms. Information on the patient's nationality and the presence of perivesical, prostatic, or spermatic cord calcifications can facilitate diagnosis. Rupture of a testicular prosthesis leads to the formation of differently-sized cysts and a granulo-

Fig. 12.5 Lipomembranous fat necrosis of the spermatic cord. All membranes show strong positivity to orcein

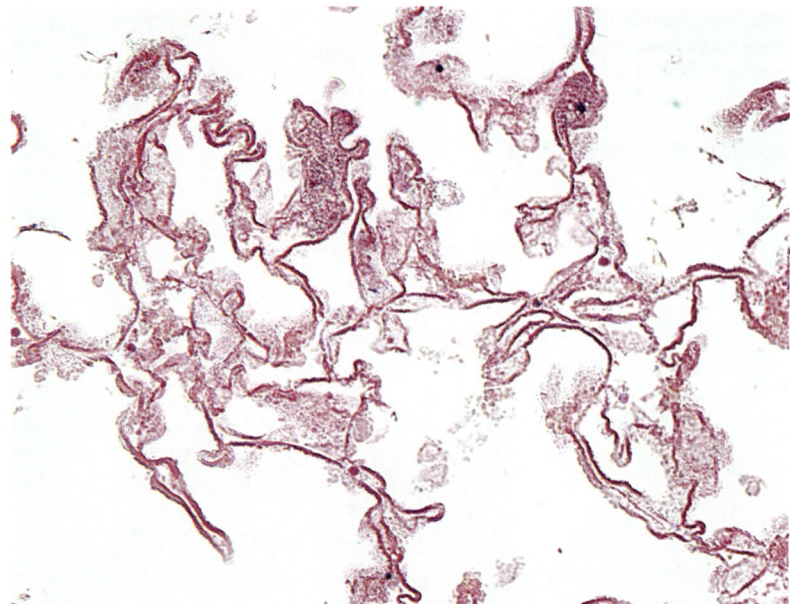

Fig. 12.6 Lipomembranous fat necrosis of the spermatic cord. Glandular, spiculated surface appearance of the membranous formations stained with Sudan black

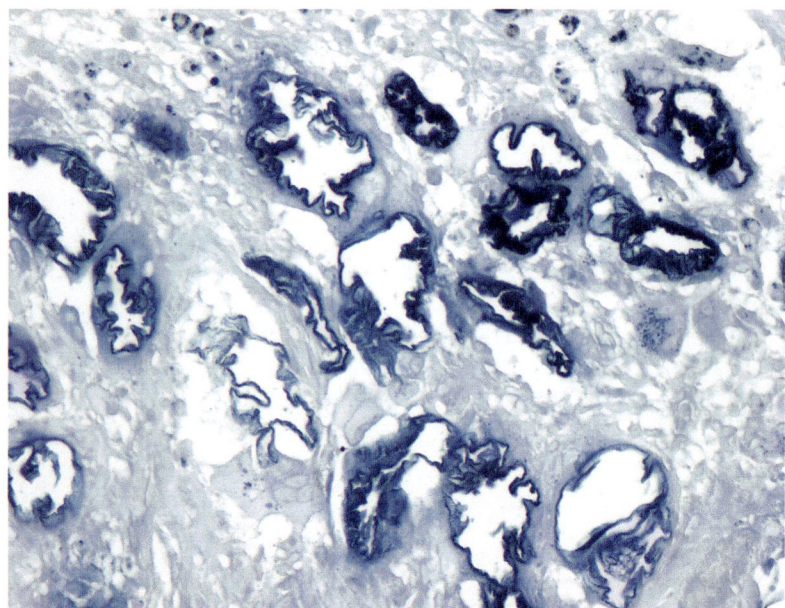

matous foreign body reaction on a refractory material. The absence of crenulated membranes and the clinical history are decisive for diagnosis. Sclerosing lipogranulomas mainly affect the scrotum but rarely the spermatic cord [22]. They consist of a rich infiltrate of foreign body giant cells together with lymphocytes and polynuclear neutrophils and eosinophils. The lesion is surrounded by a significant fibroblastic reaction.

12.2 Pseudosarcomatous Periorchitis Secondary to Testicular Torsion

In unresolved testicular torsion, the testicle atrophies, retracts, and acquires a hard consistency. A histological finding in these surgical specimens is the presence of a myofibroblastic proliferation, which, if not recognizable, may raise interesting differential diagnoses. These pseudosarcomatous changes are like those observed in other locations and are considered secondary to necrosis of the surrounding structure [23–25].

Pseudosarcomatous changes secondary to torsion are characterized by the following: (a) They are a pleomorphic lesion ranging from a xanthogranulomatous pattern to a myofibroblastic lesion depending on the time past since the ischaemic event. (b) The lesion is organized in concentric layers, with the outer part being the most fibrous (Figs. 12.7 and 12.8). In the most recent lesions, or those in contact with the necrotic remains of seminiferous tubules, there are abundant macrophages with large cytoplasm, sometimes with xanthomized cytoplasm and sometimes with eosinophilic and granular cytoplasm. The histiocytes are CD68 positive and S100 negative. Among these cells, there are lymphocytes and polynuclear and multinucleated giant cells with abundant yellowish pigment in their cytoplasm. The lesion is very similar to xanthogranulomatous lesions with different aetiologies described in other organs. On the outermost part, especially in the older lesions, there is a pro-liferation of spindle cells with marked pleomorphism and abundant mitoses presenting a storiform pattern (Figs. 12.9, 12.10, 12.11 and 12.12). Some red blood cells can be observed among the cells. This lesion may also contain lymphocytes and plasma cells. The spindle cells are vimentin positive and focally positive for smooth muscle actin and negative for S100.

The differential diagnosis, if the lesion is not studied as a whole, may consider a simple xanthogranulomatous reaction, a malignant fibrous histiocytoma or an inflammatory myofibroblastic tumour. In cases dominated by histiocytes with a clear, foamy cytoplasm due to high lipid richness, and intermingled with multinucleated giant cells and other inflammatory cells, the lesion is like xanthogranulomatous orchioepididymitis [26]. When histiocytes with large, eosinophilic, and granular cytoplasm predominate, malakoplakia must be ruled out, and this is not difficult given the absence of Michaelis-Gutmann body cells in this pseudosarcomatous reaction. If the proliferation shows a high number of mitoses and a storiform pattern, histologically it bears a strong resemblance to malignant fibrous histiocytoma [27, 28]. The macroscopic lack of tumour, the

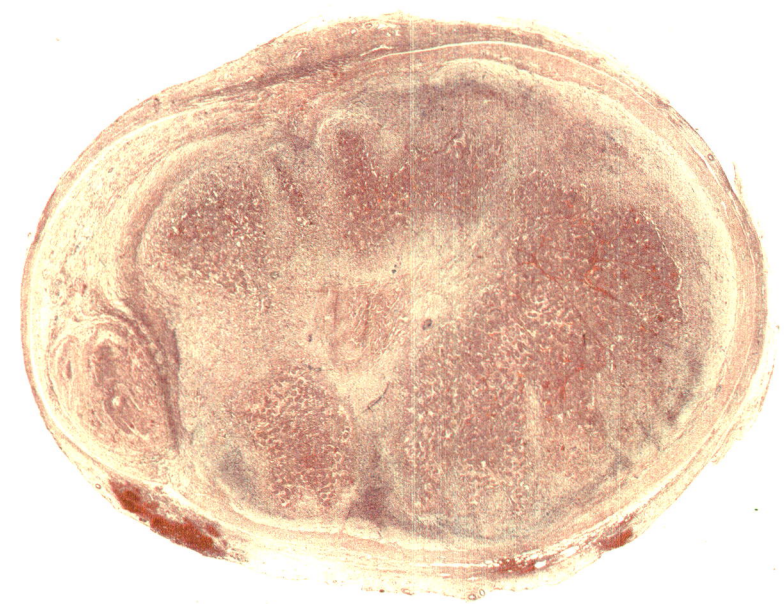

Fig. 12.7 Pseudosarcomatous periorchitis secondary to testicular torsion. Frontal section of a testicle with 2 weeks' torsion. Several nodular formations of different sizes are incompletely separated by thick septa

Fig. 12.8 Pseudosarcomatous periorchitis secondary to testicular torsion. The outlines of the necrotic seminiferous tubules are still recognizable in the centre of the nodular formations. In continuity with a very thickened albuginea, a thick band of very cellular tissue extends into the necrotic parenchyma

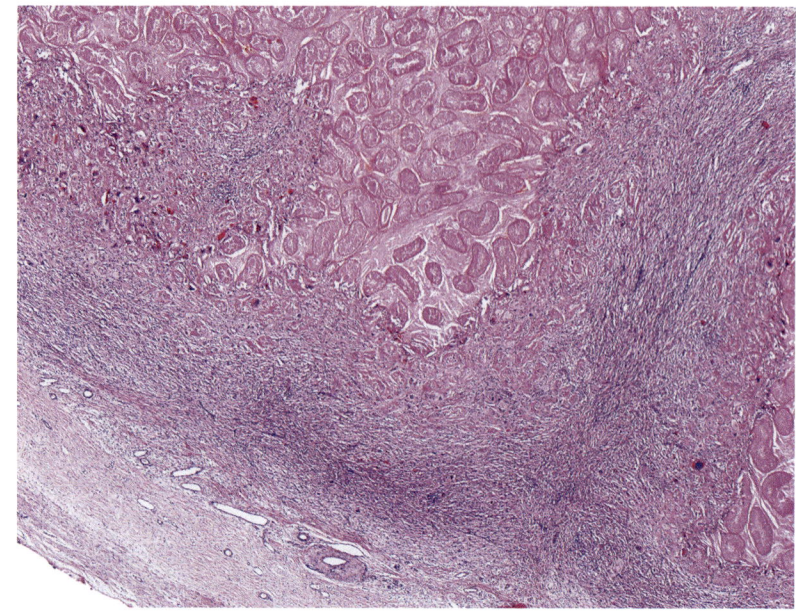

Fig. 12.9 Pseudosarcomatous periorchitis secondary to testicular torsion. Note the proliferation of spindle-shaped cells including some lymphocytes and macrophages with haematic pigment

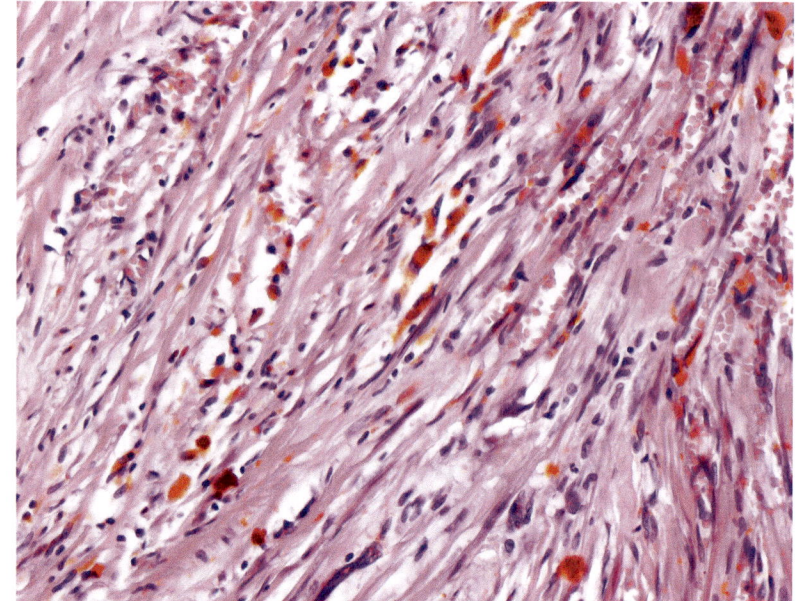

zonal architecture of the lesion, the absence of atypical mitoses, together with the assessment of the clinical data can rule out the diagnosis of a malignant fibrous histiocytoma.

Regarding the differential diagnosis with inflammatory myofibroblastic tumour, it would only be considered in cases in which the xanthomized histiocytic cell component is miss-

Fig. 12.10 Pseudosarcomatous periorchitis
secondary to testicular
torsion. The morphology
of the cells varies from
one area to another.
Cells with a spherical or
slightly oval nucleus
with prominent
nucleolus and pale
cytoplasm predominate.
Some have mitoses,
others haematic material

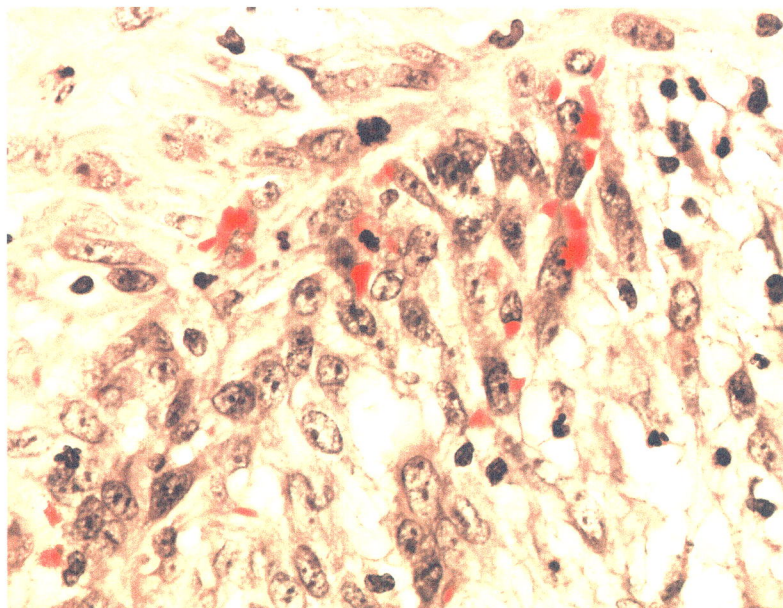

Fig. 12.11 Pseudosarcomatous periorchitis
secondary to testicular
torsion. A compact
proliferation of
fibroblastic spindle cells
with moderate aniso-
karyosis in a patient
with a history of
longstanding torsion

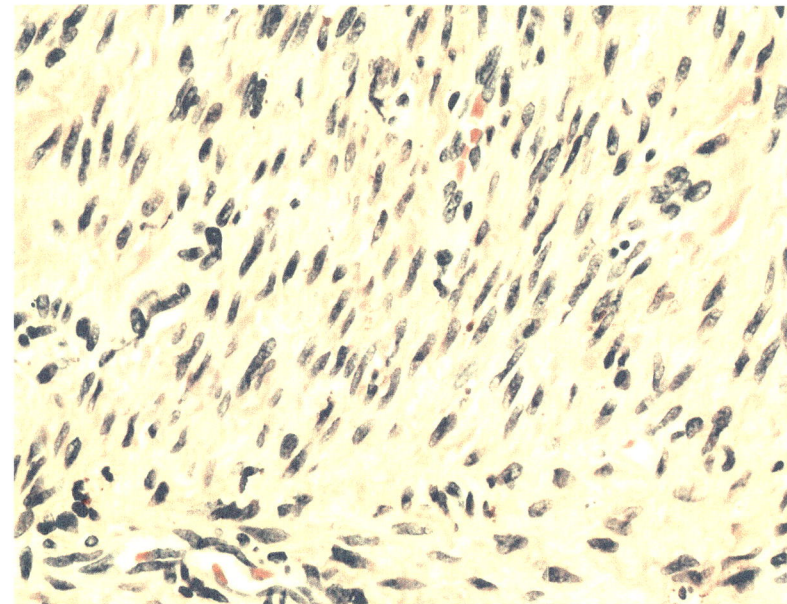

ing, and other findings of testicular torsions
such as foci of lipomembranous fat necrosis or
macrophages with remnants of haematic pigment or dystrophic calcifications were not
observed. It is noteworthy that the spindle or
stellate cells of this tumour, consisting of a
proliferation of myofibroblasts and inflammatory cells, express, in addition to actin and desmin, anaplastic lymphoma kinase (ALK) in
50% of cases [29].

Fig. 12.12 Pseudosarcomatous periorchitis secondary to testicular torsion. The visible remnants of membranous formations indicate the reactive nature of the fibroblastic proliferation

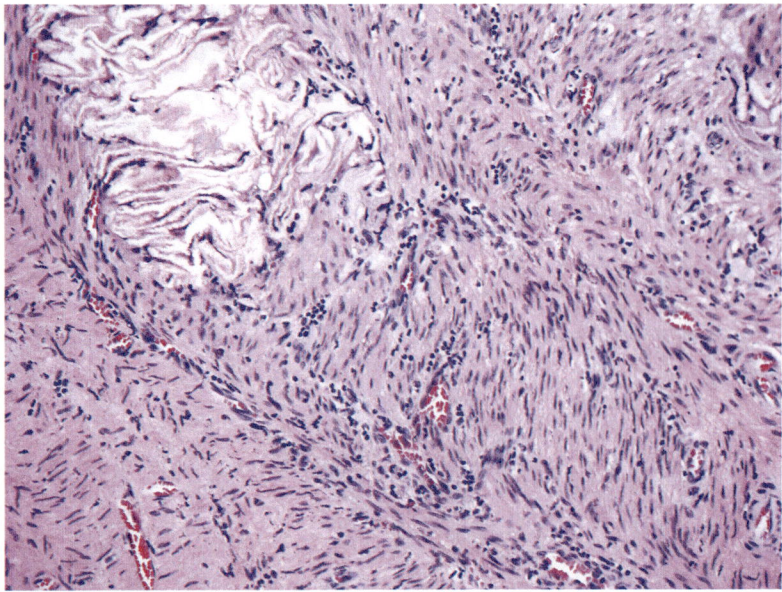

12.3 Lymphoma-Like Orchitis Secondary to Transient Testicular Torsion

The term lymphoma-like orchitis is proposed for a testicular lesion reminiscent of both tumoural (leukaemic infiltration or lymphoma) and non-tumoural lesions (testicular pseudolymphoma, idiopathic granulomatous orchitis, and certain non-specific orchitis). It is observed in some patients with a history of intermittent testicular torsion or in patients who have undergone detorsion but whose parenchyma did not recover, and in whom, due to testicular enlargement and pain, an orchiectomy has been performed [30].

The testicles show an increase in size and consistency suggestive of a tumour. The surface shows purplish areas next to other normal areas. In section, haemorrhagic areas alternate with others of normal appearance. The haemorrhages are preferentially located under the albuginea, where very congestive vessels are also observed (Figs. 12.13 and 12.14). Histologically, although the lesion is diffuse, it is markedly accentuated in some lobules. There is a dense lymphoid infiltrate that does not form a tumour mass and widely separates the seminiferous tubules. This infiltrate

consists mainly of small round cells, mostly T lymphocytes. These cells infiltrate and form intramural accumulations in the vein walls and, to a lesser extent, the walls of the seminiferous tubules (Figs. 12.15 and 12.16). In more advanced lesions, B lymphocytes and macrophages are seen. The B lymphocytes are scarce and isolated, both in the interstitium and among the remaining cells of the seminiferous epithelium. Macrophages are more abundant, especially in the wall of the most affected tubules, where they form aggregates that protrude into the tubule (Fig. 12.17). Isolated CD68-positive multinucleated giant cells are seen in some tubules (Fig. 12.18). No plasma cells are seen in the lymphoid infiltrates. In the less affected tubules, the lymphocytic infiltrates are located only in the interstitium and the seminiferous epithelium shows complete spermatogenesis. There is only a slight dilatation of the lumen in these tubules. The epididymis and spermatic cord show only congestive vessels.

Histologically, this lesion may suggest differential diagnosis with lymphomas and leukaemic infiltrates and orchitis with lymphocyte-rich infiltrates (chronic non-specific orchitis, testicular pseudolymphoma, and primary autoimmune orchitis).

Fig. 12.13 Lymphoma-like orchitis secondary to transient testicular torsion. The intense lymphoid infiltrates preferentially affect one testicular lobule. The seminiferous tubules of the less affected lobule are ectasic

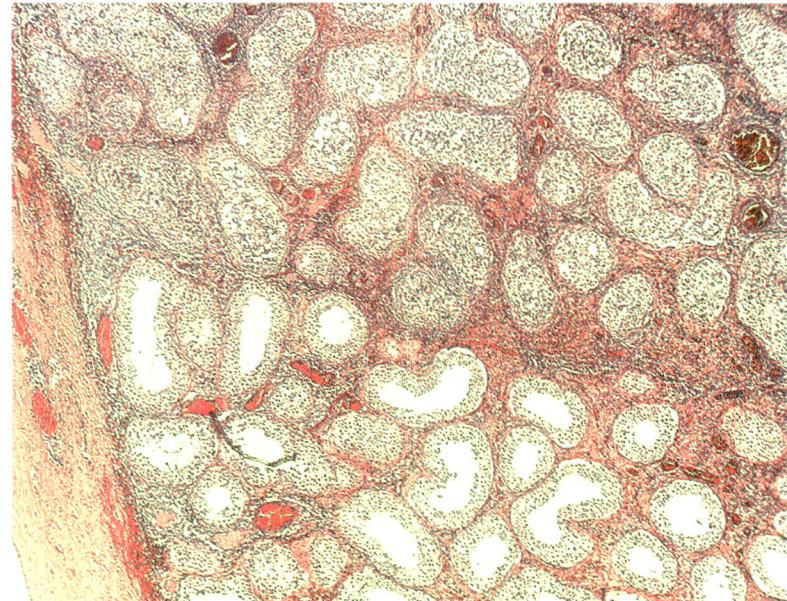

Fig. 12.14 Lymphoma-like orchitis secondary to transient testicular torsion. Observe the dense intertubular lymphoid infiltrates in sheets suggesting a leukaemic infiltrate or lymphoma

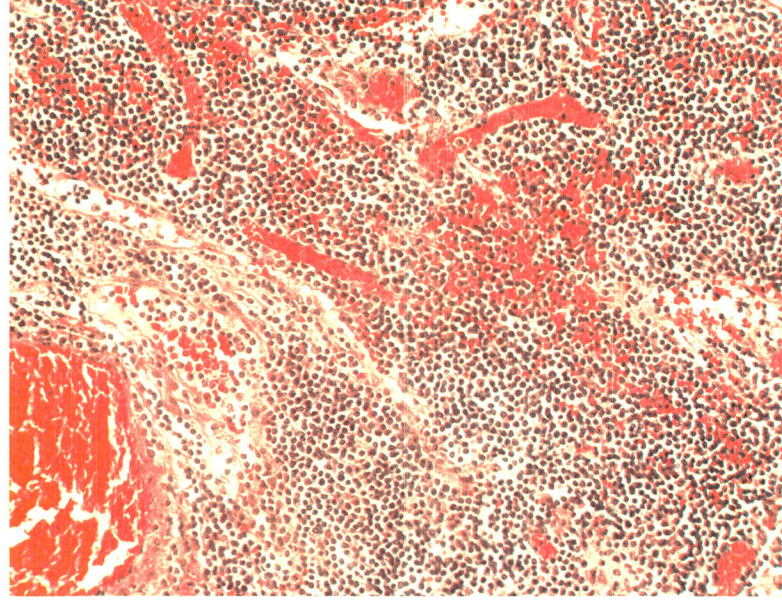

Lymphoma-like orchitis secondary to a transient testicular torsion share with testicular lymphomas and leukaemias the fact that their infiltrates consist of a preferentially T-lymphocyte population, and the manner in which they infiltrate the interstitium and vessel wall. The most important clinical differences lie in age - primary testicular lymphomas are characteristic of elderly males- and the type of lymphoma, as the most frequent testicular lymphomas (80–90%) are of the diffuse large B-cell type [31–33]. T-lymphomas in the testis are very rare [34–37]. The presence of clusters of macrophages in the wall of some tubules and even giant cells within those tubules is more suggestive of a reactive lesion than a lymphoma.

Fig. 12.15 Lymphoma-like orchitis secondary to transient testicular torsion. The wall of the intraparenchymal vein is infiltrated by lymphoid cells. The infiltrates also extend to the wall of a seminiferous tubule

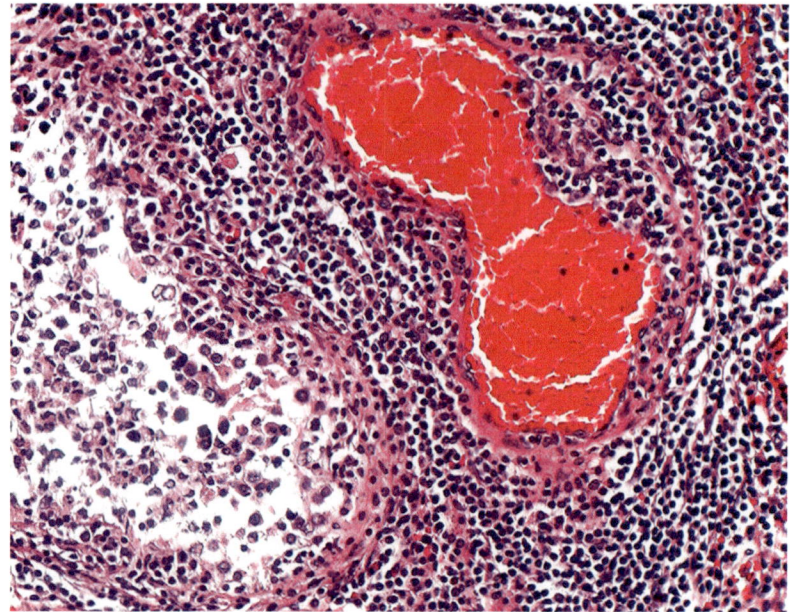

Fig. 12.16 Lymphoma-like orchitis secondary to transient testicular torsion. Most of the lymphoid cells in the intertubular interstitium are T lymphocytes (CD3 immunostaining)

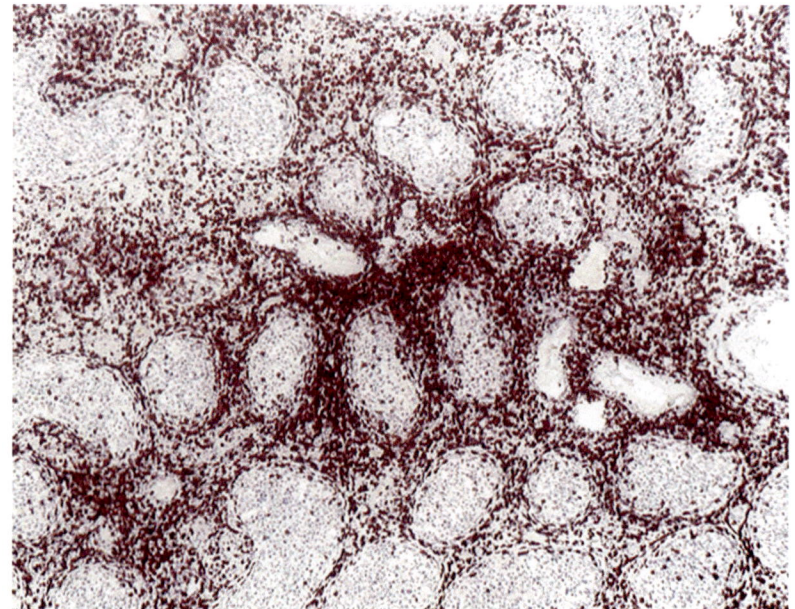

In chronic non-specific orchitis, the seminiferous tubules appear atrophic and the markedly fibrous interstitium is marked by polymorphous infiltrates with plasma cells, macrophages and lymphocytes. In some cases, the lesion is reminiscent of idiopathic granulomatous interstitial orchitis. The term lymphocytic orchitis has been used in these cases to emphasize the exuberance of the inflammatory infiltrates, which may even form lymphoid follicles [38].

Testicular pseudolymphoma is a reactive lesion that has been described in non-lymphoid organs such as the gastrointestinal tract, lung, breast, skin, spleen, kidney, and testis. It simulates a tumour and more specifically, a lymphoma. It is characterized by the presence of an

Fig. 12.17 Lymphoma-like orchitis secondary to transient testicular torsion. Isolated B lymphocytes are present preferentially in the interstitium and wall of the seminiferous tubules (CD20 immunostaining)

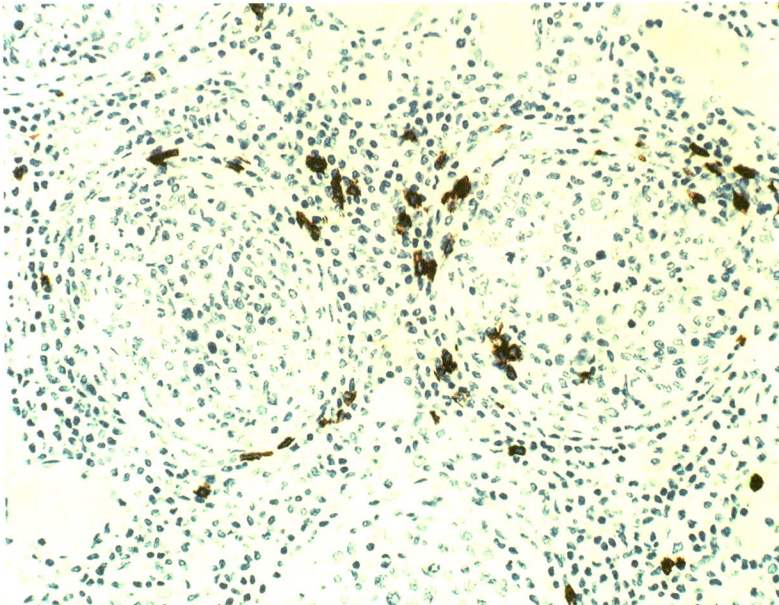

Fig. 12.18 Lymphoma-like orchitis secondary to transient testicular torsion. Clusters of macrophages located in the tubular wall protrude into the seminiferous tubules (immunostaining with CD68)

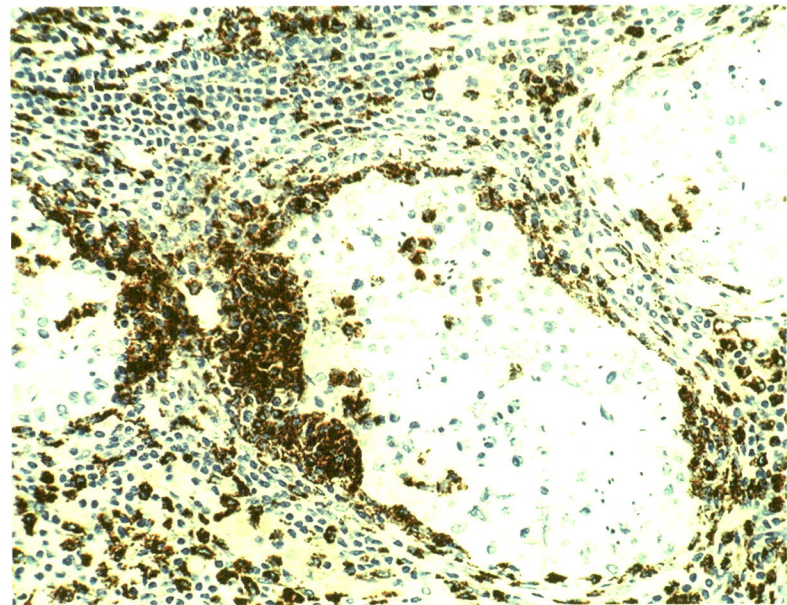

infiltrate made up of abundant mature lymphocytes of polyclonal type and plasma cells that partially or completely destroy the testicular parenchyma. It has been reported in some cases associated with epididymitis and/or orchitis [39, 40].

The lymphoma-like orchitis lesion does not fit the histological patterns of the most frequent bacterial or viral orchitis (mumps, HIV, ZIKV), and it shows some characteristics that could relate it to an initial stage in the development of an autoimmune orchitis [41]. A history of several short-lived testicular torsions, which resolve spontaneously, may lead to ischaemic lesions of the testicle. Moreover, 30–61% of cases are a precursor to testicular torsion [42]. Ischaemia causes a reaction that affects all the testicular structures involved in maintaining the delicate balance that governs testicular immune privilege. The infiltrate consisting almost exclusively of T lymphocytes, an interstitial cell otherwise normally present in small numbers, would be the tip of the iceberg of the changes occurring in the blood-testicular barrier, with infiltration by endothelial cells, myoid cells, Leydig cells, germ cells and macrophages [43]. Although there are no data on the evolution of lymphoma-like orchitis testes, if left untreated, it is likely that the immune process would lead towards idiopathic granulomatous orchitis. In this regard, although the interstitial infiltrate lacks plasma cells, multinucleated giant cells with a histiocytic nature have already been identified within the most atrophic tubules [44].

References

1. Järvi OH, Lauttamus LL, Solonen KA. Membranous reticulin dysplasia of bone. Probably a new disease entity. In: Proceedings of the 14th Scandinavian Congress of Pathology and Microbiology. Universitetsforlaget, Oslo; 1964. p. 51.
2. Nasu T, Tsukahara Y, Terayama K, Mamiya N. An autopsy case of "membranous lipodystrophy" with myeloosteopathy of long bones and leucodystrophy of the brain (in Japanese). Tokyobyourisyuudankaikiroku; 1970. p. 10–13.2.
3. Nasu T. Tsukahara Y Terayama K: a lipid metabolic disease-'membranous lipodystrophy'-an autopsy case demonstrating numerous peculiar membrane-structures composed of compound lipid in bone and bone marrow and various adipose tissues. Acta Pathol Jpn. 1973;23:539–58.
4. Hakola HPA, Järvi OH, Sourander P. Osteodysplasia polycystica hereditaria combined with sclerosing leucoencephalopathy. Acta Neurol Scand Suppl. 1970;43:79–80.
5. Hakola HP, Partanen VS. Neurophysiological findings in the hereditary presenile dementia characterized by polycystic lipomembranous osteodysplasia and sclerosing leukoencephalopathy. J Neurol Neurosurg Psychiatry. 1983;46:515–20.
6. Paloneva J, Manninen T, Christman G, Hovanes K, Mandelin J, Adolfsson R, Bianchin M, Bird T, Miranda R, Salmaggi A, et al. Mutations in two genes encoding different subunits of a receptor signaling complex result in an incidental disease phenotype. Am J Hum Genet. 2002;71:656–62.
7. Errichiello E, Dardiotis E, Mannino F, Paloneva J, Mattina T, Zuffardi O. Phenotypic expansion in Nasu-Hakola disease: immunological findings in three patients and proposal of a unifying pathogenetic hypothesis. Front Immunol. 2019;10:1685.
8. Matsukuma S, Matsunaga A, Takahashi O, Ogata S. Lipomembranous fat necrosis: a distinctive and unique morphology (review). Exp Ther Med. 2022;24:759.
9. Alegre VA, Winkelmann RK, Aliaga A. Lipomembranous changes in chronic panniculitis. J Am Acad Dermatol. 1988;19:39–46.
10. Machinami R. Membranous lipodystrophy-like changes in ischemic necrosis of the legs. Virchows Arch A Pathol Anat Histopathol. 1983;399:191–205.
11. Ramdial PK, Madaree A, Singh B. Membranous fat necrosis in lipomas. Am J Surg Pathol. 1997;21:841–6.
12. Takahashi M, Kawano H, Ishihara T, Uchino F, Takihara H, Baba Y. Membranocystic lesion in sclerosing lipogranuloma of the scrotum: an ultrastructural study. Ultrastruct Pathol. 1992;16:641–9.
13. Snow JL, Su WP. Lipomembranous (membranocystic) fat necrosis. Clinicopathologic correlation of 38 cases. Am J Dermatopathol. 1996;18:151–5.
14. Nistal M, González-Peramato P, Paniagua R. Lipomembranous fat necrosis in three cases of testicular torsion. Histopathology. 2001;38:443–7.
15. Machinami R. Incidence of membranous lipodystrophy-like change among patients with limb necrosis caused by chronic arterial obstruction. Arch Pathol Lab Med. 1984;108:823–6.
16. Segura S, Pujol RM. Lipomembranous fat necrosis of the subcutaneous tissue. Dermatol Clin. 2022;26:509–17.
17. Coyne JD, Parkinson D, Baildam AD. Membranous fat necrosis of the breast. Histopathology. 1996;28:61–4.
18. Ramdial PK, Chetty R. Vasculitis-induced membranous fat necrosis. J Cutan Pathol. 1999;26:405–10.
19. Poppiti RJ Jr, Margulies M, Cabello B, Rywlin AM. Membranous fat necrosis. Am J Surg Pathol. 1986;10:62–9.
20. Diaz-Cascajo C, Borghi S. Subcutaneous pseudo-membranous fat necrosis: new observations. J Cutan Pathol. 2002;29:5–10.
21. Matsukuma S, Takeo H, Kono T, Sato K. Fat cells and membranous fat necrosis of aortic valves: a clinico-pathological study. Pathol Int. 2013;63:345–52.
22. Marzouk E. Spontaneous localized lipogranuloma of the spermatic cord. Ital J Surg Sci. 1989;19:261–4.
23. Kubosawa H, Yano K, Oda K, Shiobara M, Ando K, Nunomura M, Sarashina H. Xanthogranulomatous gastritis with pseudosarcomatous changes. Pathol Int. 2007;57:291–5.
24. Tanaka T, Ueda T, Yokoyama T, Harada S, Hatakeyama K, Yoshimura A. Pseudosarcomatous myofibroblastic proliferation of the appendix with an abdominal abscess due to diverticulum perforation: a case report. Surg Case Rep. 2020;6:144.
25. Bale TA, Benhamida J, Roychoudury S, Villafania L, Wrzolek MA, Bouffard JP, Bapat K, Ladanyi M, Rosenblum MK. Infarction with associated pseudo-sarcomatous changes mimics anaplasia in otherwise grade I meningiomas. Mod Pathol. 2020;33:1298–306.
26. Nistal M, Gonzalez-Peramato P, Serrano A, Regadera J. Xanthogranulomatous funiculitis and orchiepididy-

mitis: report of 2 cases with immunohistochemical study and literature review. Arch Pathol Lab Med. 2004;128:911–4.

27. Nistal M, Regadera J, Jareño E, Paniagua R. Inflammatory malignant fibrous histiocytoma of the spermatic cord. Urol Int. 1988;43:188–92.

28. Xu LW, Yu YL, Li GH. Malignant fibrous histiocytoma of the spermatic cord: case report and literature review. J Int Med Res. 2012;40:816–23.

29. Aydemir H, Budak S, Kahyaoglu Z, Kumsar S. Inflammatory myofibroblastic tumor of the spermatic cord: two cases and review of the literature. Ann Saudi Med. 2020;40:66–71.

30. Nistal M, González-Peramato P, Serrano A. Interpretation of testicular non-granulomatous lymphoid infiltrates. In: Clues in the diagnosis of non-tumoral testicular pathology. Cham: Springer; 2017. p. 229–39.

31. Al-Abbadi MA, Hattab EM, Tarawneh M, Orazi A, Ulbright TM. Primary testicular and paratesticular lymphoma: a retrospective clinicopathologic study of 34 cases with emphasis on differential diagnosis. Arch Pathol Lab Med. 2007;131:1040–60.

32. King RL, Goodlad JR, Calaminici M, Dotlic S, Montes-Moreno S, Oschlies I, Ponzoni M, Traverse-Glehen A, Ott G, Ferry JA. Lymphomas arising in immune-privileged sites: insights into biology, diagnosis, and pathogenesis. Virchows Arch. 2020;476:647–65.

33. Pollari M, Leivonen SK, Leppä S. Testicular diffuse large B-cell lymphoma-clinical, molecular, and immunological features. Cancers (Basel). 2021;13:4049.

34. Liang DN, Yang ZR, Wang WY, et al. Extranodal nasal type natural killer/T-cell lymphoma of testis:

report of seven cases with review of literature. Leuk Lymphoma. 2012;53:1117–23.

35. Haroon S, Ahmed A. Peripheral T-cell lymphoma presenting as testicular mass; a diagnostic challenge. World J Surg Oncol. 2013;11:68.

36. AbdullGaffar B, Seliem RM, AlAmir A. Primary high-grade peripheral T-cell lymphoma of the testis clinically confused with scrotal abscess. Urology. 2019;127:e3–5.

37. Wang Y, Li J, Fang Y. Primary testicular T-lymphoblastic lymphoma in a child: a case report. Medicine (Baltimore). 2020;99(26):e20861.

38. Agarwal V, Li JK, Bard R. Lymphocytic orchitis: a case report. Hum Pathol. 1990;21:1080–2.

39. Algaba F, Mikuz G, Boccon-Gibod L, Trias I, Arce Y, Montironi R, Egevad L, Scarpelli M, Lopez-Beltran A. Pseudoneoplastic lesions of the testis and paratesticular structures. Virchows Arch. 2007;451:987–97.

40. Ganzer R, Burger M, Woenckhaus M, Wieland WF, Blana A. A patient with testicular pseudolymphoma—a rare condition mimicking malignancy: a case report. J Med Case Rep. 2007;1:71.

41. Silva CA, Cocuzza M, Carvalho JF, Bonfá E. Diagnosis and classification of autoimmune orchitis. Autoimmun Rev. 2014;13:431–4.

42. Patoulias D, Farmakis K, Kalogirou M, Patoulias I. Transient testicular torsion: from early diagnosis to appropriate therapeutic intervention (a prospective clinical study). Folia Med Cracov. 2017;57:53–62.

43. Qu N, Ogawa Y, Kuramasu M, Nagahori K, Sakabe K, Itoh M. Immunological microenvironment in the testis. Reprod Med Biol. 2019;19:24–31.

44. Roy S, Hooda S, Parwani AV. Idiopathic granulomatous orchitis. Pathol Res Pract. 2011;207:275–8.

13.1 Clinical Evaluation of Varicocele

Varicocele consists of an abnormal dilatation of the veins of the pampiniform plexus and testicular veins with continuous or intermittent retrograde blood flow in the spermatic veins [1] (Figs. 13.1, 13.2 and 13.3). Rare in childhood (< 1% before the age of 10 years), it is the most common andrological disorder among adolescents and adults [2]. The incidence increases as puberty progresses (8% between 11 and 14 years, 14% between 15 and 19 years). In healthy adults, it varies from 15% [3] to 18% of adults over 40 years of age [4]. Another important point is the high frequency in which a unilateral varicocele can also affect the opposite testis. About 35% to 40% of patients with palpable left-sided varicocele are found to have a contralateral varicocele on Döppler ultrasound examination.

The relationship between varicocele and infertility is well established [5, 6]. If we take a seminogram as a basis, 12% of patients with normal seminal parameters have varicocele, while 25.4% of patients with lower sperm concentration, motility, and abnormal morphology of spermatozoa are carriers of varicocele. Varicocele is present in 40% of patients with primary infertility and in 80% of patients with secondary infertility [7, 8].

Depending on the diagnostic method, varicoceles are divided into clinical and subclinical varicoceles. A clinical varicocele is diagnosed with a simple examination in a patient in orthostatic position by performing a Valsalva manoeuvre. A subclinical varicocele requires Döppler echocardiography to demonstrate the presence of blood reflux through the internal spermatic vein without palpable enlargement of the pampiniform plexus. The incidence of subclinical varicocele varies markedly depending on the diagnostic techniques used and the diagnostic centre ranging from 21% to 80% [9].

Clinically, varicoceles are classified into grades [10]. Grade 1, varicoceles are only palpable with a Valsalva manoeuvre. Grade 2, varicoceles that are palpable without a Valsalva manoeuvre. Grade 3, varicoceles that are visible through the scrotal wall. Varicocele can be primary or secondary. Primary varicocele is mainly due to blood reflux to the pampiniform plexus resulting from valve incompetence in the internal spermatic vein and is more frequent on the left side. Secondary varicocele is caused by compression of the testicular veins by abdominal and retroperitoneal neoplasia, hydronephrosis, or a compression of the left renal vein between the superior mesenteric artery and the aorta (nutcracker phenomenon) [11].

Although left-sided varicoceles are more frequent and larger in size, up to 50% of varicoceles are bilateral [12]. Isolated right-side varicoceles are rare and are frequently associated with retroperitoneal tumours or situs inversus [13]. Subclinical varicoceles do not produce altera-

M. Nistal, P. González-Peramato, *Testicular Vascular Lesions*,
https://doi.org/10.1007/978-3-031-57847-2_13

Fig. 13.1 Cross section of a normal spermatic cord. In the spermatic compartment, three sections of veins showing a thick wall are prominent. The other vessels in both the deferential and spermatic compartments are smaller in size and thin-walled

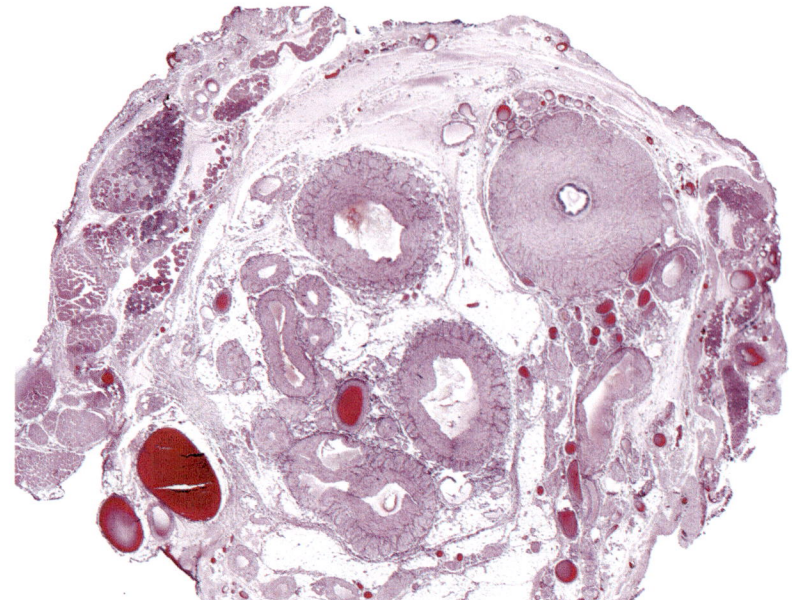

Fig. 13.2 Varicocele. Intense dilatation of several veins of the spermatic cord. The veins show relatively thin walls (Masson's trichrome)

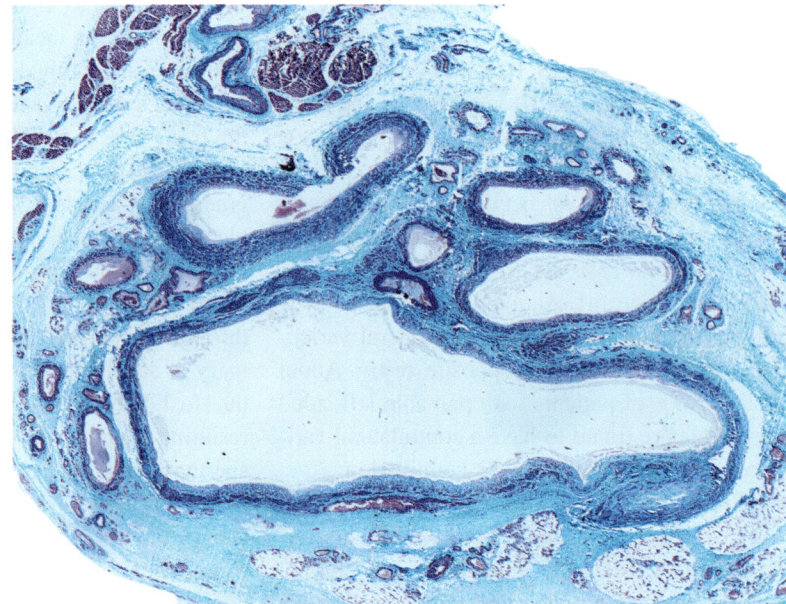

tions in fertility so do not require therapeutic measures [14].

Different imaging modalities have been used for varicocele evaluation: thermography, venography, and/or scintigraphy. Some of these methods have been relegated by other less invasive and easier-to-perform methods such as ultrasound and Döppler [15]. Ultrasonography is currently the most widely used method with a sensitivity of 97% and specificity of 94% in clinical varicoceles and a sensitivity of 83–95% in subclinical varicoceles [16]. Characteristic findings of varicocele are the presence of multiple, serpiginous tubular structures in the superior and lateral part of the testis, with intermittent or continuous flow with the Valsalva manoeuvre [17–19]. The presence of veins larger than 2 mm in diameter has a 95% sensitivity [20]. Another

Fig. 13.3 Varicocele. The pampiniform plexus, to which most of the extratesticular cavities correspond, is markedly dilated. At the level of the testicular mediastinum, there are also several dilated veins between the rete testis and the parenchyma

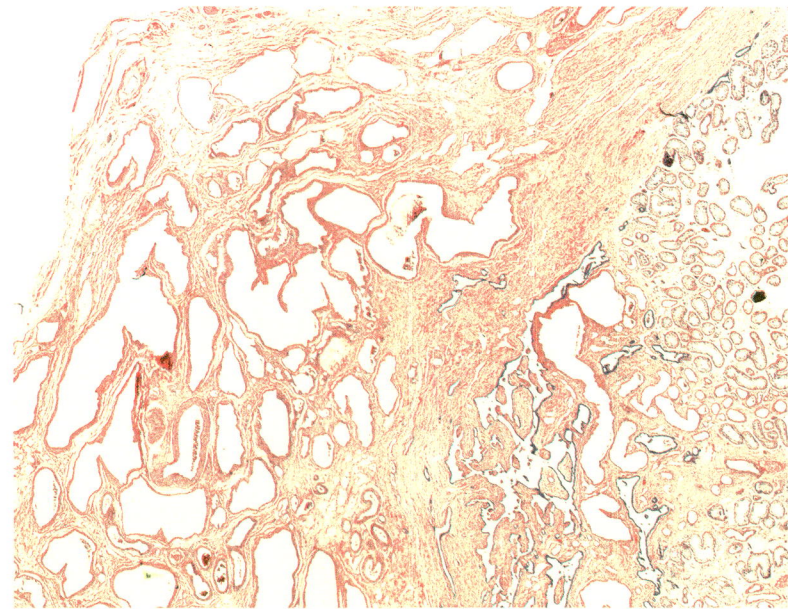

ultrasound technique introduced more recently is Shear wave elastography, which could be useful, not only for the diagnosis of varicocele, but also for the selection of patients in whom treatment is fully justified [21].

The negative effects of varicocele on the testis begin to be observed at puberty. However, it is necessary to be very cautious in assessing certain data, in particular testicular size, as testicular size asymmetry is very common at this age [22]. Adolescent varicocele is associated with decreased testicular volume and decreased sperm density, motility, and maturation [23]. Diagnosis may be delayed, because although it produces an increase in scrotal volume, this may be masked, in many cases, by ipsilateral testicular hypotrophy. Study with colour Döppler ultrasound (US) can detect the presence of reflux, measure the diameter of the spermatic vein and testicular volume; it is required to assess the severity of the varicocele and to select an early therapy [24]. Based on data provided by US, the diameter of the spermatic vein is under discussion, since diameters smaller than 2 mm can be associated with reflux. On the other hand, differences in testicular size ≥15% tend to reduce without treatment during puberty [25], although this does not necessarily ensure good testicular function. About 66% of patients with an initial size difference have, at the end of puberty, a low total motile sperm count [26].

13.2   The Diversity of Pathogenetic Mechanisms

The mechanism by which varicocele affects spermatogenesis is probably multifactorial [27]; alterations in testicular thermoregulation, hypoxia, toxic effects of metabolites of renal or adrenal origin, oxidative stress, hormonal imbalance, altered blood flow due to increased venous pressure, gonad toxins, increased apoptosis, alterations in the vascularization of the epididymis and its function, and negative effects on the contralateral testis are all possible factors [27–30]. The different mechanisms and factors involved are summarized in the algorithm (Fig. 13.4).

Fig. 13.4 Algorithm of
the pathogenic
mechanisms of testicular
lesions in varicocele

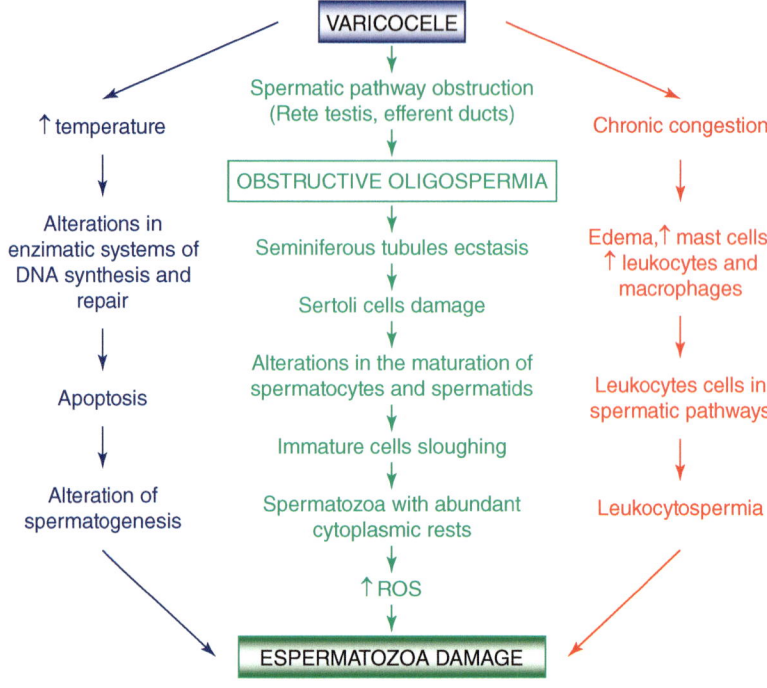

13.3   Value of Testicular Biopsy in Fertility Studies

Histological studies in varicocele are scarce since histological examination is not usually recommended. But, in the past, not only have they been very useful to know the nature of testicular lesions, but they have also demonstrated that testicular volume does not seem to be the best means to estimate fertility potential. Testicular volume and semen concentration are independent variables, which confirms the old suspicion that a percentage of seminiferous tubules is incapable of developing normal spermatogenesis in patients with varicocele. Histological studies performed in adolescents with varicocele reveal sloughing of immature germ cells, variable degrees of hypospermatogenesis, peritubular fibrosis and sclerosis of small vessel walls [31].

In biopsies performed in adults, the variability of the lesions is striking, not only from one individual to another, but also in the same sample. Schematically the lesions of the seminiferous tubules can be classified as diffuse or focal. Diffuse lesions are characterized by increased apoptosis, preferentially in first order spermato-

cytes, and probably secondary to thermal stress and hypoxia. Focal lesions can be of two types: ductal ectasia and mixed atrophy. Ductal ectasia lesions are observed in clusters of seminiferous tubules close to each other, probably belonging to the same lobule, and are characterized by great variation in tubular diameter ranging from markedly dilated to sclerosed tubules. The former have abundant desquamated immature cells in their wide lumina and vacuolisation of Sertoli cells (Fig. 13.5). The remaining sclerosed tubules show variable thickening of the tubular wall, progressive loss of germ cells and dedifferentiation of myoid cells as tubular atrophy advances [32]. These lesions are characteristic of an obstruction and are especially observed when the varicocele has an intratesticular component [33]. Mixed atrophy is a primary lesion in which, next to tubules with normal spermatogenesis, there is another group of seminiferous tubules, generally of smaller diameter, showing only Sertoli cells. It is probably also a coincident primary lesion to find a group of tubules with hypospermatogenesis can also be found next to normal tubules.

Interstitial lesions observed with varicocele affect all components and include interstitial

Fig. 13.5 Varicocele. Marked dilatation of intraparenchymal veins. The seminiferous tubules have a normal calibre, complete spermatogenesis, and desquamation of immature cells in the lumen

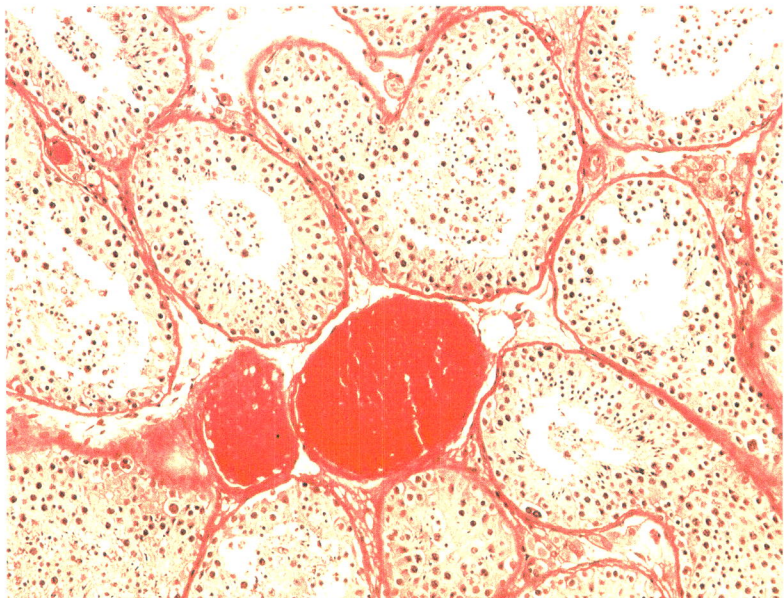

Fig. 13.6 Varicocele. Cluster of seminiferous tubules of slightly decreased calibre surrounded by an oedematous interstitium with several congestive veins

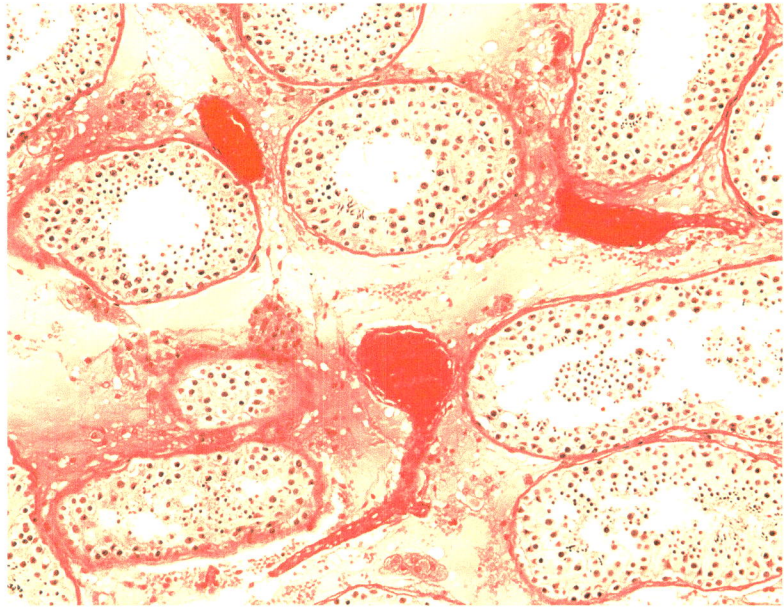

oedema, ectasia of the lymphatic vessels, blood stagnation in the small vessels, and thickening and fibrosis of the wall of the larger blood vessels and the interstitium [34] (Fig. 13.6). Leydig cells show hyperplasia ranging from 22% [35] to 39% [36], and atrophy in 4% [37] to 10% of the testis [38] (Fig. 13.7). After varicocelectomy, an improvement in germ cell maturation [39], decrease of meiotic abnormalities and normaliza-

tion of the number of Leydig cells has been observed [40]. Thickening of the tubular basement membrane and changes in the vessel wall do not regress.

Varicocele is the most common treatable cause of infertility, although there is no consensus on what should be the treatment of choice (surgical repair, percutaneous embolization) [41, 42]. In most cases, an improvement in testicular function

Fig. 13.7 Varicocele.
Leydig cell hyperplasia.
The seminiferous
tubules located in the
periphery show marked
germ cell depletion

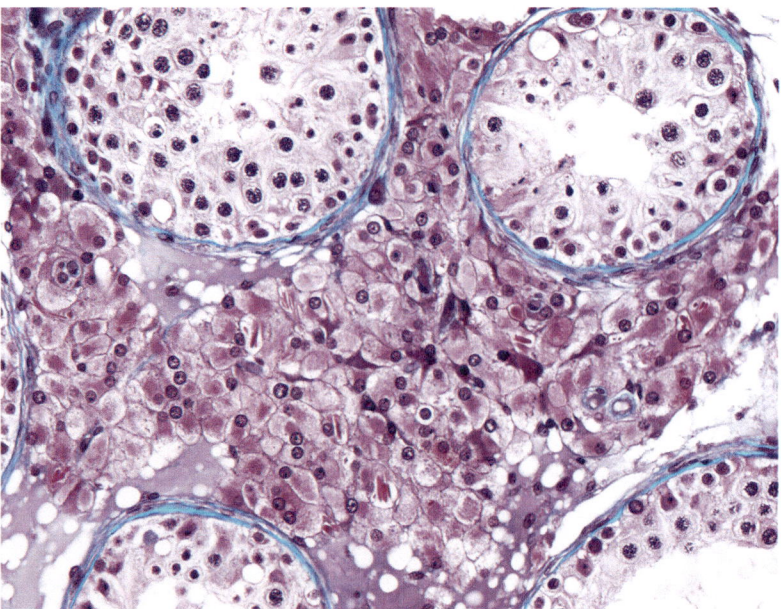

is observed. A significant increase and decrease in FSH and LH levels respectively is observed when mean serum testosterone, inhibin B, and sperm concentration levels after surgical repair are compared with the preoperative levels [43].

The most recommended treatment for varicoceles during puberty is percutaneous sclerotherapy, which achieves not only a bilateral increase in testicular volume, but also an increase in total sperm count and sperm morphology; it seems to increase the capacity to produce spermatozoa per unit of testicular volume [44]. Long-term results of patients operated early offer much better outcomes than those operated in adulthood, with the former reaching normal paternity rates [45]. Microsurgical varicocelectomy remains the gold standard in patients with severe oligozoospermia as it improves all semen parameters and pregnancy rates, although many men require IVF-ICSI afterward [46–48] and to restore normal elevated LH levels which to maintain optimal serum testosterone rates had compensated the pituitary [49]. Varicocelectomy is not only indicated to preserve or improve fertility but is a useful resource to treat testicular pain, when other causes of orchialgia have been excluded, or the patient presents with androgen deficiency hypogonadism [50–52].

13.4 Peculiarities of Intratesticular Varicocele

This rare entity is an incidental discovery during an exploration for testicular pain or infertility [53]. Its incidence is estimated at 1.3–2% of the general population compared to the 15%–20% rate of extratesticular varicocele. In 72% of cases, intra-and extratesticular varicocele coexist. Intratesticular varicocele can be uni-or bilateral [54] and is diagnosed by ultrasound [55] (Figs. 13.8, 13.9, 13.10 and 13.11). It produces hypoechoic lesions of tortuous course, cystic or tubular, multiple, radiating towards the testicular mediastinum, or, in a subalbuginea situation, or both, with spontaneous colour flow on Döppler imaging. The size of the veins is a matter of discussion, it having been suggested that if the above premises are met, the venous diameter is not important [56]. The differential diagnosis arises with hypoechoic lesions such as cystic transformation of the rete testis, segmental infarction, focal orchitis or tumour. In principle, any venous structure, regardless of its size, that shows reflux with the Valsalva manoeuvre and presents spontaneous venous flow on colour Döppler is considered characteristic of intratesticular varicocele [57].

Fig. 13.8 Section of the epididymal body and collapsed pampiniform plexus. This venous plexus appears surrounding an artery

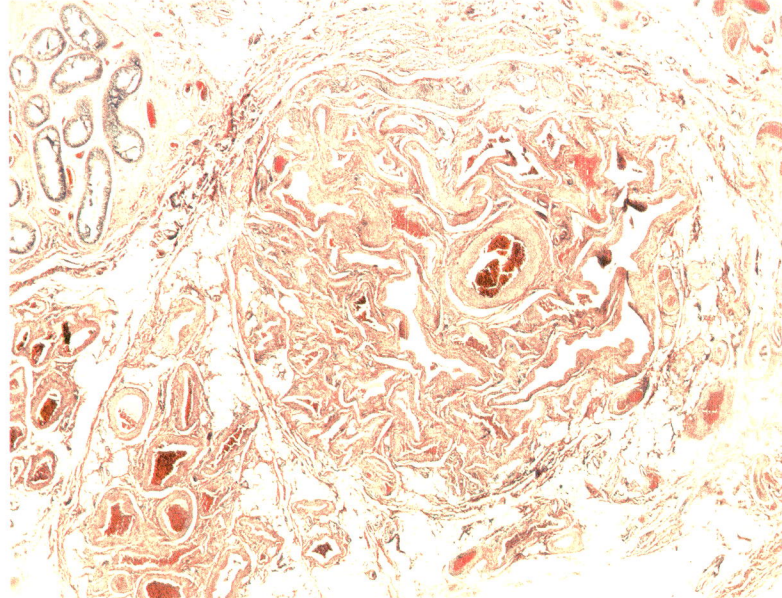

Fig. 13.9 Extratesticular varicocele. The testicular mediastinum is traversed by centripetal veins that run perpendicular to the cavities of the rete mediastinum as they leave the testis

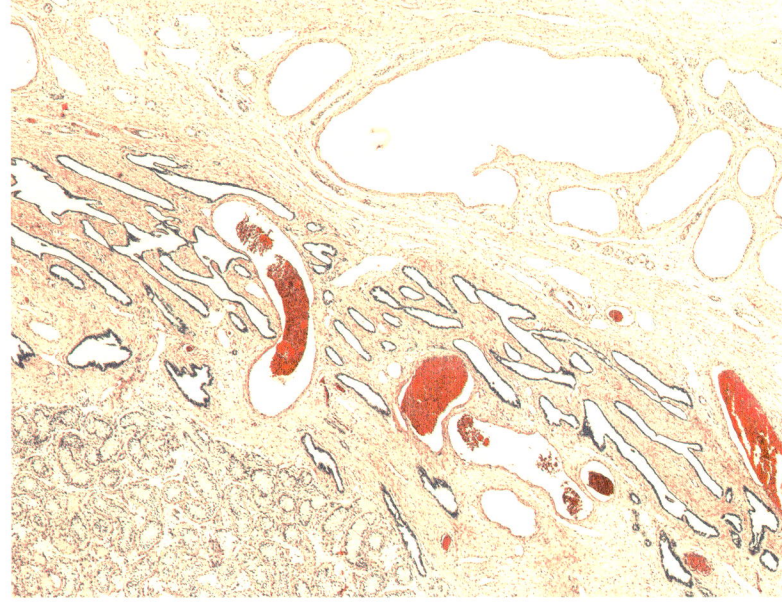

Patients show oligozoospermia and asthenozoospermia, which can be explained, at least in part, by the obstructive process of the spermatic pathway that occurs in the mediastinum and proximal parenchyma. In this area, which is not very extendable, there is a conflict of space between the dilated veins and the fine ducts of the septal rete testis that evacuate the fluid from the seminiferous tubules. Due to the pressure from the dilated veins, the straight tubules collapse and their trajectory is distorted. The seminiferous tubules present alterations in spermatogenesis of an obstructive character, which vary from one lobule to another, from tubules with only slight ectasia and normal spermatogenesis to others that are completely atrophic depending on the difficulties in the drainage of the tubular fluid [33] (Figs. 13.12 and 13.13). Testicular atrophy is common when treatment is delayed [58]. In some cases, atrophy has been observed associated with thrombosis of intratesticular varicoceles [56].

Fig. 13.10 Varicocele.
Large, dilated, and
tortuous veins at the
level of the tunica
vasculosa

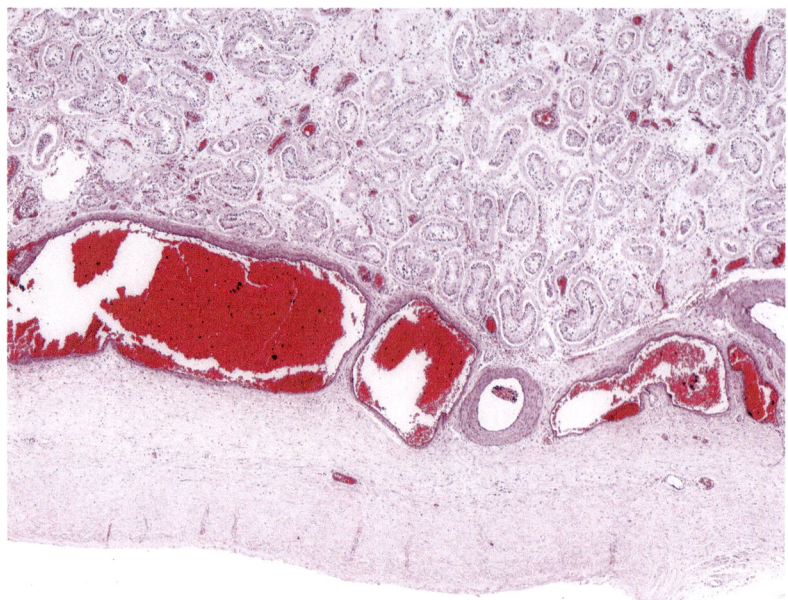

Fig. 13.11 Varicocele.
Cross section of several
dilated lumen veins
located below the
albuginea and partially
surrounded by
seminiferous tubules of
decreased diameter and
slightly dilated lumen

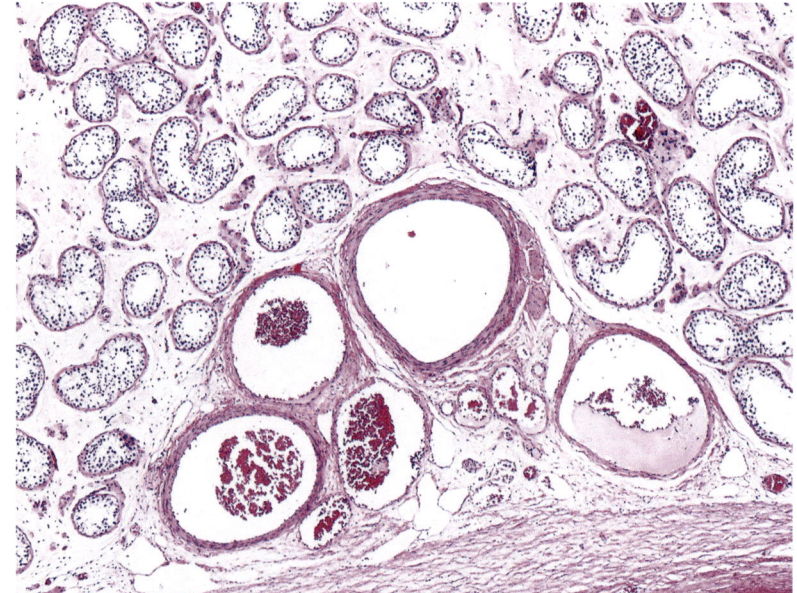

Fig. 13.12 Intratesticular varicocele. Numerous markedly dilated veins in the full testicular mediastinum distorting the cavities of the rete testis

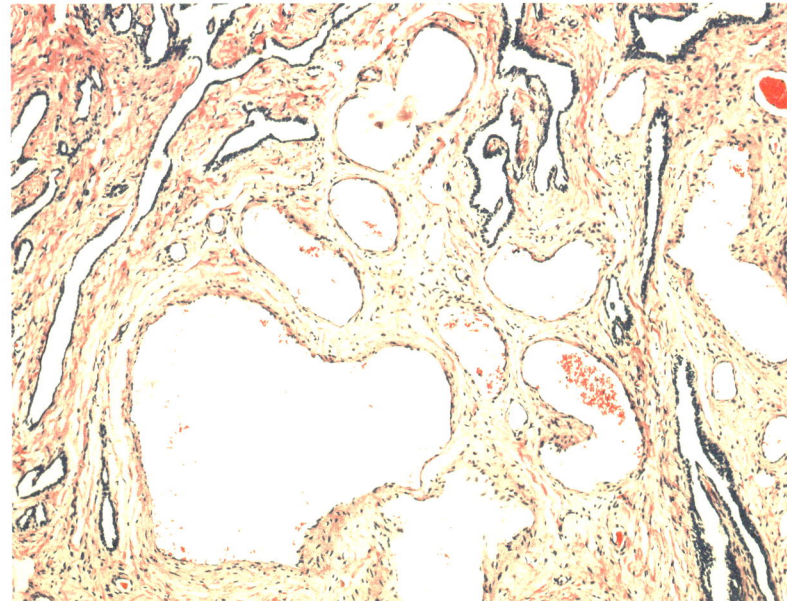

Fig. 13.13 Intratesticular varicocele. In the central part there is a group of seminiferous tubules, probably belonging to the same lobule, that are atrophic with some being completely hyalinized. The remaining seminiferous tubules have complete spermatogenesis and marked dilatation of the lumen

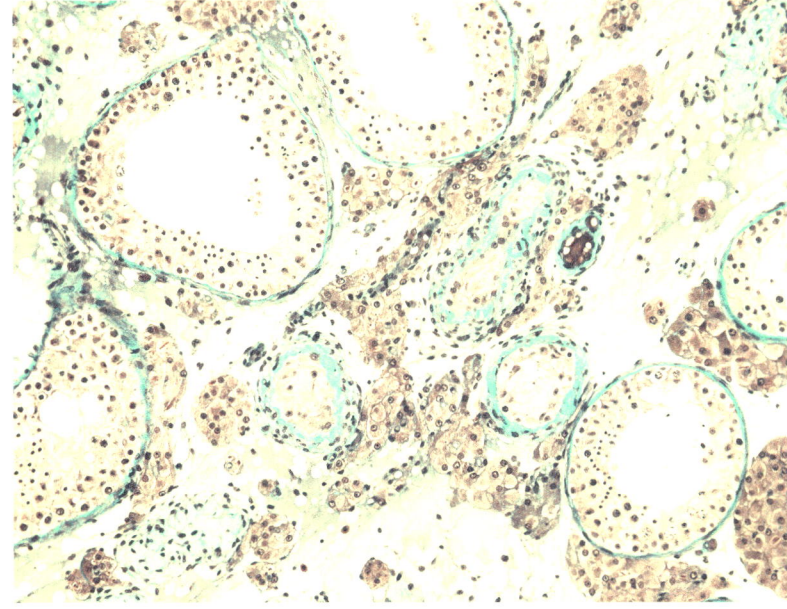

References

1. Baazeem A, Belzile E, Ciampi A, Dohle G, Jarvi K, Salonia A, Weidner W, Zini A. Varicocele and male factor infertility treatment: a new meta-analysis and review of the role of varicocele repair. Eur Urol. 2011;60:796–808.
2. Méndez-Gallart R, García-Palacios M. Rodríguez-Barca P, Estévez-Martínez E, Bautista-Casasnovas A. 15 years' experience in the single-port laparoscopic treatment of pediatric varicocele with Ligasure® technology. Cir Pediatr. 2023;36:33–9.
3. Kim ED, Lipshultz LI. Role of ultrasound in the assessment of male infertility. J Clin Ultrasound. 1996;24:437–53.
4. Levinger U, Gornish M, Gat Y, Bachar GN. Is varicocele prevalence increasing with age? Andrologia. 2007;39:77–80.
5. Agarwal A, Esteves SC. Varicocele and male infertility: current concepts and future perspectives. Asian J Androl. 2016;18:161–2.

6. Tiseo BC, Esteves SC, Cocuzza MS. Summary evidence on the effects of varicocele treatment to improve natural fertility in subfertile men. Asian J Androl. 2016;18:239–45.

7. Jarow JP, Coburn M, Sigman M. Incidence of varicoceles in men with primary and secondary infertility. Urology. 1996;47:73–6.

8. Damsgaard J, Joensen UN, Carlsen E, Erenpreiss J, Blomberg Jensen M, Matulevicius V, Zilaitiene B, Olesen IA, Perheentupa A, Punab M, Salzbrunn A, Toppari J, Virtanen HE, Juul A, Skakkebæk NE, Jørgensen N. Varicocele is associated with impaired semen quality and reproductive hormone levels: a study of 7035 healthy young men from six European countries. Eur Urol. 2016;70:1019–29.

9. Rotker K, Sigman M. Recurrent varicocele. Asian J Androl. 2016;18:229–33.

10. Dubin L, Amelar RD. Varicocele size and results of varicocelectomy in selected subfertile men with varicocele. Fertil Steril. 1970;21:606–9.

11. Gulleroglu K, Gulleroglu B, Baskin E. Nutcracker syndrome. World J Nephrol. 2014;3:277–81.

12. Almekaty KM, Elsharkawy AM, Zahran MH, Ragab MM, Rashed AS, Soliman MM, Salem KA, Ghaith AF. Bilaterality of varicocele: the overlooked culprit in male infertility. Case series study. Arch Ital Urol Androl. 2023;95:11580.

13. Alsaikhan B, Alrabeeah K, Delouya G, Zini A. Epidemiology of varicocele. Asian J Androl. 2016;18:179–81.

14. Kohn TP, Ohlander SJ, Jacob JS, Griffin TM, Lipshultz LI, Pastuszak AW. The effect of subclinical varicocele on pregnancy rates and semen parameters: a systematic review and meta-analysis. Curr Urol Rep. 2018;19:53.

15. Tsili AC, Xiropotamou ON, Sylakos A, Maliakas V, Sofikitis N, Argyropoulou MI. Potential role of imaging in assessing harmful effects on spermatogenesis in adult testes with varicocele. World J Radiol. 2017;9:34–45.

16. Belay RE, Huang GO, Shen JK, Ko EY. Diagnosis of clinical and subclinical varicocele: how has it evolved? Asian J Androl. 2016;18:182–5.

17. Pauroso S, Di Leo N, Fulle I, Di Segni M, Alessi S, Maggini E. Varicocele: Ultrasonographic assessment in daily clinical practice. J Ultrasound. 2011;14:199–204.

18. Kim YS, Kim SK, Cho IC, Min SK. Efficacy of scrotal Doppler ultrasonography with the Valsalva maneuver, standing position, and resting-Valsalva ratio for varicocele diagnosis. Korean J Urol. 2015;56:144–9.

19. Lehner K, Ingram C, Bansal U, Baca C, Balasubramanian A, Thirumavalavan N, Scovell JM, Rajanahally S, Pollard M, Lipshultz LI. Color Doppler ultrasound imaging in varicoceles: is the difference in venous diameter encountered during Valsalva predictive of palpable varicocele grade? Asian J Urol. 2023;10:27–32.

20. Gonda RL Jr, Karo JJ, Forte RA, O'Donnell KT. Diagnosis of subclinical varicocele in infertility. AJR Am J Roentgenol. 1987;148:71–5.

21. Jedrzejewski G, Osemlak P, Wieczorek AP, Nachulewicz P. Prognostic values of shear wave elastography in adolescent boys with varicocele. J Pediatr Urol. 2019;15(3):223.e1–5.

22. Lourdaux PJ, Vaganée D, Leysen C, De Wachter S, De Win G. Evolution of testicular asymmetry during puberty in adolescents without and with a left varicocele. BJU Int. 2023;131:348–56.

23. Keene DJ, Sajad Y, Rakoczy G, Cervellione RM. Testicular volume and semen parameters in patients aged 12 to 17 years with idiopathic varicocele. J Pediatr Surg. 2012;47:383–5.

24. Liguori G, Trombetta C, Garaffa G, Bucci S, Gattuccio I, Salamè L, Belgrano E. Color Doppler ultrasound investigation of varicocele. World J Urol. 2004;22:378–81.

25. Kolon TF, Clement MR, Cartwright L, Bellah R, Carr MC, Canning DA, Snyder HM 3rd. Transient asynchronous testicular growth in adolescent males with a varicocele. J Urol. 2008;180:1111–4.

26. Christman MS, Zderic SA, Canning DA, Kolon TF. Active surveillance of the adolescent with varicocele: predicting semen outcomes from ultrasound. J Urol. 2014;191:1401–6.

27. Nistal M, Redondo E. Varicocele, histología y etiopatogenia. In: En: III Congreso Nacional de Andrología. Zaragoza: ASESA; 1987. p. 59–92.

28. Nistal M, González-Peramato P, Serrano A, Regadera J. Physiopathology of the infertile testicle. Etiopathogenesis of varicocele. Arch Esp Urol. 2004;57:883–904.

29. Shiraishi K, Matsuyama H, Takihara H. Pathophysiology of varicocele in male infertility in the era of assisted reproductive technology. Int J Urol. 2012;19:538–50.

30. Nistal M, González-Peramato P, Serrano A. Clues to the analysis of testicular lesions in infertile patients with varicocele. In: Clues in the diagnosis of Non-tumoral testicular pathology. Cham: Springer; 2017. p. 191–4.

31. Jones MA, Sharp GH, Trainer TD. The adolescent varicocele. A histopathologic study of 13 testicular biopsies. Am J Clin Pathol. 1988;89:321–8.

32. Santamaría L, Martín R, Nistal M, Paniagua R. The peritubular myoid cells in the testes from men with varicocele: an ultrastructural, immunohistochemical and quantitative study. Histopathology. 1992;21:423–33.

33. Nistal M, Paniagua R, Regadera J, Santamaria L. Obstruction of the tubuli recti and ductuli efferentes by dilated veins in the testes of men with varicocele and its possible role in causing atrophy of the seminiferous tubules. Int J Androl. 1984;7:309–23.

34. North MO, Lellei I, Rives N, Erdei E, Dittmar A, Barbet JP, Tritto G. Reversible meiotic abnormalities

in azoospermic men with bilateral varicocele after microsurgical correction. Cell Mol Biol (Noisy-le-Grand). 2004;50:281–9.

35. McFadden MR, Mehan DJ. Testicular biopsies in 101 cases of varicocele. J Urol. 1978;119:372–4.

36. Agger P, Johnsen SG. Quantitative evaluation of testicular biopsies in varicocele. Fertil Steril. 1978;29:52–7.

37. Etriby A, Girgis SM, Hefnawy H, Ibrahim AA. Testicular changes in subfertile males with varicocele. Fertil Steril. 1967;18:666–71.

38. Dubin L, Hotchkiss RS. Testis biopsy in subfertile men with varicocele. Fertil Steril. 1969;20:51–7.

39. Johnsen SG, Agger P. Quantitative evaluation of testicularbiopsies before and after operation for varicocele. Fertil Steril. 1978;29:58–63.

40. Abdelrahim F, Mostafa A, Hamdy A, Mabrouk M, el-Kholy M, Hassan O. Testicular morphology and function in varicocele patients: pre-operative and postoperative histopathology. Br J Urol. 1993;72:643–7.

41. Esteves SC, Roque M, Agarwal A. Outcome of assisted reproductive technology in men with treated and untreated varicocele: systematic review and meta-analysis. Asian J Androl. 2016;18:254–8.

42. Halpern J, Mittal S, Pereira K, Bhatia S, Ramasamy R. Percutaneous embolization of varicocele: technique, indications, relative contraindications, and complications. Asian J Androl. 2016;18:234–8.

43. Tian D, Yang C, Xie B, Li H, Li J, Yang D, Zhu Z. Effects of varicocele surgical repair on serum hormone and inhibin B levels for patients with varicocele: a systematic review and meta-analysis. Am J Mens Health. 2023;17(5):15579883231199400.

44. Mancini M, Carrafiello G, Melchiorre F, Pelliccione F, Andreassi A, Mantellassi G, Ahmed Said Z, Pecori Giraldi F, Banderali G, Folli F. Early varicocelectomy by percutaneous scleroembolization improves seminiferous tubules spermatozoa release in the adolescent phase of testicular growth. Andrologia. 2019;51(7):e13286.

45. Pajovic B, Radojevic N. Prospective follow up of fertility after adolescent laparoscopic varicocelectomy. Eur Rev Med Pharmacol Sci. 2013;17:1060–3.

46. Kirby EW, Wiener LE, Rajanahally S, Crowell K, Coward RM. Undergoing varicocele repair before assisted reproduction improves pregnancy rate and live birth rate in azoospermic and oligospermic men with a varicocele: a systematic review and meta-analysis. Fertil Steril. 2016;106:1338–43.

47. Najari BB. Varicocele repair in men with severe Oligospermia: NYU case of the month, February 2019. Rev Urol. 2019;21:32–4.

48. Vu Tan L, Phuc Cam Hoang N, Ba Tien Dung M, Vinh Phu P, Martinez M, Minh DN. Spontaneous pregnancies post-microsurgical varicocelectomy in infertile men with severe oligozoospermia: a preliminary vietnamese report. Clin Ter. 2023;174:126–31.

49. Chen X, Yang D, Lin G, Bao J, Wang J, Tan W. Efficacy of varicocelectomy in the treatment of hypogonadism in subfertile males with clinical varicocele: a meta-analysis. Andrologia. 2017;49(10):e12778.

50. Pagani RL, Ohlander SJ, Niederberger CS. Microsurgical varicocele ligation: surgical methodology and associated outcomes. Fertil Steril. 2019;111:415–9.

51. Cho CL, Esteves SC, Agarwal A. Indications and outcomes of varicocele repair. Panminerva Med. 2019;61:152–63.

52. Kalantan M, Vienney N, Guillot Tantay C, Roupret M, Akakpo W. Résultats des cures de varicocèles microchirurgicales sous-inguinales [Results of subinguinal microsurgical varicocelectomy]. Prog Urol. 2023;33:481–7.

53. Dhamija E, Das CJ, Razik A. Intratesticular varicocele: a rare cause of male factor infertility. BMJ Case Rep. 2018;2018:bcr2018224547.

54. Das KM, Prasad K, Szmigielski W, Noorani N. Intratesticular varicocele: evaluation using conventional and Doppler sonography. AJR Am J Roentgenol. 1999;173:1079–83.

55. Weiss AJ, Kellman GM, Middleton WD, Kirkemo A. Intratesticular varicocele: sonographic findings in two patients. AJR Am J Roentgenol. 1992;158:1061–3.

56. Ünal E. Thrombotic and nonthrombotic types of Intratesticular varicoceles: value of sonography for the diagnosis. J Ultrasound Med. 2017;36:2355–60.

57. Kessler A, Meirsdorf S, Graif M, Gottlieb P, Strauss S. Intratesticular varicocele: gray scale and color Doppler sonographic appearance. J Ultrasound Med. 2005;24:1711–6.

58. MacLachlan LS, Nees SN, Fast AM, Glassberg KI. Intratesticular varicoceles: are they significant? J Pediatr Urol. 2013;9:851–5.

14.1 Phlebosclerosis of the Intraparenchymal Veins

Phlebosclerosis of the intraparenchymal veins is a rare finding in testicular biopsies. Testicular phlebosclerosis is defined as a venous lesion characterized by circumferential collagen deposition in the intima and media of the veins, not associated with obstruction, thrombi, or inflammation. Histologically, it is like idiopathic phlebosclerosis of the mesentery [1, 2]. The material is fibrillar and very poor in cells. Smooth muscle cells in the vessel media dedifferentiate or are pushed back in a crescent shape within the vessel wall. Even between these cells there is abundant collagen. The adventitia shows no alterations. The lumen of the vein is dilated, probably due to the fibrous ring into which the wall is transformed, preventing its collapse. Not only the centripetal and centrifugal veins are affected, but also the intraparenchymal veins, which are easily identifiable as they are not located in the interlobular septa, are not accompanied by arteries and nerves, and are directly surrounded by the seminiferous tubules. This pathology does not affect the arteries or the lymphatic vessels (Figs. 14.1, 14.2, 14.3, 14.4 and 14.5).

Most of the time, the testicular parenchyma has a certain degree of ectasia of the seminiferous tubules and sloughing of the most mature germ cells (characteristics of obstructive processes in the spermatic pathway). Some oedema is observed in the interstitium with the presence of abundant perilymphatic spaces. In cases where intratesticular varices are observed, testicular atrophy is important and large areas of hyalinized tubules can be observed.

The differential diagnosis with phlebectasias does not usually present problems, however, it must be considered that in amyloidosis an eosinophilic and acellular material also accumulates extracellularly in the vessel wall. Masson's trichrome blue staining of the vein wall with phlebosclerosis and negative Congo red staining can rule amyloidosis out.

The aetiology of phlebosclerosis is unknown. In none of the six cases in our series, there was a history of the use of sclerosing agents, such as those used in the treatment of some varicoceles or the consumption of certain beverages. In two cases, there was a history of surgery, vasectomy in one case and varicocelectomy in the other [3]. In another case, the condition was observed in the peripheral vessels of a more than 10 year old Leydig cell tumour. In the other three cases, no pertinent data had been recorded in the history.

The pathogenesis of the lesions is uncertain. The ectasia of the veins with a fibrotic wall suggest that they had been subjected to increased hydrostatic pressure for a long time. The abnormalities in the seminiferous tubules suggest an obstructive process, which could well have been caused within the testicle by compression of the cavities of the rete testis by dilated, fibrous-walled venous vessels or from outside the testicle as the result of a surgical intervention.

© The Author(s), under exclusive license to Springer Nature Switzerland AG 2024
M. Nistal, P. González-Peramato, *Testicular Vascular Lesions*,
https://doi.org/10.1007/978-3-031-57847-2_14

Fig. 14.1 Phlebosclerosis of intraparenchymal veins. Cross section of an intraparenchymal vein surrounded by several seminiferous tubules. The vein stands out compared to the seminiferous tubules due to its large size, thick wall, and dilated lumen

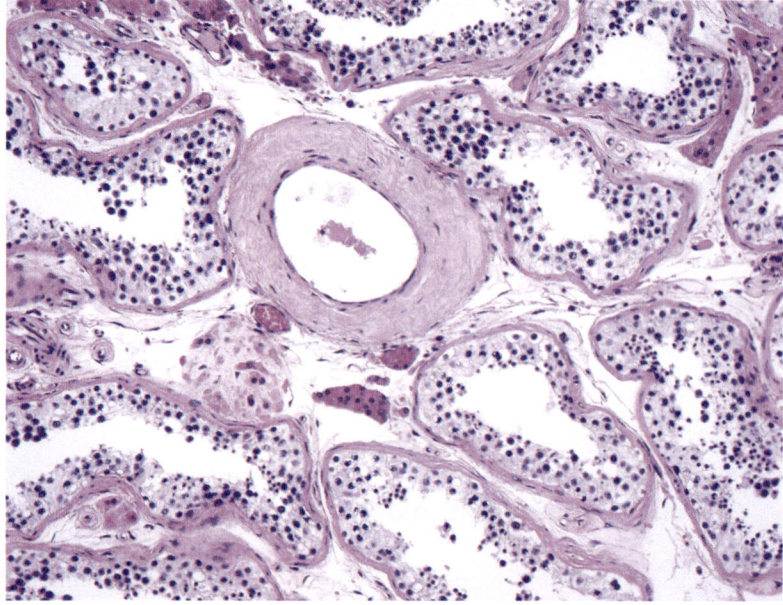

Fig. 14.2 Phlebosclerosis of intraparenchymal veins. Cross sections of two veins. Of note is the marked thickening of the media and the presence of eosinophilic material protrusions into the adventitia that simulate the presence of amyloid. The neighbouring seminiferous tubules show hypospermatogenesis

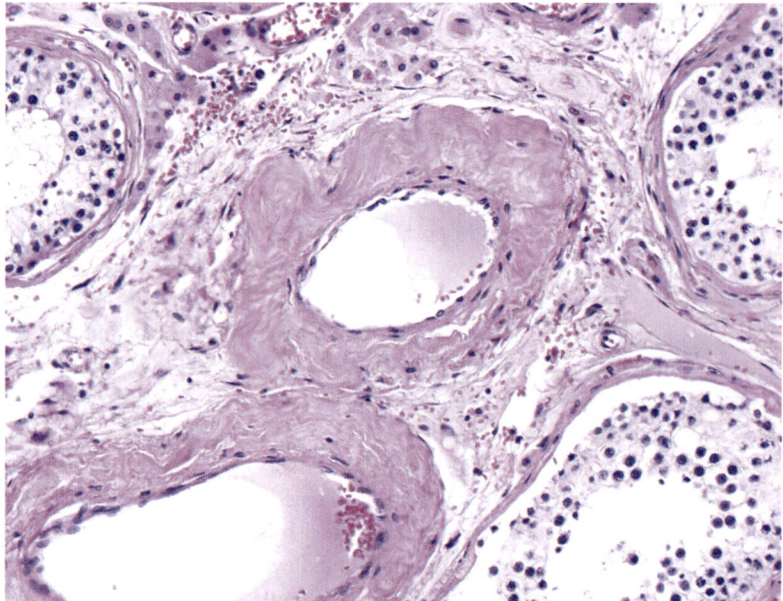

Fig. 14.3 Phlebosclerosis of intraparenchymal veins. Ecstatic intraparenchymal vein. In the thickened wall, preferably in the middle layer, there are abundant collagen fibres arranged circumferentially between the few smooth muscle cells. The adventitia is unaltered

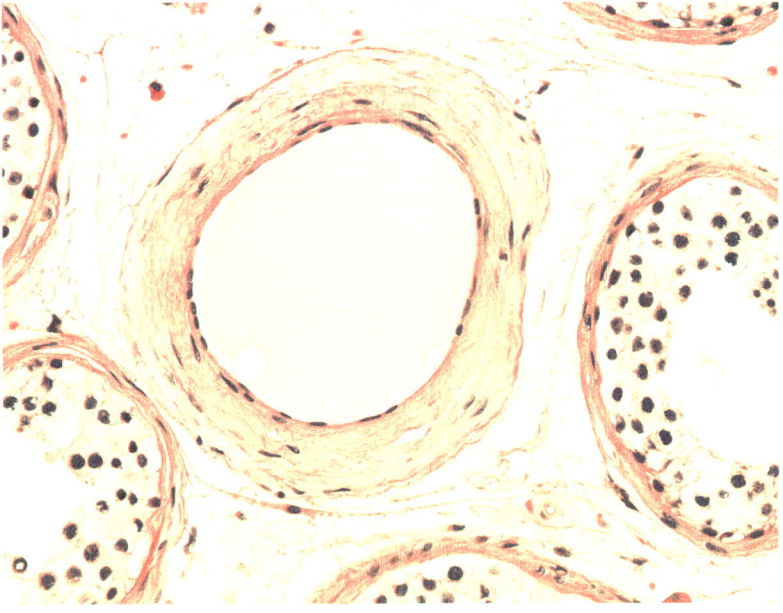

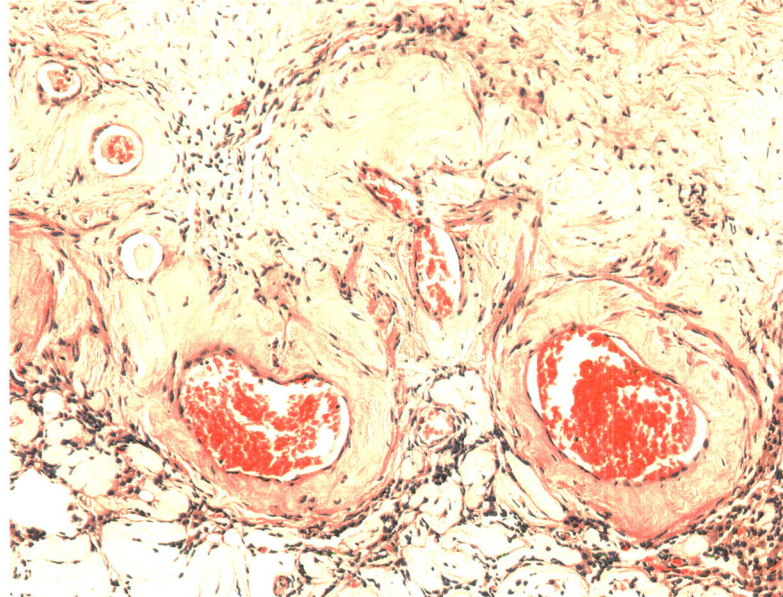

Fig. 14.4 Phlebosclerosis of intraparenchymal veins. The subalbugineal veins show a tortuous course with marked thickening of the middle layer and adventitial fibrosis. Sclerosis of the seminiferous tubules and a decrease in Leydig cells

Fig. 14.5 Phlebosclerosis of intraparenchymal veins. Transverse section of a subalbugineal vein. Apart from the thickening of the wall and the marked dilatation of the lumen, the irregular distribution of the smooth muscle cells of the middle layer stands out, while muscle cells are not recognizable in some areas but are abundant in others

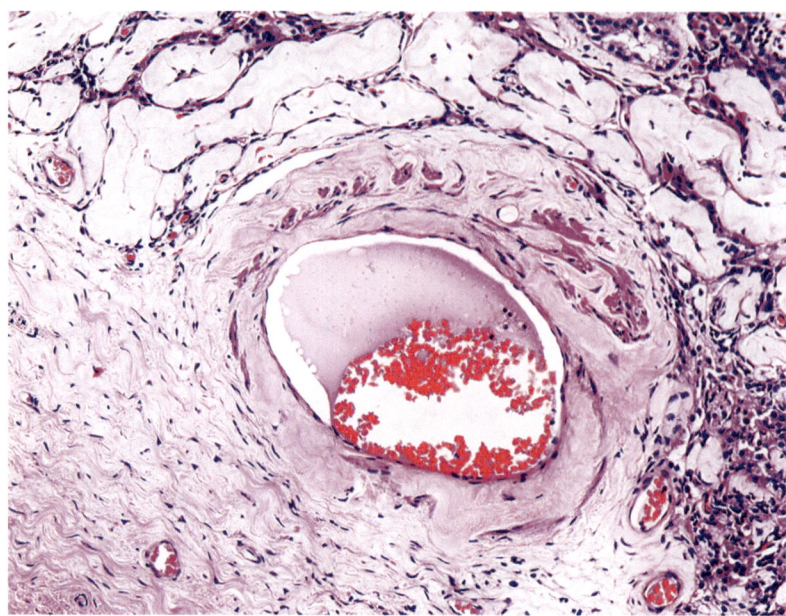

14.2 Hypertrophic Fibrosis of the Adventicia of the Intratesticular Veins

The intratesticular venous architecture obeys two patterns. Most of the veins that collect blood from the deepest 2/3 of the parenchyma drain into the testicular mediastinum (centripetal veins) forming the larger calibre veins that run between the cavities of the rete testis before leaving the testicle through the hilum to join the pampiniform plexus. The peripheral third of the testicular parenchyma drains through veins that go towards the tunica vasculosa (centrifugal veins) where they form other larger calibre veins and leave the testicle near the lower pole, from which they also join the pampiniform plexus.

The structure of the venous wall of the small and medium-sized intraparenchymal veins is very simple. The endothelium is supported by the basement membrane and one or two layers of smooth muscle cells in the middle. The adventitia is thin and poorly collagenized.

The lesion for which the name hypertrophic fibrosis of the adventitia is proposed is characterized by the following. (a) It affects many intraparenchymal vessels with a calibre between 30 and 60 microns, although vessels up to 200 microns wide may be affected. (b) The lesion preferentially affects the tunica adventitia. (c) The deep part of the adventitia and sometimes also its middle layer are made up of a concentric, collagen-rich cell-poor ring. The outermost part of the adventitia is always the thickest layer and is formed by thick longitudinal or helical collagen bundles. Few fibroblasts are arranged on the outside of the bundles. (d) The lesion can appear both in the veins between the seminiferous tubules as well as within the thick interlobular and intralobular septa. (e) Lesions are seen in pubertal and adult testes. (f) They are characteristic of androgen insensitivity syndrome. Affected veins are seen both in the parenchyma and in Sertoli-Leydig hamartomas or within Sertoli cell adenomas. (g) The number of affected vessels is proportional to the degree of fibrosis of the interstitium. (h) Neither the arteries nor the nerves are usually affected. (i) In some testicles the seminiferous tubules focally present the same type of fibrosis (Figs. 14.6, 14.7, 14.8, 14.9 and 14.10).

Hypertrophic fibrosis of the intratesticular vein adventitia is considered part of the hamartomatous process that the testicles of patients with androgen insensitivity frequently present in adulthood [4, 5].

Fig. 14.6 Adventitial hypertrophic fibrosis of intratesticular veins. A 13-year-old patient with complete androgen insensitivity and inguinal testicles. The central vessel shows concentric rings of collagen in the adventitia. The seminiferous tubules contain only Sertoli cells with spherical nuclei. In the interstitium, there are clusters of Leydig cells

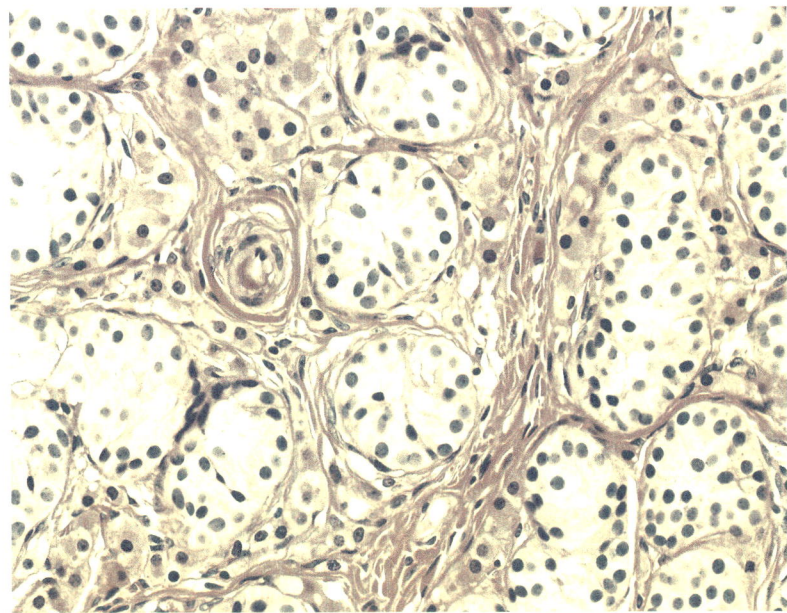

Fig. 14.7 Adventitial hypertrophic fibrosis of intratesticular veins. Oblique section of an intraparenchymal vein with thick wall at the expense of the adventitia. Longitudinally arranged collagen bundles predominate at this level. Among them, the nuclei of the fibroblasts are notable. Several Leydig cell clusters surround the vessel

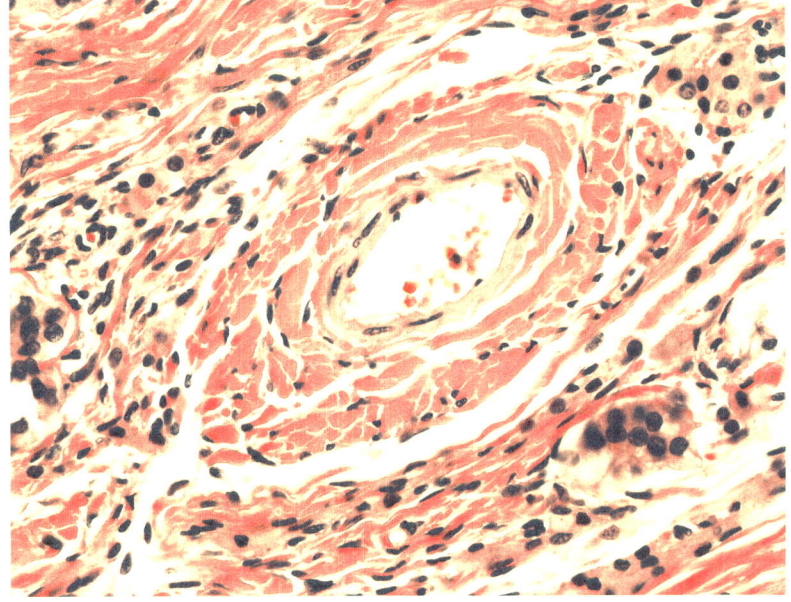

Fig. 14.8 Adventitial hypertrophic fibrosis of intratesticular veins. A 48-year-old patient with CAIS. In the periphery of a Sertoli cell adenoma (seminiferous tubules show prepubertal development without germ cells, with thick basement membranes and scarce interstitium without Leydig cells), the transverse section of a vein shows thickening of the adventitia (Masson's trichrome)

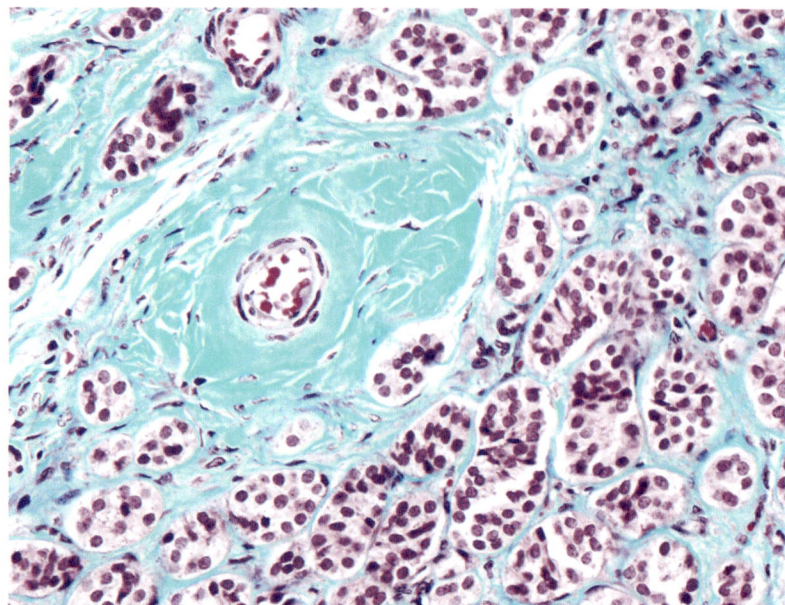

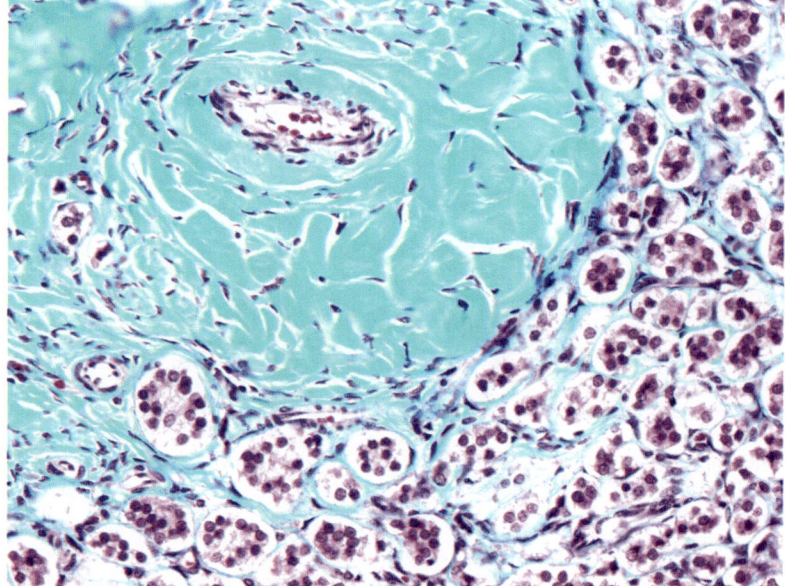

Fig. 14.9 Adventitial hypertrophic fibrosis of intratesticular veins. Section of a vein within a Sertoli cell adenoma. The adventitia has a geographical appearance due to the separation of the longitudinal bundles of collagen. Fibroblasts are arranged in the periphery of the bundles (Masson's trichrome)

Fig. 14.10 Adventitial hypertrophic fibrosis of intratesticular veins. Partially collapsed small vein. The intima shows no alterations, the media is formed by isolated muscle cells. At the level of the adventitia, there are two enormously thickened layers: an internal, circular, acellular layer and an external layer with thick bundles of longitudinally arranged collagen. Externally, note the characteristic tubular formations of a Sertoli cell adenoma

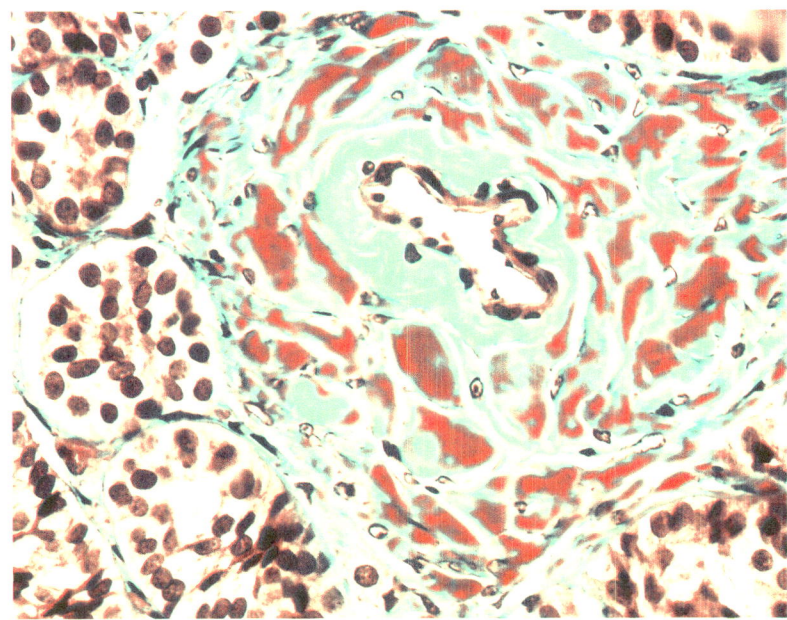

14.3   Adventitial Smooth Muscle Hyperplasia of Intratesticular Veins

The characteristics of the wall of the veins in the human body are related to the difficulties of returning blood to the heart. The supradiaphragmatic veins, despite their calibre, have a wall formed only by an intima and isolated muscle cells in the adventitia. For their part, infradiaphragmatic veins have a wall structured in three well-defined layers: intima; media, with several layers of circular smooth muscle cells; and adventitia in which, apart from connective and elastic tissue, there are thick bundles of longitudinal muscle cells. In the extremities, especially in the lower ones, many valves are added. The internal spermatic vein also shows a well-developed layer of longitudinal bundles of smooth muscle cell bundles in the adventitia [6].

The wall of the normal intratesticular veins is very thin, being made up of endothelium supported by a basal lamina surrounded by collagen fibres and isolated smooth muscle cells preferably arranged in a circular fashion. In larger veins, the smooth muscle cell layer is complete. Externally, the adventitia, made of connective tissue, joins the vessel to the remaining structures of the testis. This structure is maintained both in the veins that drain towards the hilum (centripetal veins), which are the majority, and those that drain towards the albuginea (centrifugal veins). Both follow the interlobular septa [7].

The condition that we have defined as adventitial smooth muscle hyperplasia of intratesticular veins (ASMHV) has been observed in three elderly patients with hydrocele and a large hernial sac. ASMHV is morphologically characterized by the fact that the wall structure of the intraparenchymal veins resembles that of the thicker subdiaphragmatic veins. The thick wall of the intratesticular veins is due to the longitudinal smooth muscle cell bundles of the adventitia. In some veins, these bundles are few in number, but in other vessels, they form several layers with hardly any connective tissue between them. Between the bundles, vasa vasorum are observed. The middle and intimal layers are unchanged. The lumen of these hyperplasic veins is much reduced compared to that of their accompanying arteries, with no evidence of thrombi or inflammatory phenomena (Figs. 14.11, 14.12, 14.13, 14.14, 14.15 and 14.16).

Muscular hyperplasia of the vein wall has also been described in the entity known as idiopathic myointimal hyperplasia of the mesenteric veins

Fig. 14.11 Adventitial smooth muscle hyperplasia of intratesticular veins. An 89-year-old patient with a large hydrocele and inguino-scrotal hernia. This and the following figures correspond to the orchiectomy specimen. In the thickness of the interlobular septum, sections of two arteries, small veins, and solid cross-sectioned cords stand out

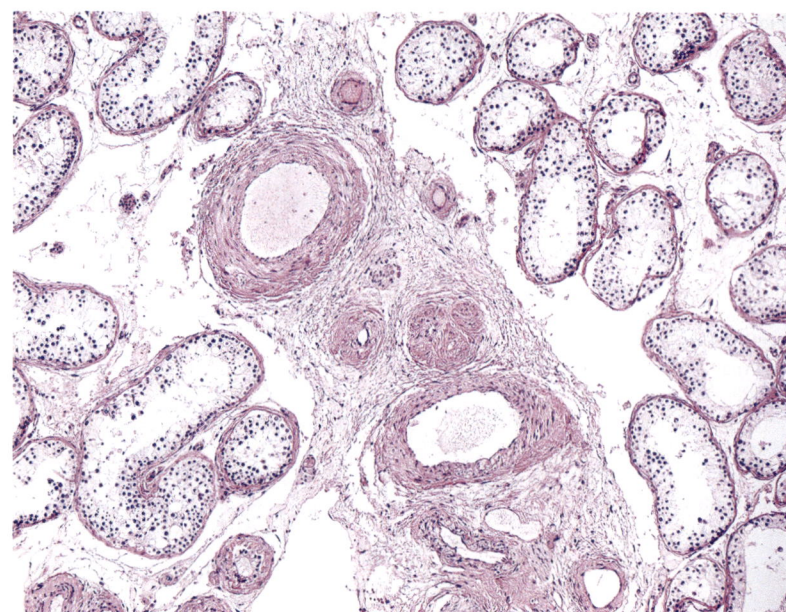

Fig. 14.12 Adventitial smooth muscle hyperplasia of intratesticular veins. Next to two seminiferous tubules with deficient spermatogenesis, there is a tubular formation with a small lumen and a thick wall

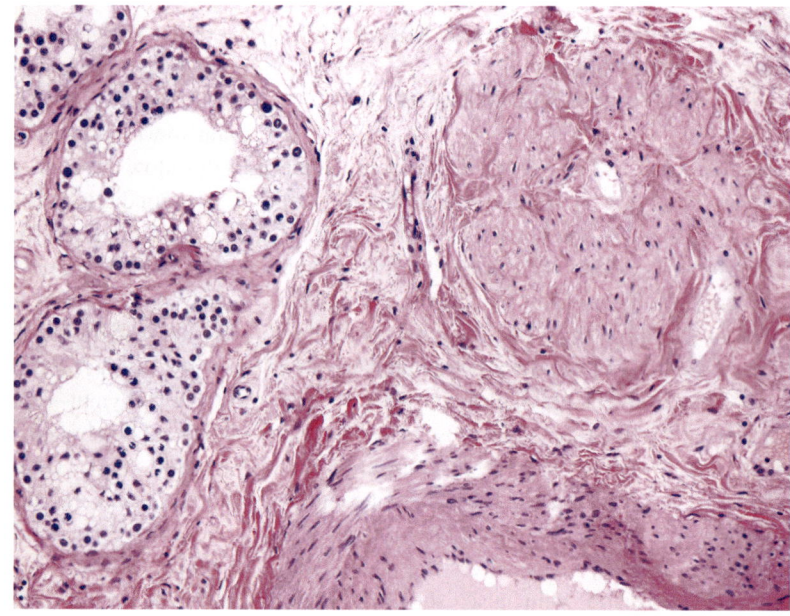

(IMHMV) [8]. A rare, non-inflammatory, non-thrombotic veno-occlusive disease affecting patients in mid-life, it can lead to chronic ischaemia of the colon refractory to medical treatment and require colectomy [9, 10]. However, muscular hyperplasia and ASMHV/they do not appear to have anything in common either clinically or histologically. In the ASMHIV described here, although it histologically shows a veno-occlusive, non-thrombotic, and non-inflammatory pathology, there is none of the myointimal proliferation characteristic of IMHMV, while the muscular proliferation that is present only affects the adventitia and is arranged longitudinally.

The aetiology and pathogenesis of the lesions are unknown. None of the patients had

Fig. 14.13 Adventitial smooth muscle hyperplasia of intratesticular veins. The central part is occupied by a cell-poor, well-defined nodular formation with a lobular architecture. Nearby there are several arterioles and in the opposite area, another, smaller, nodular formation

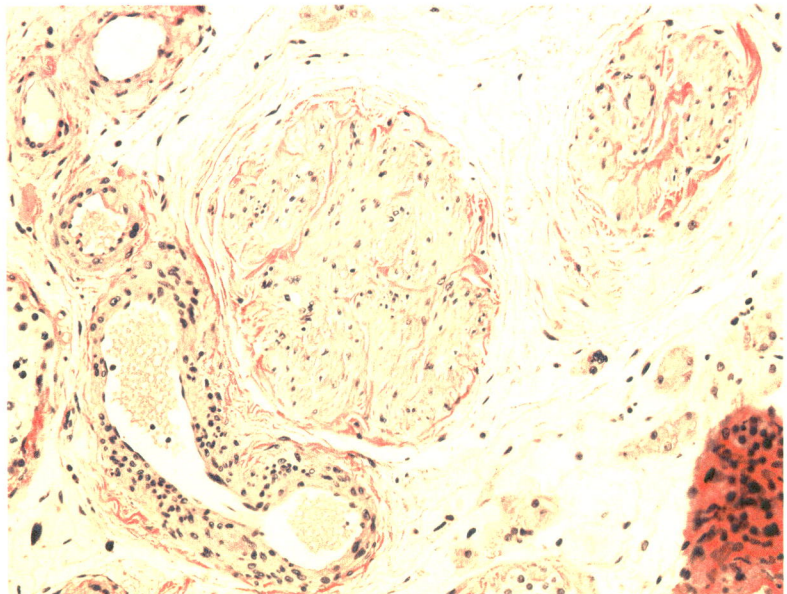

Fig. 14.14 Adventitial smooth muscle hyperplasia of intratesticular veins. Note the small calibre vessels with a thick wall in the vicinity of an artery that is only partially included in the figure

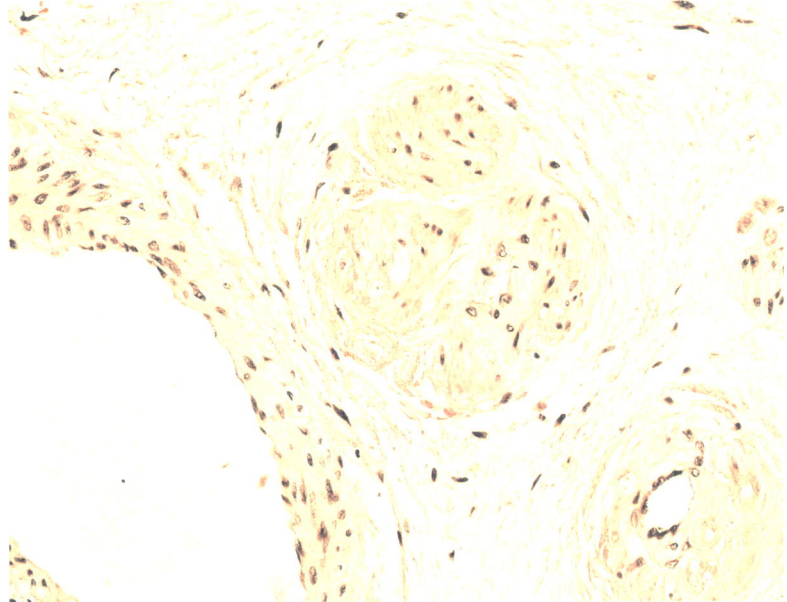

previous pathology or a history of drug use. Although the mission of the smooth muscle bundles in the adventitia of the subdiaphragmatic veins is to propel blood towards the heart, and so overcome the force of gravity, it does not seem that this could be a logical explanation for their presence in intratesticular veins. On the one hand, arterial flow of these testicles is greatly reduced by arteriosclerosis, and, on the other, large hydroceles are accompanied by atrophic testicles. One possibility is that this longitudinally arranged smooth muscle hyperplasia is related to hormonal changes that occur with age [11].

Fig. 14.15 Adventitial smooth muscle hyperplasia of intratesticular veins. Cross section of a seminiferous tubule, a vein, and an artery. Actin immunostaining reveals the myoid cells of the seminiferous tubule, the muscle cells of the middle layer of the artery, and in the central part, a small vein surrounded by longitudinal bundles of smooth muscle cells

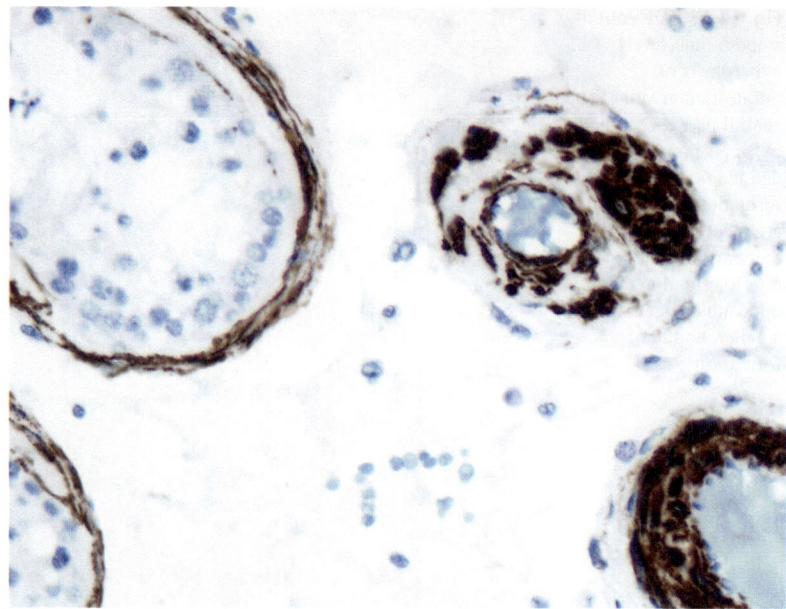

Fig. 14.16 Adventitial smooth muscle hyperplasia of intratesticular veins. Cross section of an intraparenchymal vein. The intima and medial layer are unaltered. The adventitia consists of well-individualized longitudinal fascicles of smooth muscle cells (actin immunostaining)

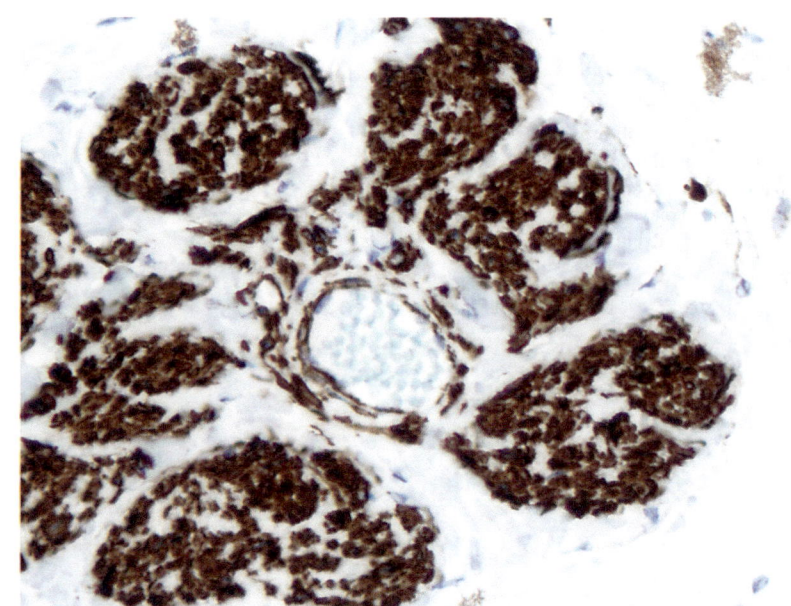

References

1. Wang J, Shao J, Lu H, Wang B, Chen J. Idiopathic mesenteric phlebosclerosis: one case report and systematic literature review of 240 cases. Am J Transl Res. 2021;13:13156–66.
2. Takasaki T, Motomura Y, Shioya K. Idiopathic mesenteric Phlebosclerosis. Clin Gastroenterol Hepatol. 2022;20:A19.
3. Nistal M, González-Peramato P, Serrano A. Clues to the analysis of testicular lesions in infertile patients with varicocele. In: Clues in the diagnosis of nontumoral testicular pathology. Cham: Springer; 2017a. p. 191–4.
4. Regadera J, Martínez-García F, Paniagua R, Nistal M. Androgen insensitivity syndrome: an immunohistochemical, ultrastructural, and morphometric study. Arch Pathol Lab Med. 1999;123:225–34.

5. Nistal M, González-Peramato P, Serrano A. Usefulness of histological studies in patients with the androgen insensitivity syndrome. In: Clues in the diagnosis of non-tumoral testicular pathology. Cham: Springer; 2017b. p. 41–8.

6. Tilki D, Kilic E, Tauber R, Pfeiffer D, Stief CG, Tauber R, Ergün S. The complex structure of the smooth muscle layer of spermatic veins and its potential role in the development of varicocele testis. Eur Urol. 2007;51:1402–9.

7. Kormano M, Suoranta H. Microvascular organization of the adult human testis. Anat Rec. 1971;170:31–9.

8. Genta RM, Haggitt RC. Idiopathic myointimal hyperplasia of mesenteric veins. Gastroenterology. 1991;101:533–9.

9. Rozner R, Gisriel S, Damianos J, Grimshaw AA, Rizwan R, Nawaz A, Chan K, Wan D, Pantel H, Bhutta AQ, Fenster M, Brandt LJ, Barbieri A, Robert ME, Feuerstadt P, Li DK. Idiopathic myointimal hyperplasia of the mesenteric veins: a systematic review and individual patient data regression analysis. J Gastroenterol Hepatol. 2023;38:1040–6.

10. Lincango EP, Cheong JY, Prien C, Connelly TM, Hernandez Dominguez O, Tursun N, Liska D, Lipman J, Lightner A, Kessler H, Valente MA, Hull T, Steele SR, Holubar SD. Idiopathic myointimal hyperplasia of the mesenteric veins: a systematic review of surgical management. Surgery. 2023;174:473–9.

11. Hogg ME, Vavra AK, Banerjee MN, Martinez J, Jiang Q, Keefer LK, Chambon P, Kibbe MR. The role of estrogen receptor α and β in regulating vascular smooth muscle cell proliferation is based on sex. J Surg Res. 2012;173(1):e1–10.

Venous Thrombosis. Segmental Infarction and Polypoid Granulomatous Endophlebitis

15

15.1 Venous Thrombosis

15.1.1 Spermatic Vein Thrombosis

This rare situation counts less than 30 cases published and has the following characteristics: It can affect all ages, being less frequent in the paediatric age group (6% of cases) [1]; it is generally a unilateral process, although metachronous and bilateral affectations have been described [2]; the left spermatic vein is most frequently affected, and the symptomatology is nonspecific. The preferential involvement of the left spermatic vein would be related to the compression produced by the superior mesenteric artery on the former vein (nutcracker syndrome) [3].

Clinically the most frequent symptoms are pain, which can be acute or chronic, and swelling. Given these symptoms, the following pathologies must be ruled out: epididymitis, incarcerated hernia, torsion of the spermatic cord, varicocele, spermatocele, hydrocele, and testicular tumour [4, 5]. Diagnosis requires a Döppler ultrasound examination to confirm there is no flow in the thrombosed spermatic vein. Intratesticular vascularisation is not affected. In most cases, the aetiology cannot be determined. It has been related to: varicocele, trauma, inguinal region injury, heavy exercise, prolonged sexual activity, long-hour flights, obstruction of venous drainage by a renal tumour, coagulopathies, protein C or S deficiency, factor V Leiden mutation [6], cardiac

catheterisation complications, COVID-19 infection, the manifestation of an occult cancer [7–9], the use of some drugs [10], Henoch-Schönlein purpura [11], sepsis and/or autoimmune diseases [12].

The evolution of spermatic vein thrombosis ranges from resolving spontaneously to producing pulmonary embolism [13]. Standard conservative treatment includes analgesics and anti-inflammatory drugs as well as bed rest and scrotal support plus the use of anticoagulants. Surgical exploration, with or without removal of the thrombus, would allow exclusion of other pathologies such as spermatic cord torsion, incarcerated hernia, and tumours [12, 14].

The testicle, most of the time, does not present alterations. Cases of testicular infarction secondary to spermatic vein thrombosis are exceptional [15, 16].

15.1.2 Pampiniform Plexus Thrombosis

Pampiniform plexus thrombosis is a rare situation in surgical pathology with about 26 published cases. However, it is observed in 8% of adult autopsies. It may be partial or total. In most cases, thrombosis occurs on the left side due to anatomical peculiarities of venous drainage [17], such as possible meso-aortic compression of the spermatic vein and the left renal vein (nutcracker

© The Author(s), under exclusive license to Springer Nature Switzerland AG 2024
M. Nistal, P. González-Peramato, *Testicular Vascular Lesions*,
https://doi.org/10.1007/978-3-031-57847-2_15

syndrome) [18]. Right-sided thrombosis and bilateral cases, which may present metachronically, are exceptional [19].

The clinical symptoms vary from testicular discomfort to painful swelling in the inguinoscrotal region [20, 21]. On examination, an irreducible nodular formation is observed extending from the deep inguinal ring to the superior pole of the testis. The differential diagnosis arises first with an incarcerated inguinal hernia, which has led to the practice of some unnecessary surgical interventions. Other diagnoses to consider are epididymitis, torsion of the spermatic cord or testicular appendages and both benign and malignant tumours of the spermatic cord. The correct diagnosis is provided by ultrasonography with colour Döppler study.

Aetiological factors are all those that can cause spontaneous or surgical endothelial trauma such as inguinal hernia repair or following subinguinal varicocelectomy [22], vigorous work or exercise that increase intra-abdominal pressure [10], venous stasis (long-hour flights), a state of hypercoagulability (polycythaemia vera) [23], tumours of the genitourinary tract, and the use of some drugs.

Histologically, thrombosis of one or more veins produces minimal alterations of the testicular parenchyma reminiscent of those of varicocele, and both entities may even coincide [24]. Diffuse thrombosis of the pampiniform plexus may result in testicular atrophy. There is also hyalinisation of the seminiferous tubules with a decrease of Leydig cells, which accumulate abundant lipofuscins. The rete testis is reduced to collapsed channels with frequent subepithelial microliths (Figs. 15.1, 15.2, 15.3 and 15.4).

The recommended treatment, when thrombosis affects only the pampiniform plexus, is conservative. In cases where the thrombosis extends beyond the external inguinal ring or reaches the proximity of the renal vein, excision has been proposed, in addition to anticoagulant therapy to prevent pulmonary embolism.

15.1.3 Intraparenchymal Vein Thrombosis

When studying intratesticular thrombosis three situations are observed: arterial thrombosis, venous thrombosis, and thrombosis of small vessels (arterioles, venules, and capillaries.) Thrombosis of arterial vessels has already been discussed in the chapters on arterial pathology. Therefore, only intraparenchymal vein thrombo-

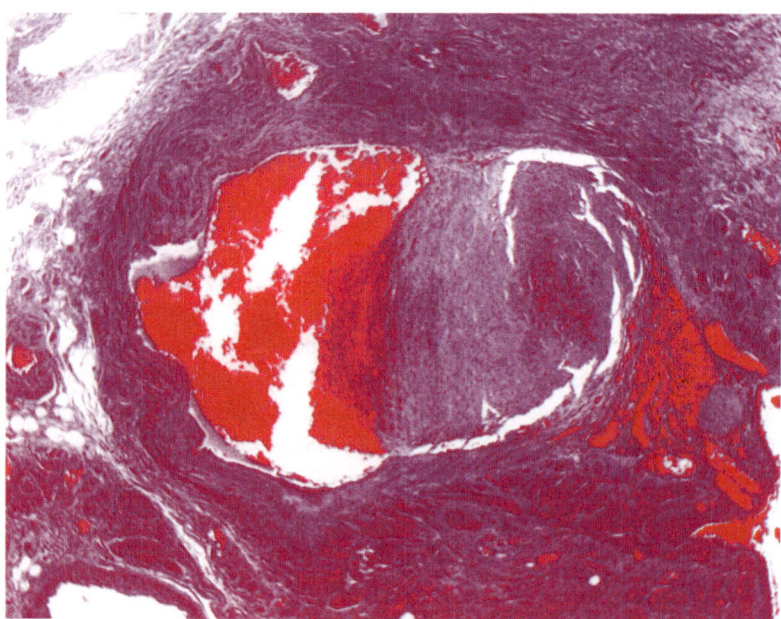

Fig. 15.1 Thrombosis of the pampiniform plexus. Vein of the pampiniform plexus with recent thrombosis. Much of the lumen is occupied by haematic material

Fig. 15.2 Old pampiniform plexus thrombosis. Most pampiniform plexus vessels show completely calcified thrombi

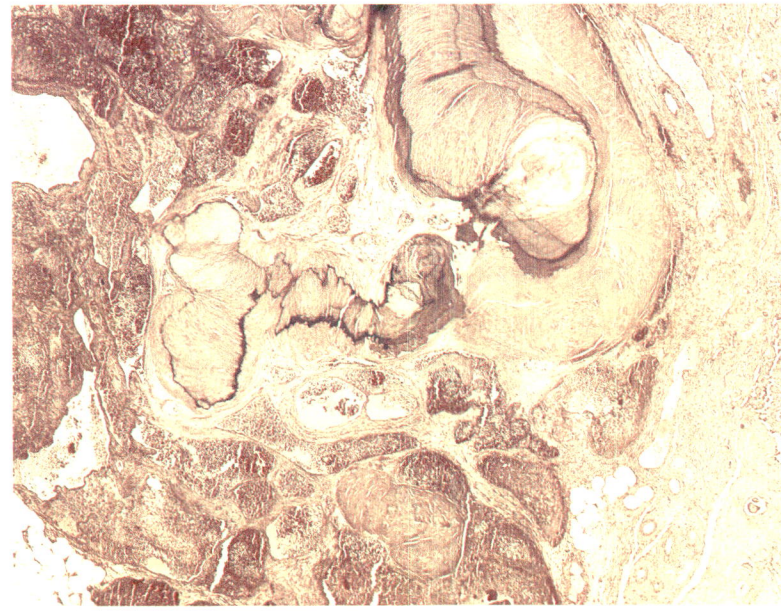

Fig. 15.3 Thrombosis of the pampiniform plexus. Sinuous aspect of the central vessel, just recognizable by the presence of a fully calcified thrombus

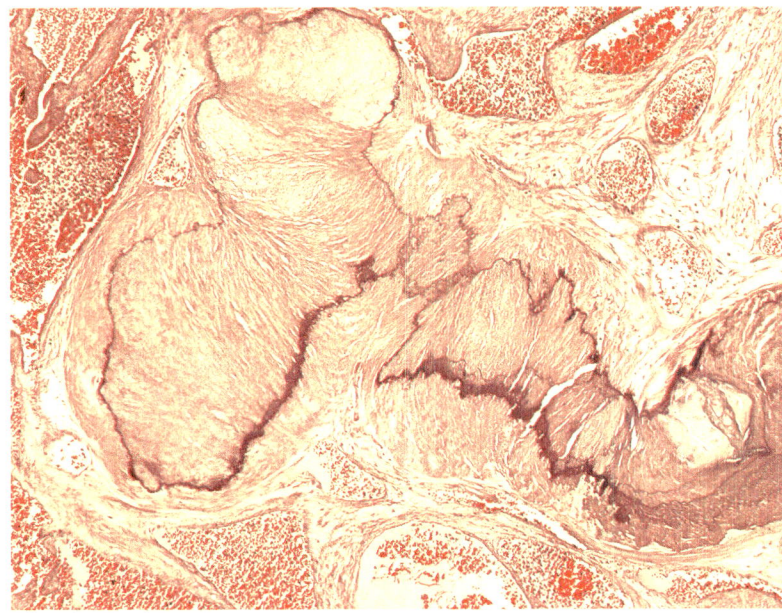

sis and small vessel thrombosis are considered in this section, two processes that have many common points in their pathogenesis.

It is well known that patients with malignant tumours such as mucosecretory adenocarcinomas and some leukaemias are carriers of a prohaemostatic state that sometimes manifests itself by venous thrombosis [25] and, at the most severe, by disseminated intravascular coagulation (DIC) [26, 27]. In solid tumours, the incidence of DIC is estimated to be 7% [28], while the figures rise in leukaemic patients from 15 to 20% in acute lymphoblastic leukaemia to 90% in those with acute promyelocytic leukaemia [29, 30]. Such high percentages are largely attributable to the deleterious effect of chemotherapy on endothelial cells [31, 32].

Fig. 15.4 Partially recanalized thrombosis in a pampiniform plexus vessel. The surrounding veins show no alterations

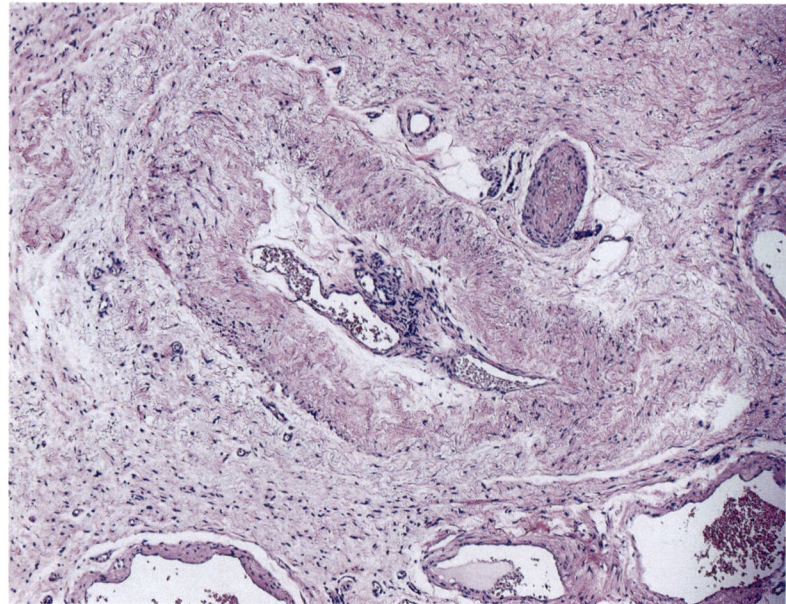

Fig. 15.5 Recanalized thrombosis of a vein with a diameter of more than 400 microns in the peritumoral parenchyma. The vessel also shows a thick fibrous wall and absence of inflammatory infiltrates

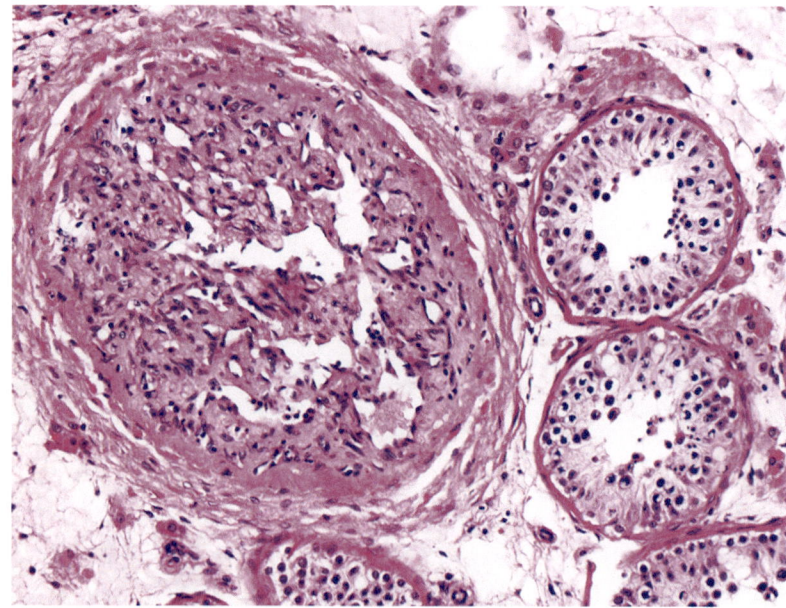

Isolated thrombosis of intraparenchymal veins. Isolated thrombosis of intraparenchymal veins, in the absence of other vascular pathology, is an exceptional event. We have only observed it in three cases in adults. In two cases, the testes were carriers of a mixed germ cell tumour. The patients had developed retroperitoneal and pulmonary metastases. The vessels affected by their calibre were centripetal or centrifugal veins and had recanalized thrombi. No pathology was recognized in smaller veins or capillaries (Figs. 15.5 and 15.6). The third case was a patient treated with androgens and antiadrogens for several years for sex change. The thrombosed veins were in the tunica vasculosa. It is possible that thrombosis is related to oestrogen treatment in which thrombosis in other organs has been reported [33].

Fig. 15.6 Recanalized thrombosis in a vein of 150 microns in diameter. The surrounding seminiferous tubules show complete but quantitatively abnormal spermatogenesis

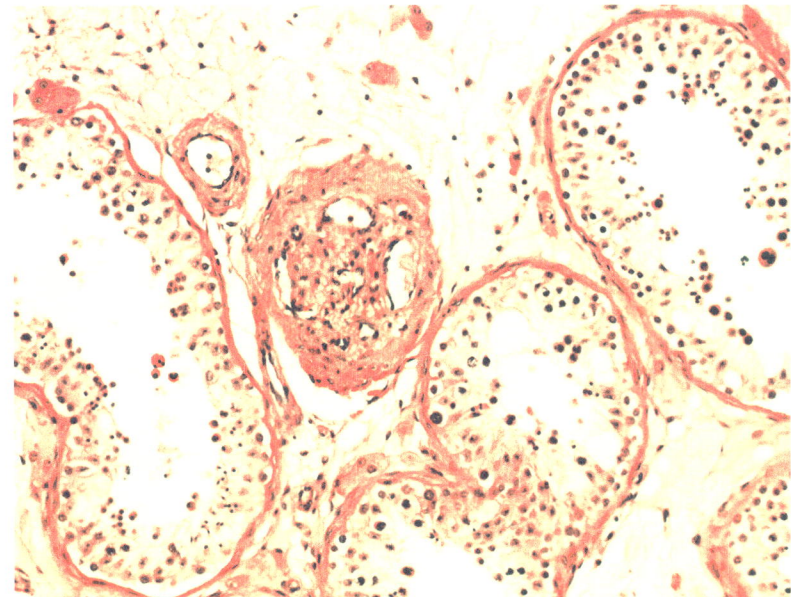

Fig. 15.7 Disseminated intravascular coagulation. Most of the small veins, distributed regularly between the seminiferous tubules, show a lumen occupied by a thrombus. There is a marked decrease in spermatogenesis

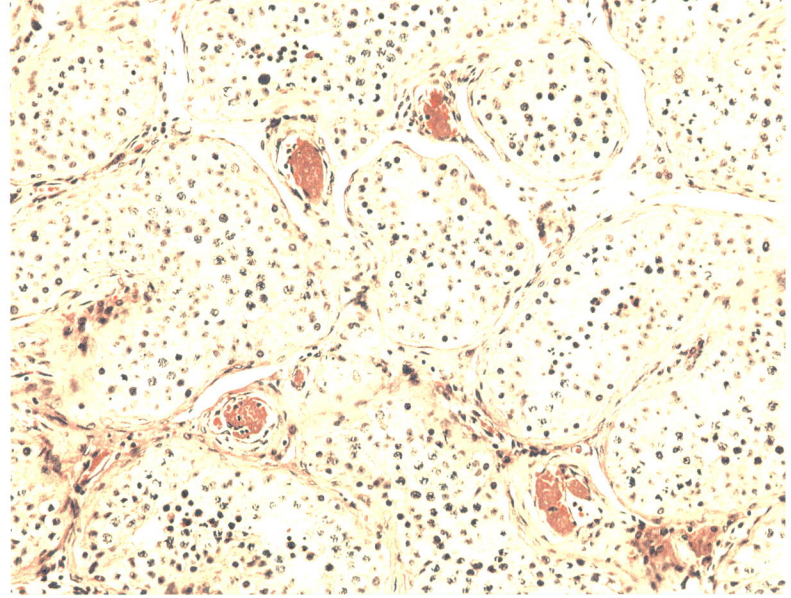

The absence of associated thromboses in paratesticular structures (epididymis, spermatic cord, testicular tunica vaginalis), although it does not rule out involvement of other organs, suggests that thrombosis would be directly related to local factors derived from tumour cells.

Thrombosis of small vessels is related to chronic forms of disseminated intravascular coagulation, whatever their aetiology, in which

thrombosis predominates over haemorrhage [34]. The thrombosed vessels are preferentially venules, capillaries, and small arterioles. The lumen is occupied by fibrino-platelet thrombi. Some thrombi are attached to the vascular wall, while others form casts in the vessel lumen and are frequently endothelialized (Figs. 15.7 and 15.8). They are not accompanied by hematic extravasation, and any inflammatory infiltrates, if

Fig. 15.8 Disseminated intravascular coagulation. Transverse and oblique sections of two completely thrombosed veins. In the neighbouring seminiferous tubules only Sertoli cells, some spermatogonia and isolated first order spermatocytes are recognized. No inflammatory infiltrates are observed

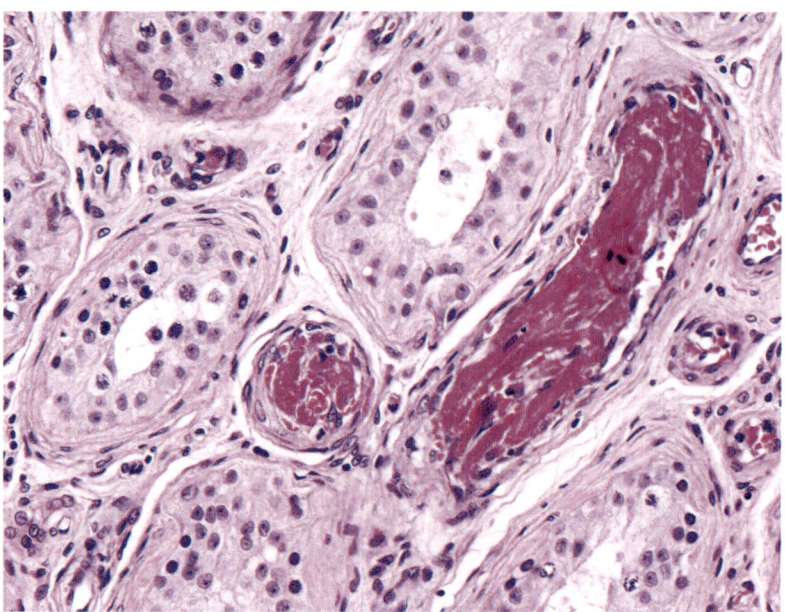

present, are minimal and focal. Multiple small, thrombosed vessels cause parenchymal ischaemia, severe seminiferous epithelial injury, and hormonal dysfunction.

15.2   Segmental Infarction

Segmental testicular infarction is rare. The left testicle is affected slightly more often due to the different vascular anatomy [35]. Even today, despite the high degree of suspicion provided by imaging techniques, a good number of cases are still diagnosed by the pathologist in the study of orchiectomy specimens.

The aetiology has been linked to infection (orchioepididymitis) [36], vasculitis, fibroplasia of the intima of the spermatic artery, previous surgery (orchidopexy, herniorrhaphy, varicocelectomy, nephrectomy) [37], sickle cell disease and polycythaemia [38], blood hypercoagulability states (such as deficiency of antithrombin III or protein S), and cholesterol thromboembolism [39]. In most cases, the exact cause is unknown and it is considered idiopathic [40, 41].

Isolated cases have been described in children, even in newborns [42], but in general, it is a pathology of young adults (20–40 years of age).

The most frequent clinical presentation is that of an acute scrotum (testicular torsion, epididymitis, orchitis, tumours, etc.). To avoid unnecessary orchiectomies, it is necessary to make a diagnostic effort. The differential diagnosis is focused on three main processes: torsion of the spermatic cord, intratesticular haematoma and testicular tumour. The imaging technique of choice is ultrasound with colour Döppler [43]. With ultrasound it is perceived as a solitary, solid, wedge-shaped or round area, with well-defined borders, of mixed or low reflectivity without predilection for an anatomical part of the testicle, which simulates a tumour [44]. The correct diagnosis is determined by the absence or decrease of Döppler flow in its interior [45].

Segmental infarction can be haemorrhagic or ischaemic depending on the venous or arterial aetiology [46] (Figs. 15.9, 15.10, 15.11 and 15.12). There is a correlation between ultrasound imaging and histology. The segmental infarcts that simulate a tumour, due to the expansive effect of the haemorrhage, are mostly venous in nature, while the most frequent cause of the others is the obstruction of an artery. These segmental arterial infarctions are preferentially located in the upper pole of the testicle, which is related with the vasculari-

Fig. 15.9 Segmental haemorrhagic infarction of the testis. Nodular, lobulated, blackish, expansive lesion occupying more than one third of the testicular parenchyma

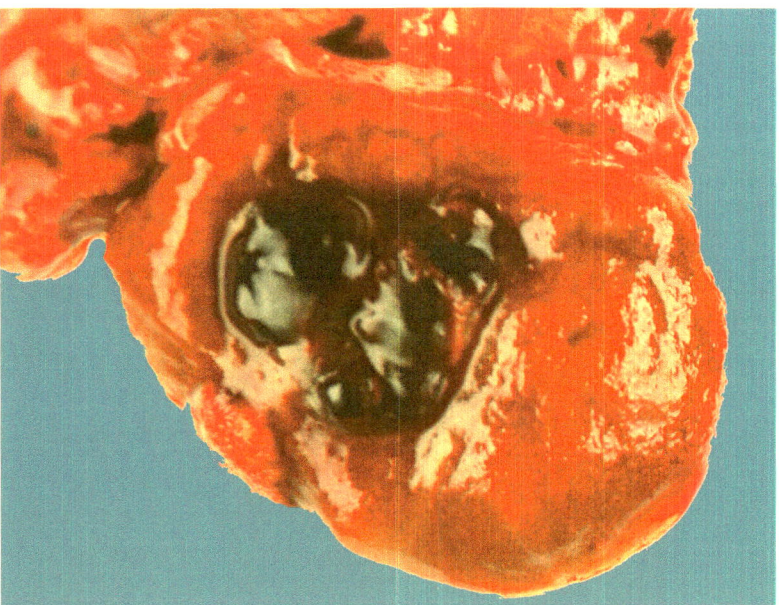

Fig. 15.10 Haemorrhagic infarction of the testicle. In the wall of the infarct, there is a zone of recent haemorrhage, a cellular area with lymphocytes and macrophages and a peripheral fibrous band. Peripherally the testicular parenchyma shows significant atrophy

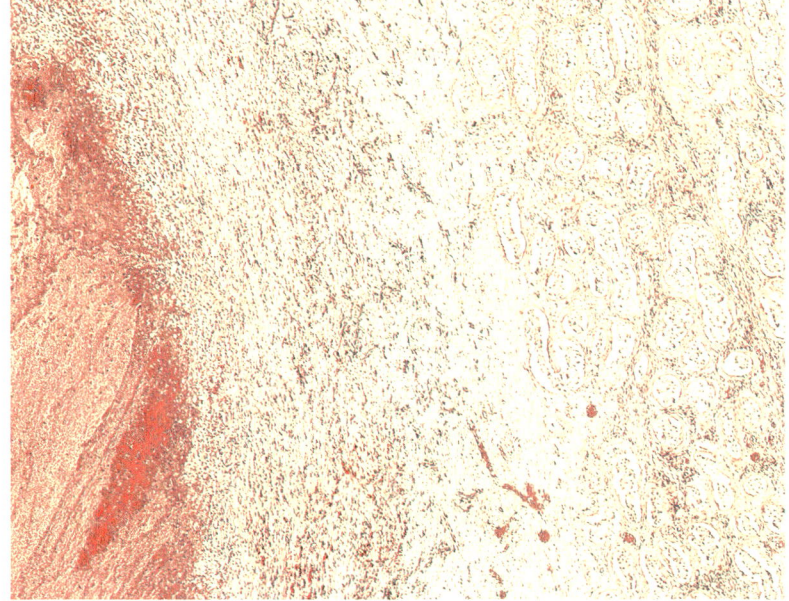

sation of the testicle. The upper pole is exclusively supplied by the testicular artery, while the lower pole receives blood from both the testicular and the deferential arteries. In this respect, it should be noted that the a single pathology, such as epididymitis, can cause both venous and arterial infarctions, and, more importantly, segmental infarctions or global infarctions of the testicle [47, 48].

Correct treatment depends on diagnostic certainty. Orchiectomy is advised in cases where malignancy cannot be excluded, with testis-sparing surgery in young patients and conservative treatment if the diagnosis is certain [49, 50]. Follow-up of conservatively treated patients at 3 months shows a decrease in infarct size [51], probably as a consequence of scar fibrosis in the infarcted area.

Fig. 15.11 Traumatic intratesticular haematoma. Subalbuginea haemorrhage with extension to a testicular lobule in a 16-year-old patient

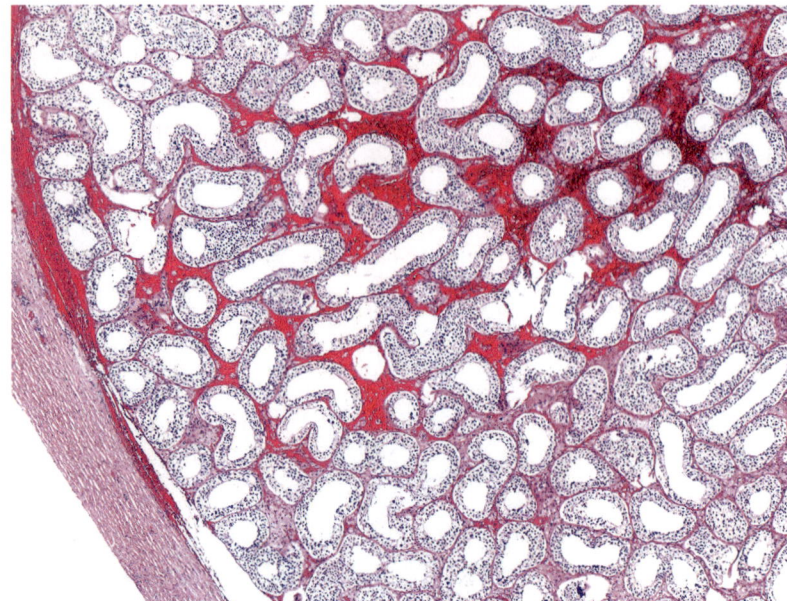

Fig. 15.12 Traumatic intratesticular haematoma. The haemorrhage extends following the interlobular septa and affecting the parenchyma of a lobule

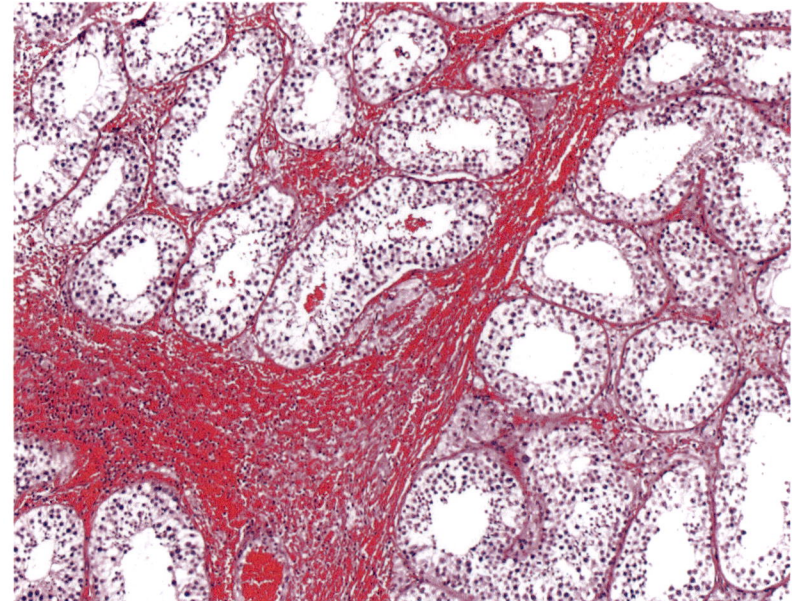

15.3 Polypoid Granulomatous Endophlebitis of the Spermatic Cord

This descriptive term refers to inflammatory vascular lesions of the veins and lymphatic vessels of the spermatic cord, preferentially associated with the presence of Schistosoma haematobium [52]. This parasite is widely distributed in the countries of the Middle East and Africa. Man is affected by bathing in water contaminated by cercariae. Cercariae penetrate through the skin and develop in the liver. Adult worms migrate to the perivesical and pelvic veins where they lay eggs and die. In some cases, he worms reach the spermatic cord and epididymis through the spermatic and deferential veins, but they do not usually reach the testicle.

At the level of the spermatic cord, they produce nodular, yellowish lesions. The testicle may suffer an infarction secondary to involvement of the testicular artery or its branches. Histologically the lesions in the spermatic cord are varied. The preferential involvement is of the veins and lymphatics. A granulomatous reaction with giant cells around the eggs predominates, but the lesion described as polypoid granulomatous endophlebitis of the spermatic cord is characteristic. Polypoid granulomatous endophlebitis is characterized by the presence of inflammatory infiltrates preferentially at the level of the intima of the spermatic veins. The infiltrates consist of polynuclear neutrophils and eosinophils and an intense multinucleated giant cell reaction. The vascular lumen appears completely obstructed most of the time; other times, the polypoid infiltrate protrudes into the vascular lumen leaving small slit-like luminae between the pedunculated inflammatory mamelons.

In some vessels, eosinophilic material is observed in relation to the inflammatory infiltrate. No eggs or worms are recognizable in most of the veins so this material could correspond to the remains of dead worms located above the lesion. Involvement of the medial and adventitial layers is limited to nonspecific infiltrates and rarely shows giant cells. Older lesions tend to become fibrotic, so that they are only recognizable as clusters of giant cells bounded peripherally by a ring of connective tissue (Figs. 15.13, 15.14, 15.15, 15.16, 15.17 and 15.18).

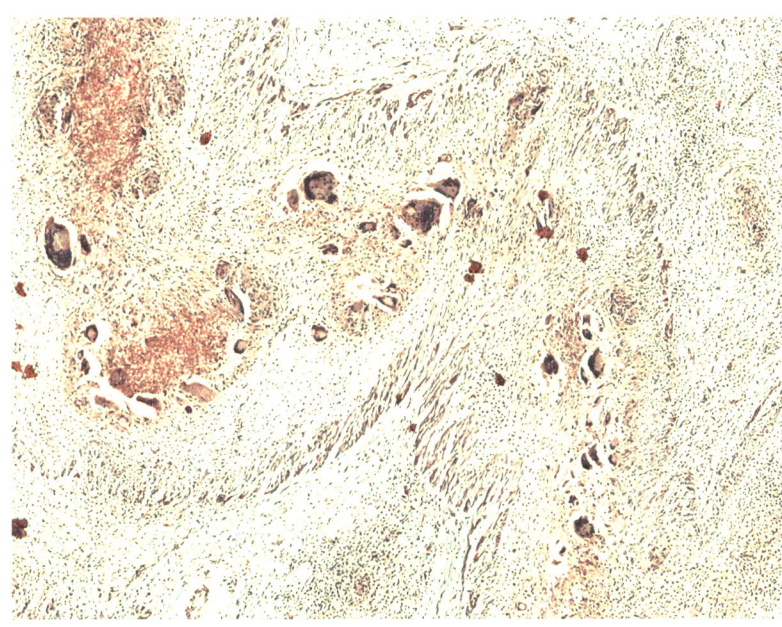

Fig. 15.13 Polypoid granulomatous endophlebitis of the spermatic cord. Venous tracts of sinuous contours show an inflammatory process in which giant cells are prominent. (Masson trichrome staining)

Fig. 15.14 Polypoid granulomatous endophlebitis of the spermatic cord. The wall of the vein occupying the centre is barely recognizable because of the intense polymorphous inflammatory infiltrate surrounding eosinophilic granular material. The inflammation also affects other vessels of the spermatic cord

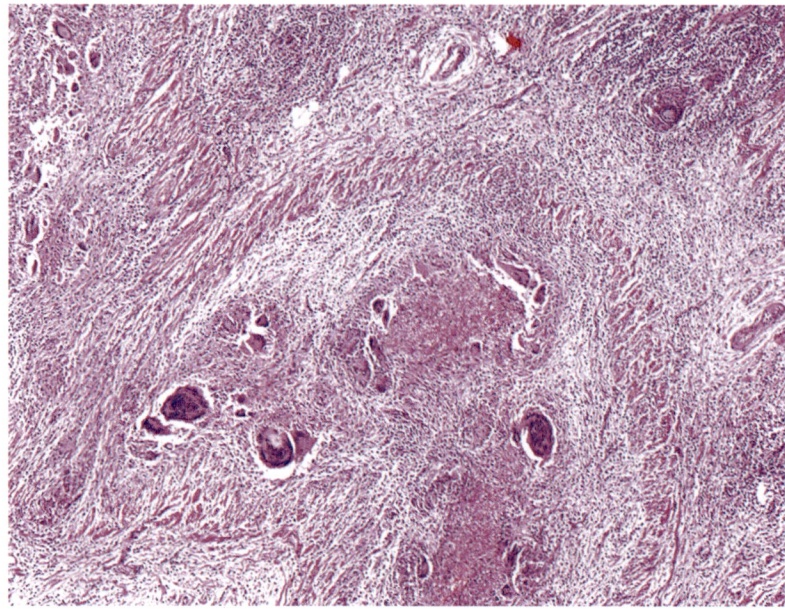

Fig. 15.15 Polypoid granulomatous endophlebitis of the spermatic cord. Cross section of a vein. The lumen is reduced to a small crescent-shaped cleft. The granulomatous inflammatory process protrudes into the lumen. The medial layer has hardly any lesions. The adventitia shows chronic nonspecific inflammation

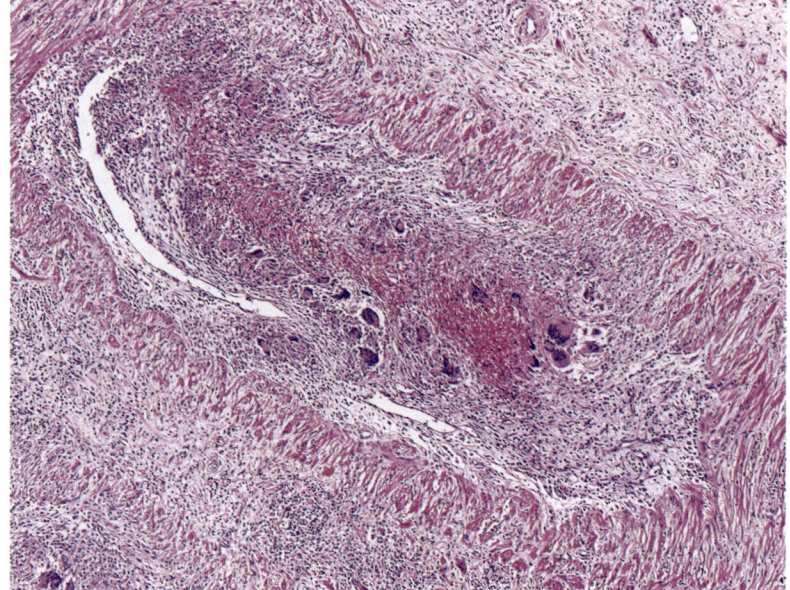

Fig. 15.16 Polypoid granulomatous endophlebitis of the spermatic cord. The lesions are centred in the intimal layer of the vein. Observe granular eosinophilic material surrounded by abundant polynuclear neutrophilic and eosinophilic leukocytes and several foreign body giant cells

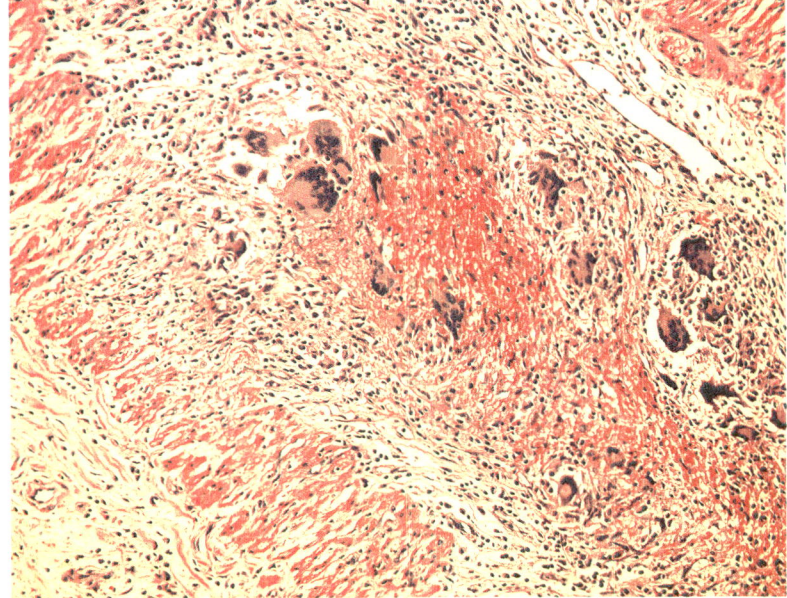

Fig. 15.17 Polypoid granulomatous endophlebitis of the spermatic cord. Cross section of a vein in the presence of inflammatory tissue involving all layers of the vessel. Foreign body giant cells are seen only in the intima

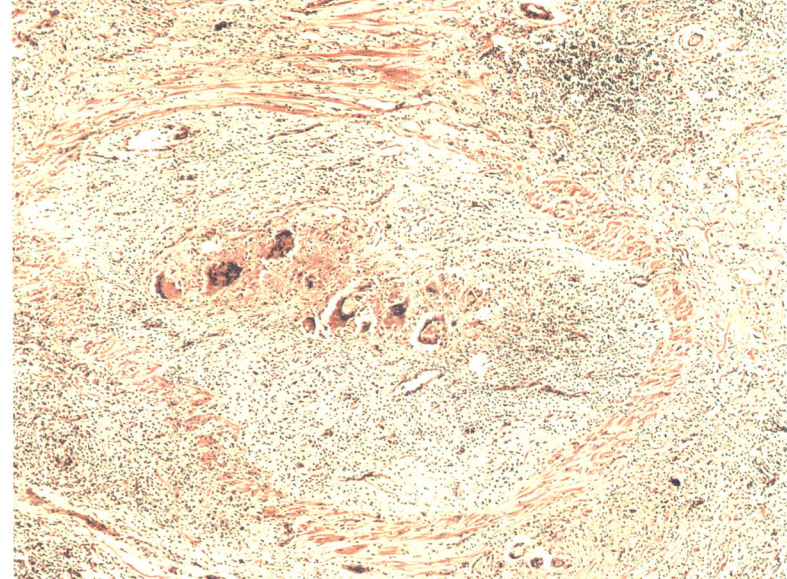

Fig. 15.18 Polypoid granulomatous endophlebitis of the spermatic cord. The presence of a granulomatous lesion with giant cells surrounded by a fibrous ring suggests an old venous lesion (Masson's trichrome staining)

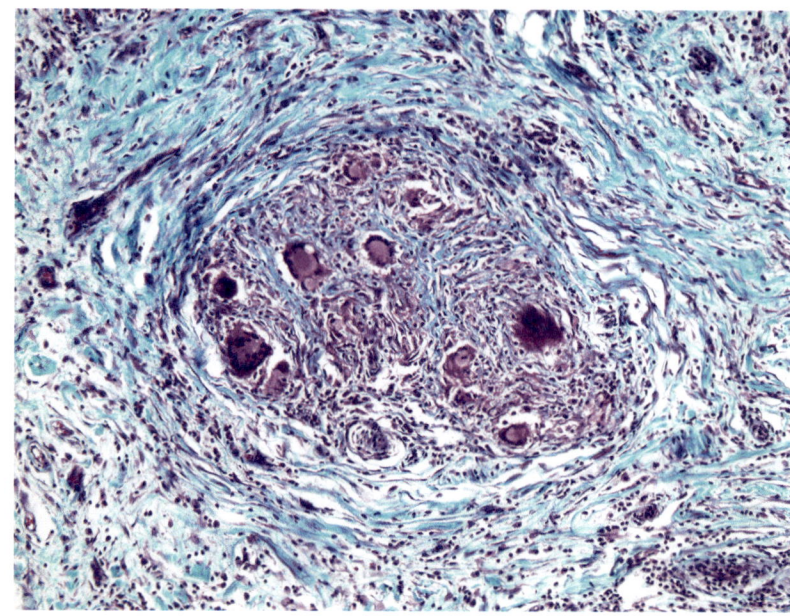

References

1. Pérez-Ardavín J, Serrano Durbá A, Miró I, Conca Baena MA, March-Villalba JA, Polo Rodrigo A, Sangüesa CC, Domínguez HC. Spontaneous spermatic vein thrombosis in pediatric patients: a condition to be considered. Cir Pediatr. 2020;33:99–101.
2. Khalil IA, Mohammed H, Aldeeb M, Hatem M, Alani A, Al-Jalham K. Metachronous bilateral spontaneous spermatic vein thrombosis: a rare cause of orchialgia. Urol Case Rep. 2022;45:102234.
3. Kurklinsky AK, Rooke TW. Nutcracker phenomenon and nutcracker syndrome. Mayo Clin Proc. 2010;85:552–9.
4. Kleinclauss F, Della Negra E, Martin M, Bernardini S, Bittard H. Thrombose spontanée d'une varicocèle gauche [spontaneous thrombosis of left varicocele]. Prog Urol. 2001;1:95–6.
5. Sigalos JT, Pastuszak AW. Chronic orchialgia: epidemiology, diagnosis and evaluation. Transl Androl Urol. 2017;6:S37–43.
6. Bolat D, Gunlusoy B, Yarimoglu S, Ozsinan F, Solmaz S, Imamoglu FG. Isolated thrombosis of right spermatic vein with underlying factor V Leiden mutation. Can Urol Assoc J. 2016;10:E324–7.
7. Gleeson MJ, McDermott M, McDonald G, McDermott TE. Spontaneous thrombosis of the left spermatic vein. Br J Urol. 1992;70:567.
8. Lenz CJ, McBane RD, Cohoon KP, Janczak DT, Simmons BS, Saadiq RA, Mimier M, Casanegra AI, Daniels PR, Wysokinski WE. Testicular vein thrombosis: incidence of recurrent venous thromboembolism and survival. Eur J Haematol. 2018;100:83–7.
9. Kolleri JJ, Abdirahman AM, Mahmood NS, Ladumor S, Hameed S. Spontaneous bilateral spermatic vein thrombosis: a rare clinical presentation. Cureus. 2021;13:e20161.
10. Kayes O, Patrick N, Sengupta A. A peculiar case of bilateral, spontaneous thromboses of the pampiniform plexi. Ann R Coll Surg Engl. 2010;92:W22–3.
11. Diana A, Gaze H, Laubscher B, De Meuron G, Tschantz P. A case of pediatric Henoch-Schönlein purpura and thrombosis of spermatic veins. J Pediatr Surg. 2000;35:1843.
12. Murthy PB, Gill BC, Khurana S, Nyame YA, Sabanegh ES, Kaouk JH. Spermatic vein thrombosis. Urology. 2018;119:32–4.
13. Castillo OA, Diaz M, Vitagliano GJ, Metrebian E. Pulmonary thromboembolism secondary to left spermatic vein thrombosis: a case report. Urol Int. 2008;80:217–8.
14. Petca RC, Popescu RI, Călin C, Budău M, Petca A, Jinga V. Left spermatic vein thrombosis—an uncommon diagnosis: a case report. Chirurgia (Bucur). 2020;115:505–10.
15. Coolsaet B, Weinberg R. Thrombosis of the spermatic vein in children. J Urol. 1980;124:290–1.
16. Maas C, Müller-Hansen I, Flechsig H, Poets CF. Acute scrotum in a neonate caused by renal vein thrombosis. Arch Dis Child Fetal Neonatal Ed. 2011;96(2):F149–50.
17. Hashimoto L, Vibeto B. Spontaneous thrombosis of the pampiniform plexus. Scand J Urol Nephrol. 2006;40:252–4.
18. Rudloff U, Holmes RJ, Prem JT, Faust GR, Moldwin R, Siegel D. Mesoaortic compression of the left renal vein (nutcracker syndrome): case reports and review of the literature. Ann Vasc Surg. 2006;20:120–9.
19. Bakshi S. Bilateral spontaneous thrombosis of the pampiniform plexus mimicking incarcerated inguinal hernia: case report of a rare condition and literature review. Surg Case Rep. 2020;6:47.

20. Tanner R, Twomey M, Maher MM, Fitzgerald E, O'Connor J. A rare cause of testicular pain: thrombosis of the Pampiniform plexus. Ir Med J. 2016;109:347–8.

21. Amador Robayna A, Rodríguez Talavera J, Ballesta Martínez B, Falcón Barroso J, Carrión Valencia A, Orribo Morales N, Santacruz Pérez M, Monllor GJ. Deep vein thrombosis: a rare cause of acute testicular pain. Case report: literature review. Urol Int. 2018;101:117–20.

22. Zampieri N, Castellani R, Mantovani A, Scirè G, Peretti M, Zampieri G, Camoglio FS. Thromboses of the pampiniform plexi after subinguinal varicocelectomy. Pediatr Surg Int. 2014;30:441–4.

23. Jacobs J, Sharma D, Vnencak-Jones C. The first report of a JAK2 V617F-positive myeloproliferative neoplasm with initial manifestation as a rare pampiniform venous plexus thrombosis and review of the literature. J Thromb Thrombolysis. 2022;53:213–7.

24. Ouanes Y, Sellami A, Chaker K, Mokhtar B, Ben Rhouma S, Nouira Y. Thrombosis of the pampiniform plexus: about a case report. Urol Case Rep. 2018;20:28–9.

25. Sack GH, Levin J, Bell WR. Trousseau's syndrome and other manifestations of chronic disseminated coagulopathy in patients with neoplasmas: clinical pathophysiologic and therapeutic features. Medicine (Baltimore). 1977;56:1–37.

26. Levi M. Disseminated intravascular coagulation in cancer patients. Best Pract Res Clin Haematol. 2009;22:129–36.

27. Levi M. Cancer-related coagulopathies. Thromb Res. 2014;133:S70–S5.

28. Sallah S, Wan JY, Nguyen NP, Hanrahan LR, Sigounas G. Disseminated intravascular coagulation in solid tumors: clinical and pathological study. Thromb Haemost. 2001;86:828–33.

29. Barbui T, Falanga A. Disseminated intravascular coagulation in acute leukemia. Semin Thromb Hemost. 2001;27:593–604.

30. Avvisati G, ten Cate JW, Sturk A, Lamping R, Petti MG, Mandelli F. Acquired alpha-2-antiplasmin deficiency in acute promyelocytic leukaemia. Br J Haematol. 1988;70:43–8.

31. Falanga A. Mechanisms of hypercoagulation in malignancy and during chemotherapy. Haemostasis. 1998;28(Suppl 3):50–60.

32. Levi M. Management of cancer-associated disseminated intravascular coagulation. Thromb Res. 2016;140:S66–70.

33. Gerstman BB, Piper JM, Tomita DK, Ferguson WJ, Stadel BV, Lundin FE. Oral contraceptive estrogen dose and the risk of deep venous thromboembolic disease. Am J Epidemiol. 1991;133(1):32–7.

34. Nistal M, González-Peramato P, Serrano A. Vascular pathology related to extracellular material accumulation. In: Clues in the diagnosis of non-tumoral testicular pathology. Springer, Cham; 2017. p. 219–22.

35. Bertolotto M, Derchi LE, Sidhu PS, Serafni G, Valentino M, Grenier N, Cova MA. Acute segmental testicular infarction at contrast-enhanced ultra sound:

36. Bird K, Rosenfield AT. Testicular infarction secondary to acute inflammatory disease: demonstration by B-scan ultrasound. Radiology. 1984;152:785–8.

37. West S, Karamsadkar S, Cross S. Segmental testicular infarction following nephrectomy. Radiol Case Rep. 2018;14:278–81.

38. Fernández-Pérez GC, Tardáguila FM, Velasco M, Rivas C, Dos Santos J, Cambronero J, Trinidad C, San MP. Radiologic findings of segmental testicular infarction. AJR Am J Roentgenol. 2005;184:1587–93.

39. Adachi S, Tsutahara K, Kinoshita T, Hatano K, Kinouchi T, Kobayashi M, Inoue H, Takada T, Hara T, Yamaguchi S. Segmental testicular infarction due to cholesterol embolism: not the first case, but the first report. Pathol Int. 2008;58:745–8.

40. Nistal M, Palacios J, Regadera J, Paniagua R. Postsurgical focal testicular infarct. Urol Int. 1986;41:149–51.

41. Gianfrilli D, Isidori AM, Lenzi A. Segmental testicular ischaemia: presentation, management and follow-up. Int J Androl. 2009;32:524–31.

42. Penson DF, Aronson WJ. Segmental testicular infarction in the neonate: a case report. J Urol. 1995;153:1992–3.

43. Dewbury KC. Scrotal ultrasonography: an update. BJU Int. 2000;86(Suppl 1):143–52.

44. Bilagi P, Sriprasad S, Clarke JL, Sellars ME, Muir GH, Sidhu PS. Clinical and ultrasound features of segmental testicular infarction: six-year experience from a single Centre. Eur Radiol. 2007;17:2810–8.

45. Sriprasad S, Kooiman GG, Muir GH, Sidhu PS. Acute segmental testicular infarction: differentiation from tumour using high frequency colour Doppler ultrasound. Br J Radiol. 2001;74:965–7.

46. Jordan GH. Segmental hemorrhagic infarct of testicle. Urology. 1987;29:60–3.

47. Eisner DJ, Goldman SM, Petronis J, Millmond SH. Bilateral testicular infarction caused by epididymitis. AJR Am J Roentgenol. 1991;157:517–9.

48. Heaney C, Friedman D, Akgul M, Rehfuss A. Epididymo-Orchitis leading to global testicular infarction in a pediatric patient—a case report. Urology. 2023;173:e26–9.

49. Shen YH, Lin YW, Zhu XW, Cai BS, Li J, Zheng XY. Segmental testicular infarction: a case report. Exp Ther Med. 2015;9:758–60.

50. Jin HL, Ma Q, Zhu J, Zang YC, Zhou YB, Xue BX, Yang DR, Sun CY, Gao J, Xu LJ, Zhang B. A case report of acute testicular pain secondary to segmental testicular infarction. BMC Urol. 2022;22:52.

51. Sentilhes L, Dunet F, Thoumas D, Khalaf A, Grise P, Pfster C. Seg mental testicular infarction: diagnosis and strategy. Can J Urol. 2002;9:1698–701.

52. Elbadawi A, Khuri FJ, Cockett AT. Polypoid granulomatous and sclerosing endophlebitis of spermatic cord: new pathologic type of schistosomal funiculitis. Urology. 1979;13:309–14.

The lymphatic vessels of the testis are preferentially located in the tunica vasculosa, interlobular septa, and mediastinum (Fig. 1). The perilymphatic spaces in the interstitium are much less developed than in other mammals such as mice, rats, guinea pigs, and ruminants, in which there are true lymphatic vessels [1, 2] (Fig. 2). In the epididymis, the lymphatic vessels are highly developed at the level of the head, between the efferent ducts, and, to a lesser degree, along the main duct of the epididymis (Fig. 3). While the wall of the intratesticular lymphatic vessels and the epididymis consists only of endothelial cells, a discontinuous basal lamina and isolated smooth muscle cells, in the spermatic cord there are collectors with a wall with abundant smooth muscle cells irregularly arranged in the medial layer and numerous

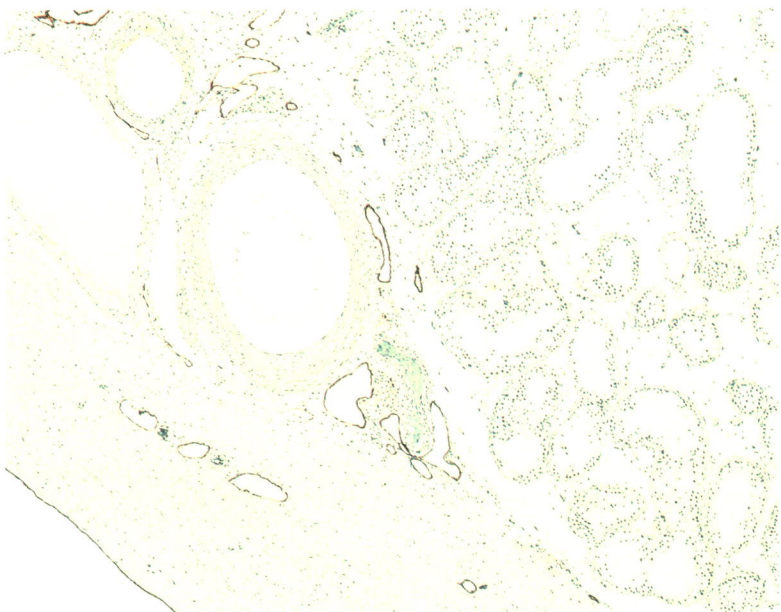

Fig. 1 Lymphatic vessels are arranged in the tunica vasculosa around arteries and veins. Others are recognized in the full thickness of the albuginea. Immunostaining of endothelial cells with D2-40 allows them to be perfectly identified

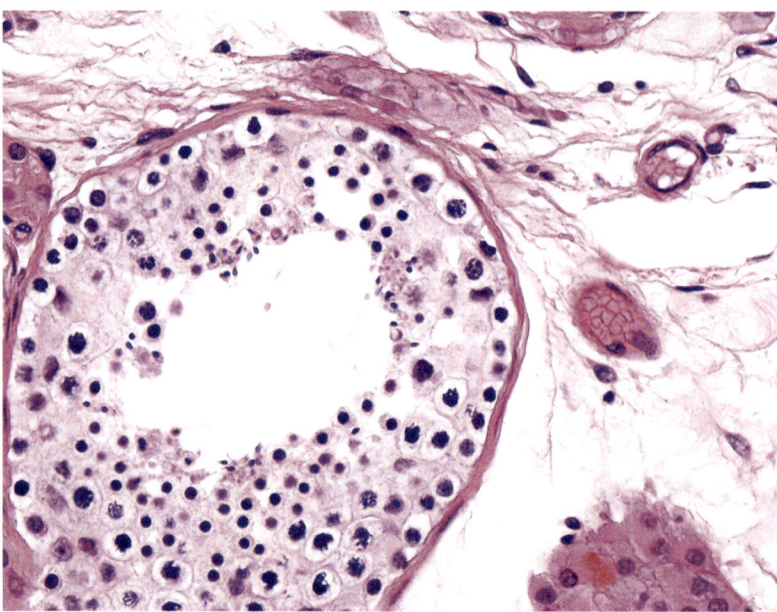

Fig. 2 Lymphatic vessels are not usually observed between the seminiferous tubules. Some of the indentations probably correspond to perilymphatic spaces

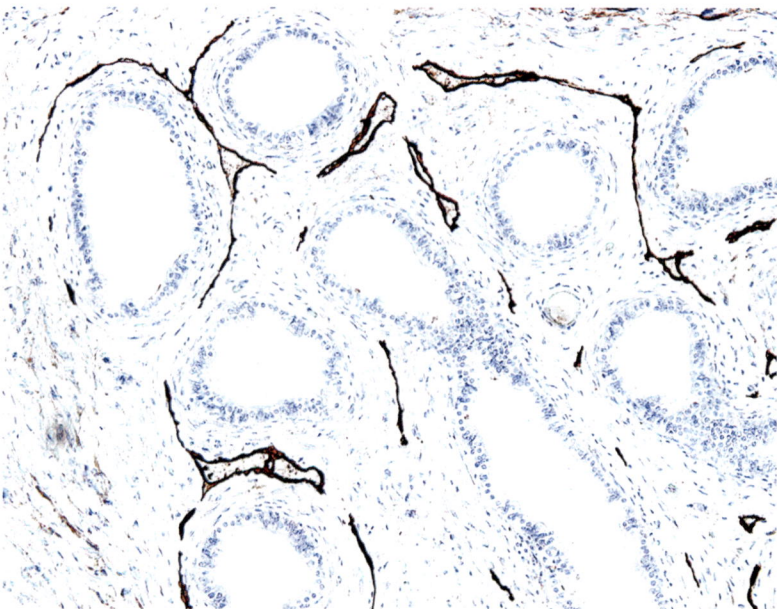

Fig. 3 The epididymal head has a rich network of lymphatic vessels distributed both around the efferent ducts and in the intertubular connective tissue (D2-40)

valves [3] (Fig. 4). Another structure containing numerous lymphatic vessels is the appendix testis (Fig. 5). The significance of this fact is unknown.

In the tunica vaginalis parietalis, the lymphatic vessels are arranged in two plexuses, a superficial one, in the submesothelial layer, and a deeper one, above the dense connective tissue plane. They are interconnected by thin vessels irregularly perpendicular to the surface (Fig. 6).

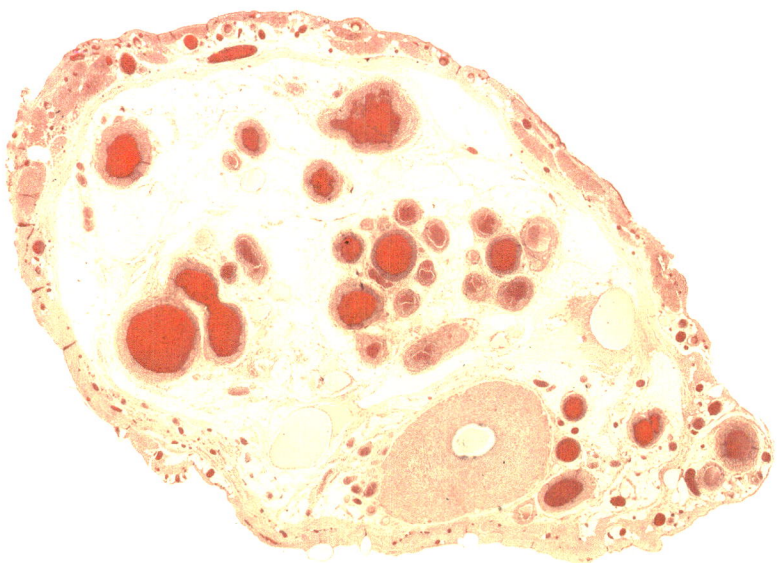

Fig. 4 Cross section of the spermatic cord. The larger lymphatic collectors are preferentially arranged in the spermatic compartment. The lymphatic vessels of the deferential and cremasteric compartments are generally scarce and smaller

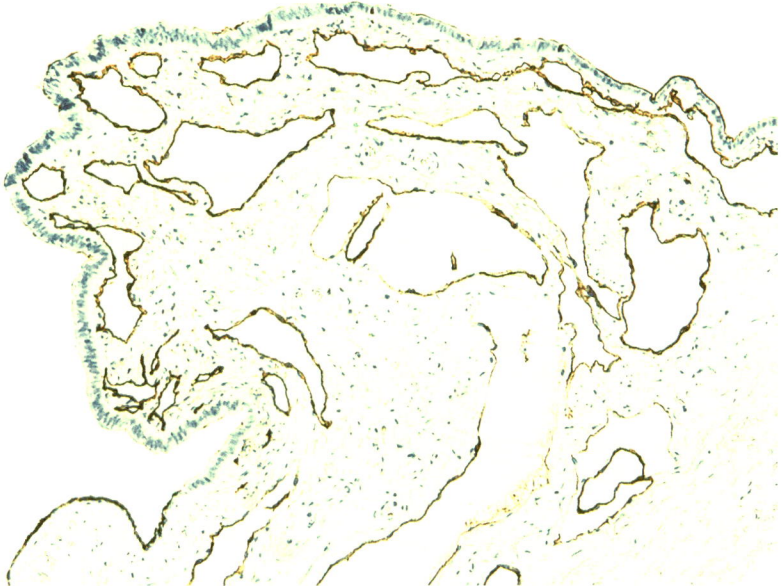

Fig. 5 The testicular appendix has numerous lymphatic vessels both under and within the epithelial lining (D2-40). Positivity for D2-40 of the normal mesothelium is observed in the lower part of the lining

The superficial plexus is closely related to the mesothelium. It is formed by specialized drainage units called lacunae, the terminal portion of the lymphatic vessels, and which are arranged parallel to the surface.

The mesothelium is lined by two different cell types. The flat mesothelial cells are the most abundant, are poor in organelles, and these are located

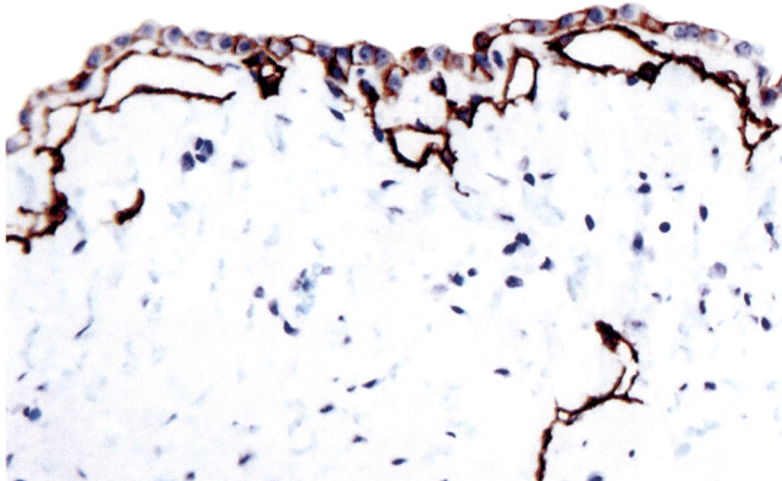

Fig. 6 The parietal sheet of the testicular tunica vaginalis has abundant lymphatic vessels. Under the mesothelium, lying parallel to it, is the submesothelial plexus. Several flattened lymphatic lacunae are observed (D-240)

in the vicinity of the nucleus, these cells have abundant microvilli. Cubic mesothelial cells are clustered together giving the mesothelial surface a paving stone-like appearance. They have a larger nucleus, a prominent nucleolus, and, in the cytoplasm, abundant mitochondria, large development of the rough endoplasmic reticulum and Golgi complex, as an expression of their increased activity. They also have abundant actin microfilaments of 5 nm in diameter. Lymphatic stomata are formed between these cubic cells [4].

The lymphatic stomata measure 1–2 microns in diameter and are partially occluded by digitating extensions of the surrounding mesothelial cells. The submesothelial connective tissue beneath the lymphatic stomata is called macula cribriformis and has a large number of perforations 3–5 microns in diameter. Cytoplasmic extensions of endothelial cells from the underlying lymphatic lacunae extend through these perforations. These cells come into contact with the mesothelial cells of lymphatic stomata [5]. Identification of lymphatic vessel endothelial cells is usually done with podoplanin (D2-40) [6], but, as this marker can also be expressed in mesothelial cells, it is convenient to use another mesothelial marker such as cytokeratin 7 (CK7) in addition. The physiological function of the lymphatic stomata is to serve as channels for the drainage of fluid from the serous cavities.

The following are included among the non-tumorous lesions in the following chapters: Hydrocele as an example of difficulties in the reabsorption of fluid from the vaginal cavity. Primary testicular lymphangiectasia as a manifestation of a congenital malformation and lymphangiectasia secondary to obstruction of lymphatic drainage as an acquired process. And for the first time, a histological picture is described and the name of pseudolymphangiectasia or of microcystic testicular oedema that simulates testicular lymphangiectasia is proposed. Tumour pathology has included lymphangioma, benign lymphangioendothelioma, and haemangiolymphangioma.

References

1. Fawcett DW, Heidger PM, Leak LV. Lymph vascular system of the interstitial tissue of the testis as revealed by electron microscopy. J Reprod Fertil. 1969;19:109–19
2. Okraszewska E, Cendrowska I, Jedrzejewski KS. The intratesticular lymphatic network in men, bulls and rams. Folia Morphol (Warsz). 1996;55:401–2.
3. Holstein AF, Orlandini GE, Möller R. Distribution and fine structure of the lymphatic system in the human testis. Cell Tissue Res. 1979;200:15–27.
4. Wang ZB, Li M, Li JC. Recent advances in the research of lymphatic stomata. Anat Rec (Hoboken). 2010;293:754–61
5. Wang J, Ping Z, Jiang T, Yu H, Wang C, Chen Z, Zhang X, Xu D, Wang L, Li Z, Li JC. Ultrastructure of lymphatic stomata in the tunica vaginalis of humans. Microsc Microanal. 2013;19:1405–9.
6. Cîmpean AM, Raica M, Izvernariu DA, Tătucu D. Lymphatic vessels identified with podoplanin. Comparison of immunostaining with three different detection systems. Rom J Morphol Embryol. 2007;48:139–43.

16.1 Chronic Hydrocele

Normally, between the two layers of the testicular tunica vaginalis, visceral, and parietal, there is a small amount of fluid that is continuously renewed; the fluid comes from the testicular parenchyma, crosses the albuginea, which behaves as a semi-permeable membrane, and is reabsorbed by the mesothelium of the parietal layer. Hydroceles are abnormal collections of this fluid between the two layers of the tunica vaginalis of the testis. The incidence of hydrocele in the general population is 1% [1]. Hydroceles can be congenital (primary) or acquired (secondary).

A congenital hydrocele is caused by failure of obliteration of the processus vaginalis. The testes begin to develop in the retroperitoneum, close to the kidney. As they descend into the scrotum through the inguinal canal, they are accompanied by a fold of peritoneum, the processus vaginalis. Normally obliteration starts from the upper portion of the vaginal process. It is usually completed in term foetuses or during the first year of life. Distally, the lower part persists as the tunica vaginalis and covers the testis on its anterior, lateral, and medial surface as well as part of the head of the epididymis.

Four types of primary hydroceles are distinguished: congenital hydrocele, infantile hydrocele, encysted hydrocele, and vaginal hydrocele. Abdomino-scrotal hydrocele is a congenital hydrocele in which there is no obliteration of the vaginal process and there is direct communication between the fluid in the abdominal cavity and the testis [2, 3]. In infantile hydrocele, there is an obliteration of the vaginal process at the level of the deep inguinal ring, thus allowing abundant fluid to accumulate distally [4]. Encysted hydrocele is the result of fluid accumulation at the level of the spermatic cord when the proximal and distal portions of the vaginal process are obliterated while the middle portion remains patent [5]. In vaginal hydrocele, the vaginal process is normally obliterated, and fluid accumulates around the testis [6].

Secondary hydroceles are related to a previous underlying pathology which may be inflammatory (filariasis, tuberculosis of the epididymis, (or) syphilis...) [7, 8], traumatic [9], a previous surgical intervention in the inguinal region or scrotum [10], testicular torsion or its embryonic appendages, tumoural [11] or hypoproteinaemia due to a systemic disease. In third world countries, the most frequent cause is parasitic diseases such as filariasis, which is responsible for the larger hydroceles.

In chronic hydroceles, mesothelial cell fluid reabsorption capacity is exceeded, and, meanwhile, the opening of the lymphatic stomata provides useful drainage channels for vaginal fluid for some time. Their diameter, normally only observable under the microscope, can reach more than 20 microns, even allowing the passage of cells like macrophages in one direction or the other, or of tumour cells, bacteria, or drugs.

Fig. 16.1 Mesothelial stomas. Patient with chronic, noninflammatory hydrocele. Parietal layer of the testicular tunica vaginalis. A lymphatic cistern is seen beneath the mesothelial lining. The central protrusion into the mesothelium corresponds to a lymphatic stoma

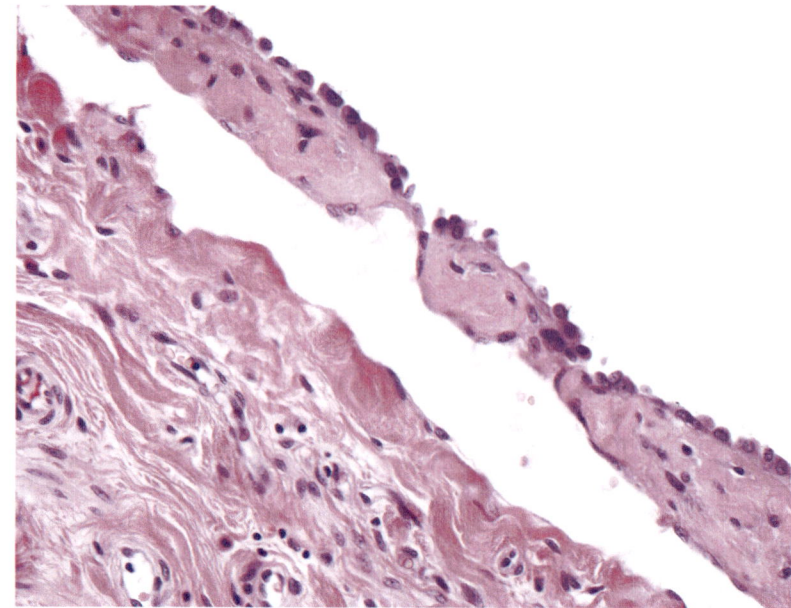

Fig. 16.2 The lymphatic stomata are in the areas of the mesothelial lining where the lymphatic stomata have a cubic appearance. In the central part the lymphatic cistern cells are separated from the mesothelial cells by a thin basal lamina

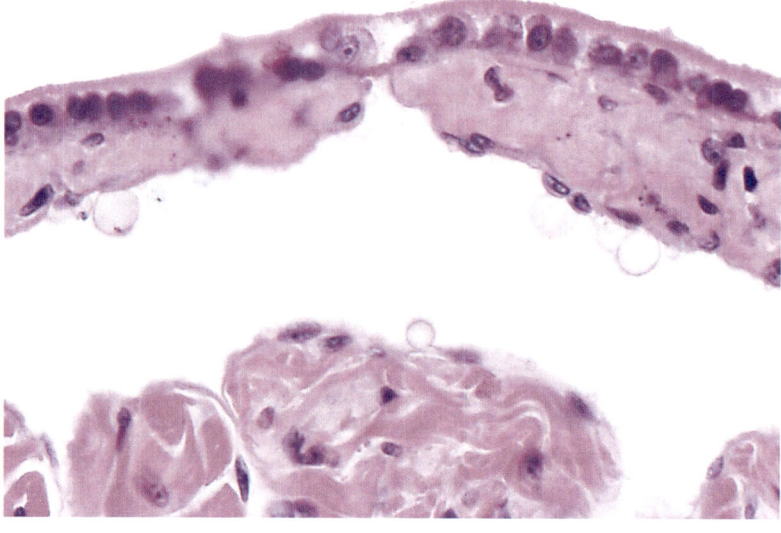

Opening and closing is regulated by cytokines, VEGF, angiotensin II and NO. But their function is lost if obstructive pathology in the lymphatic vessels of the spermatic cord or in the retroperitoneal nodes into which they drain is associated (Figs. 16.1, 16.2, 16.3, 16.4, 16.5 and 16.6).

When treating hydrocele, it is important to keep in mind the age of the patient, the size of the hydrocele and the severity of the symptoms [12]. Hydrocelectomy is the gold standard for the treatment of hydrocele. Over the years, this surgical treatment has gradually become more minimally invasive [13, 14], reducing complications such as scrotal haematoma, wound infection, persistent scrotal pain or even infertility [15].

Fig. 16.3 The mesothelium formed by cubic cells with ample eosinophilic cytoplasm and their nucleus displaced towards the surface presents a solution of continuity that contacts in the deepest part with the endothelium of the lymphatic capillaries that cross the cribriform macula (CD31)

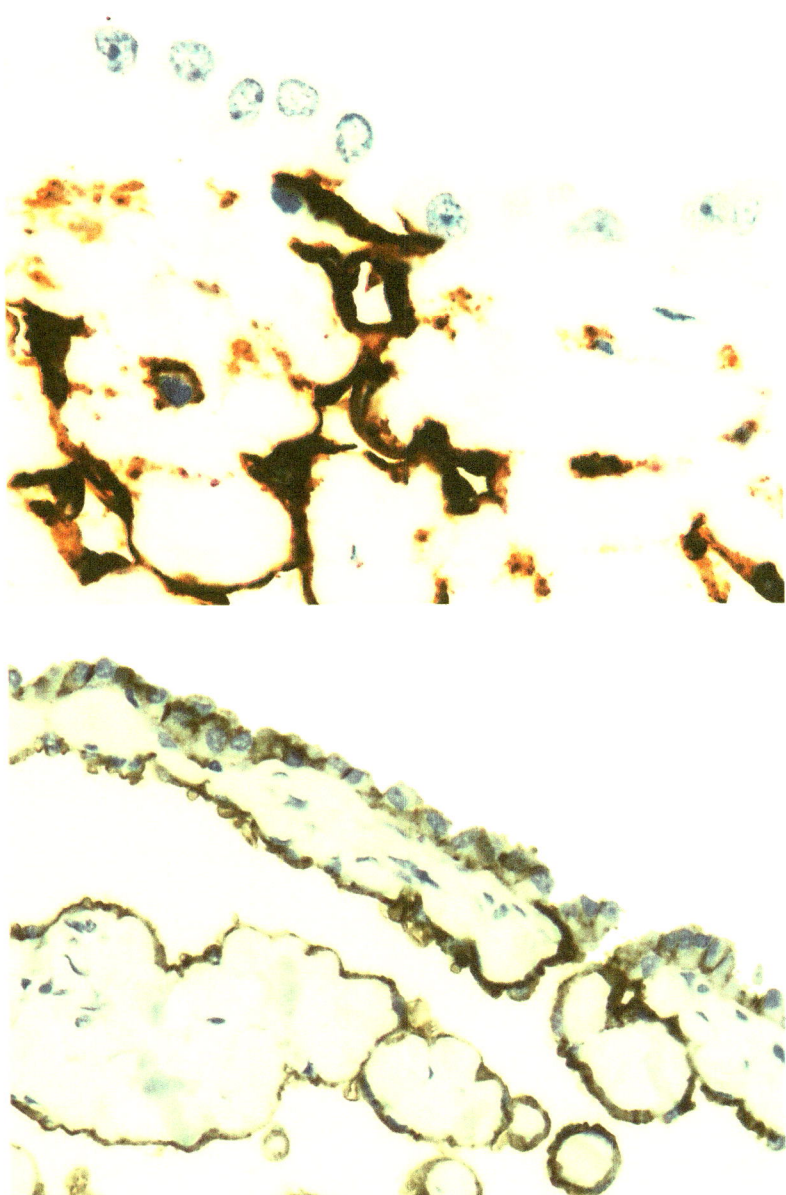

Fig. 16.4 Open lymphatic stomata. The lymphatic cisterns communicate with the vaginal cavity through a narrow channel (D2–40)

Fig. 16.5 Marked dilatation of all the lymphatic vessels of the parietal layer of the tunica vaginalis. The most superficial vessels are in continuity with the vaginal cavity through a very open lymphatic stoma (CD31)

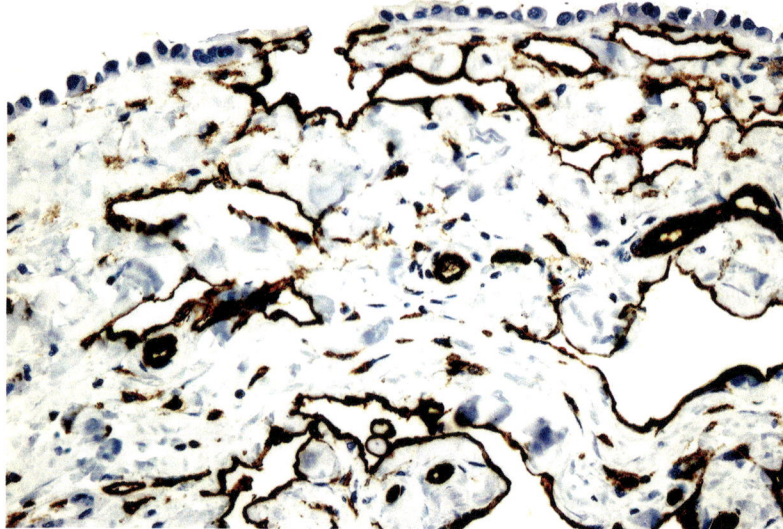

Fig. 16.6 Intense opening of a lymphatic stomata exceeding 50 microns associated with dilatations of the lymphatic lacunae and the lymphatic vessels draining them (D2–40)

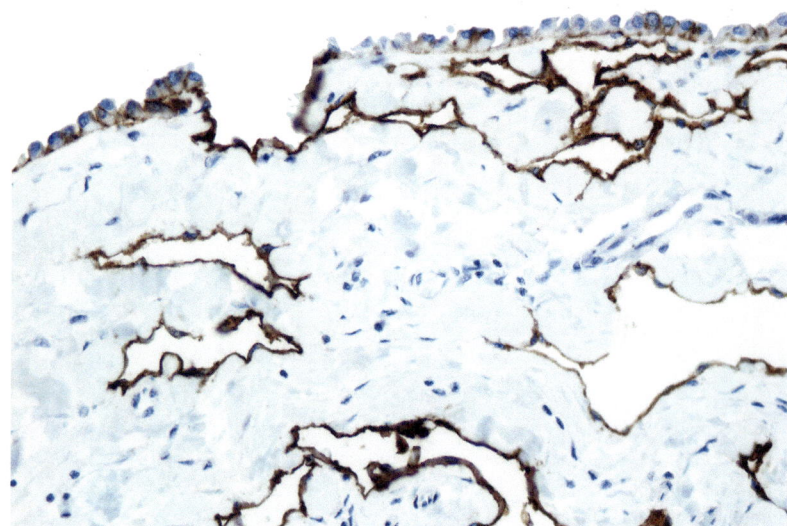

16.2   Scrotal Elephantiasis

This syndrome is characterized by enlargement of the scrotum and perineal area secondary to chronic lymphedema produced by obstruction of lymphatic drainage at any level from the testicle to the inter-aortocaval and para-caval lymph nodes where most of the collecting vessels drain. Two forms are distinguished, tropic elephantiasis and elephantiasis nostras verrucosa.

Tropic elephantiasis is the most frequent. It is caused in more than 90% of cases by infec-

tion by a nematode belonging to the Filariodidea family, Wuchereria bancrofti, or by Brugia malayi and Brugia timori in the remaining cases [16]. Infection occurs when mosquitoes transmit filarial parasites to humans [17]. The diagnosis of filariasis is based on the finding of the parasite in blood studies, preferably collected around midnight. Circulating filarial antigen detection can also be used as it shows a high degree of sensitivity (up to 96%), although there are often false positives [17].

Elephantiasis nostras was initially described to refer to elephantiasis of bacterial origin [18], but the term has now expanded to include all non-filarial forms [19, 20]. The most frequent aetiology of elephantiasis nostras is related to genital malignancies [21], lymphomas, infections such as follicular occlusion triad [22], untreated hernias [23], surgery, lymphadenectomy, radiotherapy [24], chronic venous stasis [25], and obesity. Elephantiasis nostras also includes idiopathic cases [26] and those related to hypoplasia of lymphatic vessels or genetic disorders such as Milroy's disease [27].

Patients with scrotal elephantiasis often have impaired urinary functions and social and sexual relationships. Chronic lymphatic obstruction causes accumulation of water, macromolecules, and proteins in the dermis. The protein-rich fluid induces fibroblastic proliferation and local alteration of the immune response. Fibroblast proliferation leads to fibrosis of the dermis and subcutaneous cellular tissue. The alteration of the immune response favours chronic inflammation and lymphangitis, which again produces fibrosis. Oedema, fibrosis, and inflammation are responsible for the macroscopic appearance of the skin, which varies from markedly thickened, papulo-keratotic lesions to cobblestone-like or verrucous lesions (Figs. 16.7 and 16.8).

The treatment of scrotal elephantiasis is complete excision of the affected skin and subcutaneous cellular tissue. Sometimes it will require skin grafting, lymphangioplasty and lymphatic-venous anastomosis [20, 28, 29].

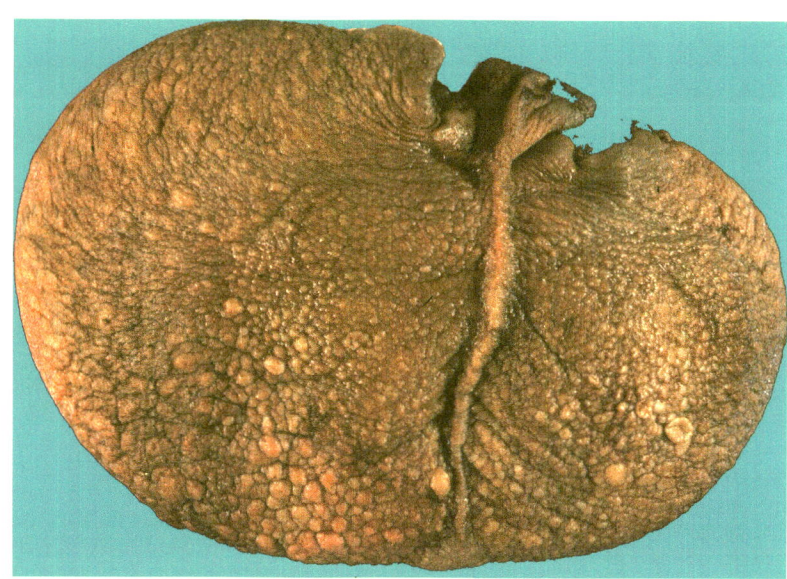

Fig. 16.7 Scrotal elephantiasis. Scrotal resection specimen showing a warty surface with involvement of both scrotal pouches

Fig. 16.8 Scrotal elephantiasis. Characteristic cobblestone appearance. The larger protrusions correspond to papules and vesicles filled with a clear fluid

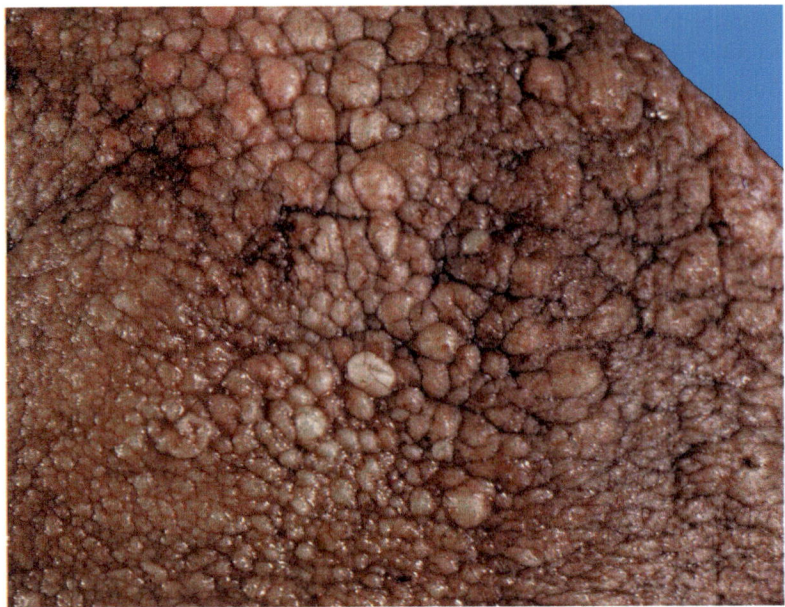

References

1. Mihmanli I, Kantarci F. Sonography of scrotal abnormalities in adults: an update. Diagn Interv Radiol. 2009;15:64–73.
2. Khalili M, Gholamzadeh Baeis M, Rouzrokh M. Abdominoscrotal hydrocele: a case report. Urol Case Rep. 2020;32:101254.
3. Hosoda T, Ishioka S, Hijikata K. Laparoscopic treatment of an abdominoscrotal hydrocele: a case report. Int J Surg Case Rep. 2022;90:106668.
4. Elhaddad A, Awad M, Shehata SM, Shehata MA. Laparoscopic management of infantile hydrocele in pediatric age group. Pediatr Surg Int. 2022;38:581–7.
5. Sugianto KY, Vijay PS. Encysted spermatic cord hydroceles in 3-year old boy, case report. Urol Case Rep. 2021;24(38):101652.
6. Lee SR. Laparoscopic hydrocelectomy with transabdominal preperitoneal hernioplasty or iliopubic tract repair for treatment of encysted spermatic cord hydrocele. Surg Endosc. 2022;36:5540–5.
7. Huang Y, Chen B, Cao D, Chen Z, Li J, Guo J, Dong Q, Wei Q, Liu L. Surgical management of tuberculous epididymo-orchitis: a retrospective study of 81 cases with long-term follow-up. BMC Infect Dis. 2021;21:1068.
8. Baykan AH, Sayiner HS, Inan I. Brucella and non-Brucella epididymo-orchitis: comparison of ultrasound findings. Med Ultrason. 2019;21:246–50.
9. Chu CB, Chen J, Shen YM, Liu SJ, Sun L, Nie YS, Liu J, Cao JX, Du HD, Zou ZY, Yuan X. Individualized treatment of pediatric inguinal hernia reduces adolescent recurrence rate: an analysis of 3006 cases. Surg Today. 2020;50:499–508.
10. Miguel PR, Reusch M, daRosa AL, Carlos JR. Laparoscopic hernia repair—complications. JSLS. 1998;2:35–40.
11. Ben Kridis W, Lajnef M, Khmiri S, Boudawara O, Slimen MH, Boudawara T, Khanfir A. Testicular leydig cell tumor revealed by hydrocele. Urol Case Rep. 2020;35:101520.
12. Cimador M, Castagnetti M, De Grazia E. Management of hydrocele in adolescent patients. Nat Rev Urol. 2010;7:379–85.
13. Bin Y, Yong-Bao W, Zhuo Y, Jin-Rui Y. Minimal hydrocelectomy with the aid of scrotoscope: a ten-year experience. Int Braz J Urol. 2014;40:384–9.
14. Lin L, Hong HS, Gao YL, Yang JR, Li T, Zhu QG, Ye LF, Wei YB. Individualized minimally invasive treatment for adult testicular hydrocele: a pilot study. World J Clin Cases. 2019;7:727–33.
15. Kiddoo DA, Wollin TA, Mador DR. A population based assessment of complications following outpatient hydrocelectomy and spermatocelectomy. J Urol. 2004;171:746–8.
16. Mathonet PY, Altdorfer A, Pirotte B. Giant scrotal elephantiasis in a migrant from Niger. Eur J Clin Microbiol Infect Dis. 2022;41:133–5.
17. WHO: Lymphatic filariasis. Fact sheet Updated October 2016 http://www.who.int/mediacentre/factsheets/fs102/en/. Accessed Oct 2016.
18. Castellani A. Elephantiasis Nostras (non-filarial elephantiasis): (section of tropical diseases and parasitology). Proc R Soc Med. 1934;27:519–24.
19. Sisto K, Khachemoune A. Elephantiasis nostras verrucosa: a review. Am J Clin Dermatol. 2008;9:141–6.

20. Judge N, Kilic A. Elephantiasis Nostras Verrucosa. Excision with full-thickness skin grafting of the penis, scrotum, and perineal area. J Dermatol Case Rep. 2016;10:32–4.

21. Taghy A, Hassam B. Scrotal elephantiasis revealing prostate cancer. Pan Afr Med J. 2014;17:190.

22. Liu JC, Liu XG, Xu C, Zhao HF, Jiang XZ. Scrotal elephantiasis associated with follicular occlusion triad: a case report and literature review. Medicine (Baltimore). 2019;98(16):e15263.

23. Miranda H, Colangelo AC, Antunes M, Schiavone M, Merigliano S, Pizzol D. Giant elephantiasis and inguino-scrotal hernia. PLoS Negl Trop Dis. 2017;11(6):e0005494.

24. Verma SB. Lymphangiectasias after penec-tomy, inguinal lymph node dissection, ure-throstomy and radiation. Acta Derm Venereol. 2006;86:175–6.

25. Tanhaeivash R, Franiel T, Grimm MO, Horstmann M. Gigantic suprapubic lymphedema: a case study. World J Mens Health. 2016;34:148–52.

26. Dianzani C, Gaspardini F, Persichetti P, Brunetti B, Pizzuti A, Margiotti K, Degener AM. Giant scrotal elephantiasis: an idiopathic case. Int J Immunopathol Pharmacol. 2010;23:369–72.

27. Butler C, Osterberg C, Horvai A, Breyer B. Milroy's disease and scrotal lymphoedema: pathological insight. BMJ Case Rep. 2016;2016:bcr2016215396.

28. Salako AA, Olabanji JK, Oladele AO, Alabi GH, Adejare IE, David RA. Surgical reconstruction of Giant Penoscrotal lymphedema in Sub-Saharan Africa. Urology. 2018;112:181–5.

29. Hattori Y, Hayata N, Nakamura K, Takahashi T, Mitsumori K, Ohnishi H. Successful surgical resec-tion and reconstruction of scrotal elephantiasis. IJU Case Rep. 2020;4:79–81.

17.1 Testicular Lymphangiectasias

Testicular lymphangiectasias consists of an abnormal development of the intratesticular lymphatic vessels [1] (Figs. 17.1, 17.2 and 17.3). A distinction is made between congenital lymphangiectasias and acquired lymphangiectasias. In congenital lymphangiectasias, the lymphatic vessels of the tunica vasculosa of the albuginea and interlobular septa appear increased in number and size and present cystic transformation. The lymphatic vessels of the testicular mediastinum are not dilated nor do the paralymphatic structures of the interstitium appear to be affected. The lymphatic vessels of the epididymis and the spermatic cord are normally developed.

Primary testicular lymphangiectasias have been observed, as an isolated event, in children, both in normally descended testes and in cryptorchid testicles (Fig. 17.4) or within a systemic pathology such as in Noonan syndrome [2] or androgen insensitivity syndrome [3] (Fig. 17.5). Lymphatic dilatation does not seem to have an impact on the parenchyma, which only shows pathology when the lymphangiectasias settle in undescended testes or the patient is a carrier of another pathology [4].

The fact that this type of lymphangiectasia has not been observed in adults suggests that the lymphatic vessels may undergo involution or be masked when tubular development occurs at puberty.

Secondary acquired lymphangiectasias are more frequent. Testicle and paratesticular structures (epididymis, testicular sheaths, and spermatic cord) may also be affected. They are produced by a defect in the normal lymphatic drainage of these structures secondary to surgical treatments on the inguinal region (Fig. 17.6), chronic inflammatory processes of the spermatic cord, or radiotherapy of the retroperitoneal lymph nodes. The lesions are very important, especially at the level of the testicular parenchyma and in the parietal layer of the testicular tunica vaginalis [5].

At the level of the testicular parenchyma, the seminiferous tubules have different degrees of atrophy of the seminiferous epithelium and there is a great increase of the interstitium due to the presence of abundant lymphatic vessels that dissect clusters of Leydig cells (Figs. 17.7 and 17.8). Since the intertubular space is poor in lymphatics, everything suggests that there has been an active lymphangiogenesis associated with the transformation of the paralymphatic spaces into true lymphatic vessels as demonstrated by immunostaining with D2–40 (Figs. 17.9 and 17.10).

At the level of the parietal layer of the tunica vaginal, there is a marked dilatation of the deep lymphatic plexus. The vessels are transformed into cavities that push the mesothelial layer

Fig. 17.1 Congenital testicular lymphangiectasias. Newborn autopsy specimen. Both testicles had the same appearance. There are cystic formations identifiable as dilated lymphatic vessels distributed irregularly throughout the parenchyma

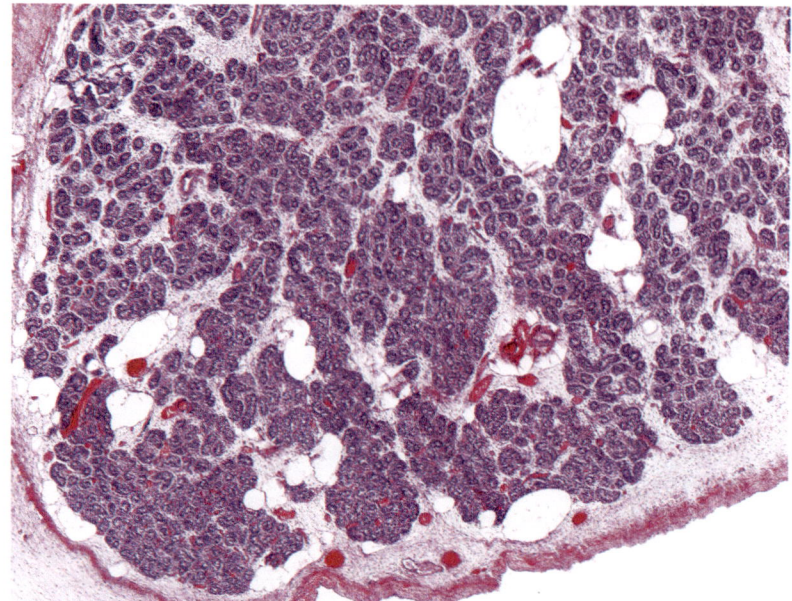

Fig. 17.2 Congenital testicular lymphangiectasias. The tunica vasculosa can be recognized in the upper part. The presence of numerous lymphatic vessels arranged side by side like the beads of a rosary is notable

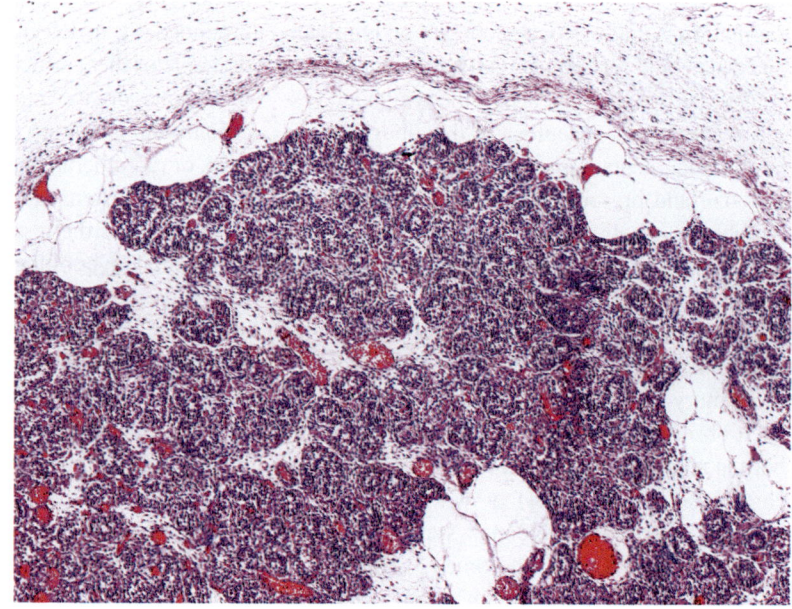

resulting in protrusions on the vaginal surface [6] (Figs. 17.11 and 17.12).

A striking fact has been observed in the study of the testes in our series of more than 50 cases of patients undergoing gender reassignment. In a quarter of the cases, there is marked dilatation of the lymphatic vessels, preferably those located in the tunica vasculosa of the albuginea and in the parietal layer of the tunica

vaginalis. This contrasts with the high frequency of arteriosclerosis lesions of the centripetal and centrifugal arteries present in more than half of these patients. This would result in a lower blood flow and consequently a reduced need for interstitial fluid return via lymphatic vessels. On the other hand, not all testes with lymphangiectasia are carriers of vasculitis lesions. And finally, none of the patients had a

Fig. 17.3 Congenital testicular lymphangiectasias. The cystic dilatations of the lymphatic vessels are preferentially located in the interlobular septa as is suggested by the small arteries that are visible between them or in their periphery

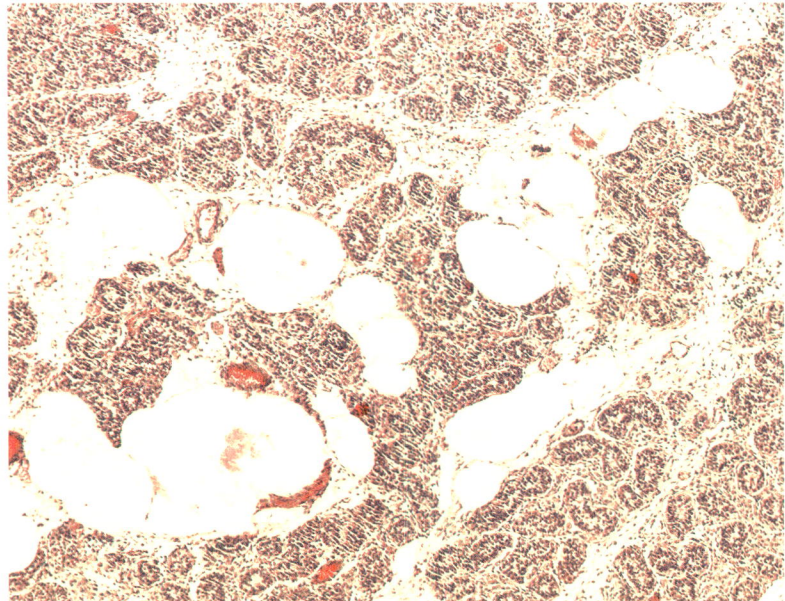

Fig. 17.4 Congenital testicular lymphangiectasias in a 4-year-old boy with cryptorchidism type III (seminiferous tubules with intense decrease in diameter, decrease in Sertoli cells number and absence of germ cells). The lymphatic vessels of the tunica vasculosa have transformed into cystic formations partially surrounding an artery

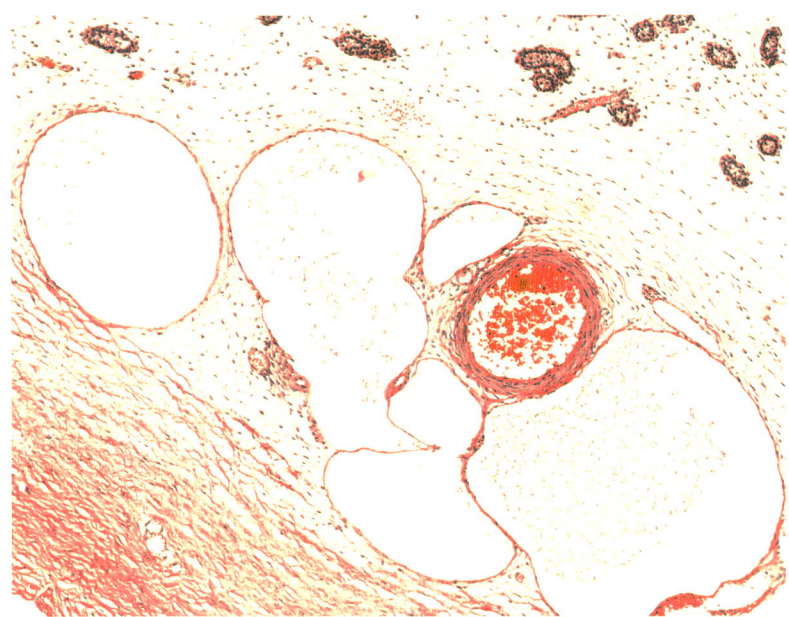

history of pathology in the inguinal or retroperitoneal region that could affect normal testicular lymphatic drainage. A possible explanation may lie in a lymphogenic effect of the high-dose oestrogen treatment that the patients had received [7].

Fig. 17.5 Congenital testicular lymphangiectasias. A 5-year-old patient with complete androgen insensitivity syndrome. Numerous lymphatic vessels in the tunica vasculosa and in the thickness of the albuginea, in which there is a longitudinally sectioned vessel with valves. The seminiferous tubules have a decreased calibre and the interstitium is greatly enlarged by a very cellular tissue

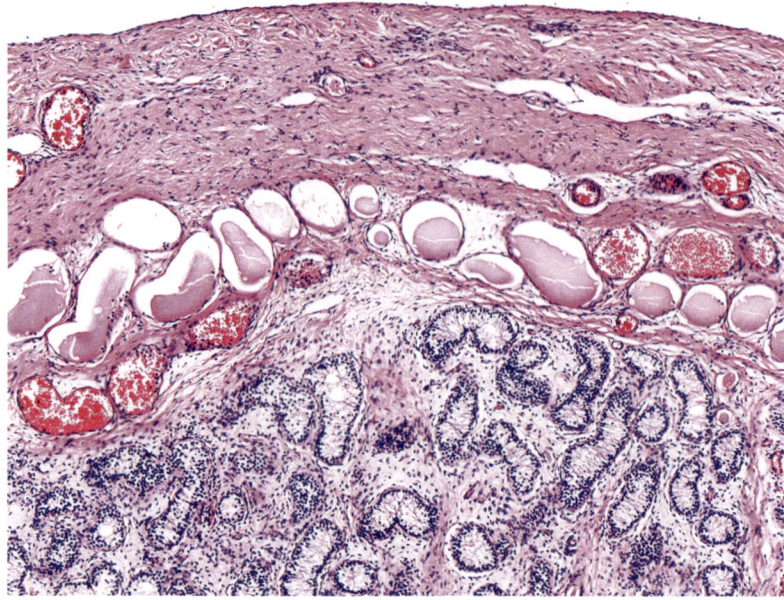

Fig. 17.6 Secondary testicular lymphangiectasias in a patient operated on for inguinal hernia who developed a large haematoma. Orchiectomy specimen. The seminiferous tubules are widely separated by thin-walled cystic formations with slightly eosinophilic contents. (Masson trichrome)

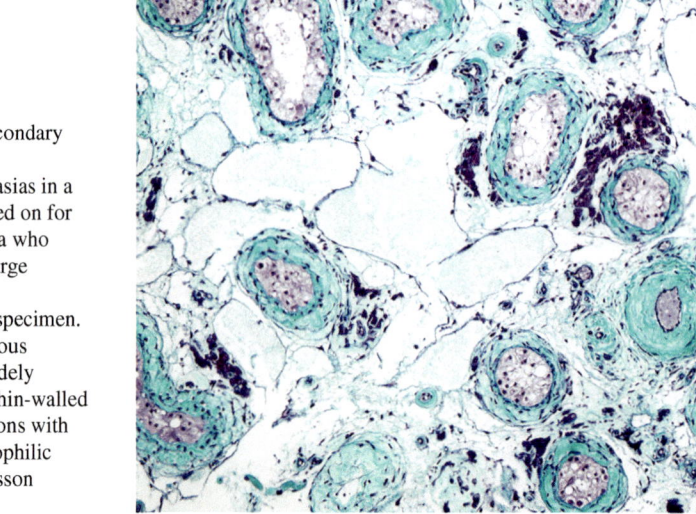

Fig. 17.7 Secondary testicular lymphangiectasias. Seminiferous tubules surrounded by lymphatic vessels with variable degrees of dilatation. The seminiferous tubules show marked atrophy, fibrosis of their wall, absence of lumen, few Sertoli cells, and isolated spermatogonia. (Masson trichrome)

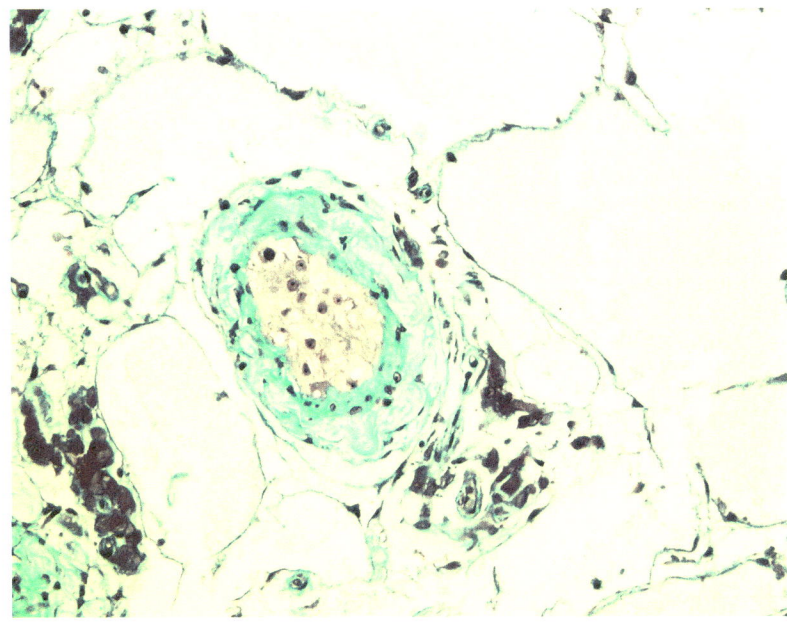

Fig. 17.8 Secondary testicular lymphangiectasias. Clusters of Leydig cells dissociated by the presence of paralymphatic spaces between their cells which remain floating inside the paralymphatic spaces. The resulting image is reminiscent of that seen in testicular metastases of some adenocarcinomas. (Masson trichrome)

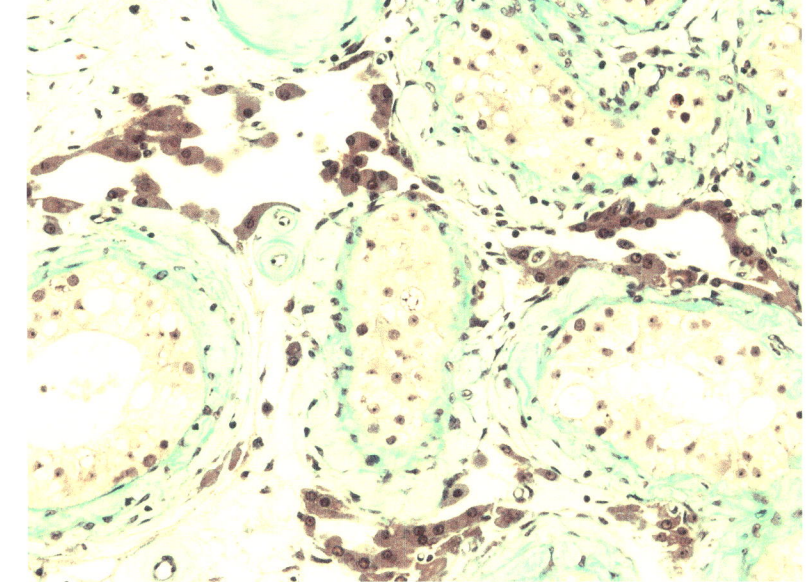

Fig. 17.9 Secondary
testicular
lymphangiectasias.
D2–40 Immunostaining
reveals the large number
of lymphatic vessels
evenly distributed in the
testicular parenchyma

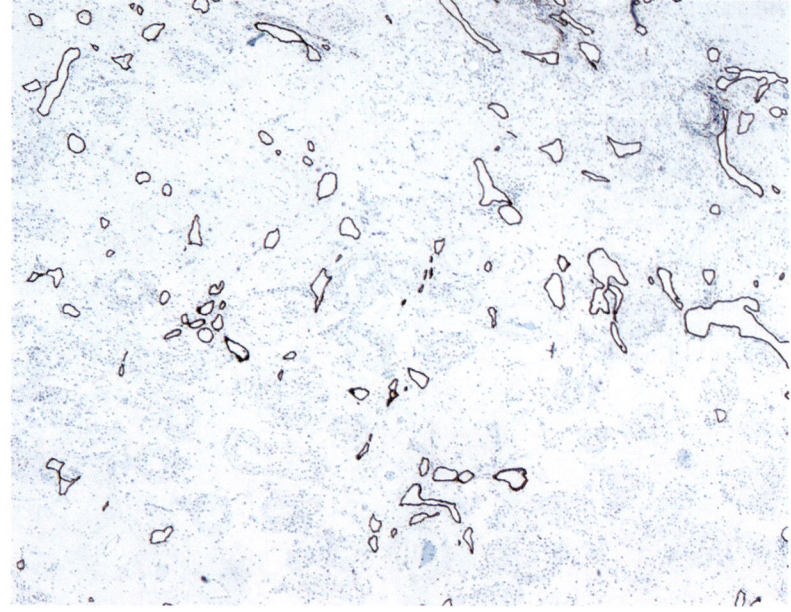

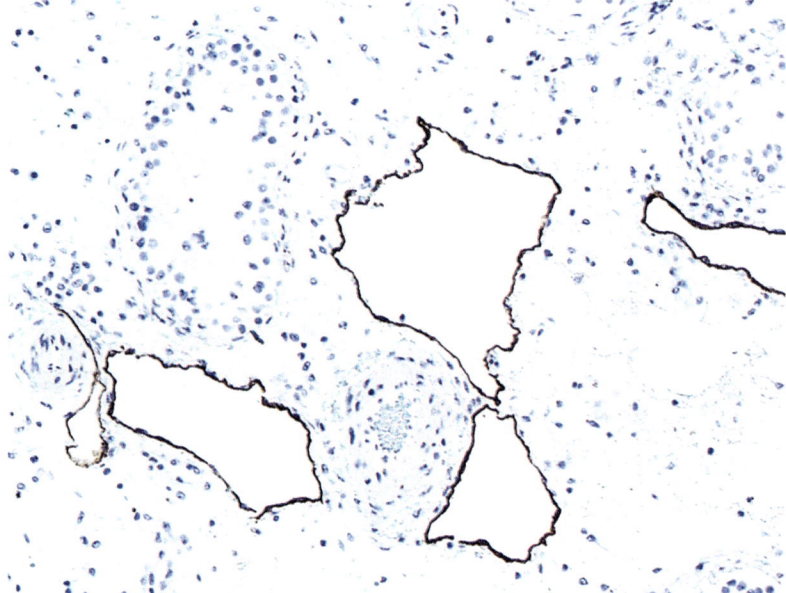

Fig. 17.10 Secondary
testicular
lymphangiectasias.
Dilated lymphatic
vessels with geographic
contours between the
seminiferous tubules
(D2–40)

Fig. 17.11 Secondary vaginal lymphangiectasias. A 37-year-old patient treated 3 years ago for a germ cell tumour in the left testicle with retroperitoneal metastases. He has developed a seminoma in the right testicle and hydrocele. The parietal layer of the testicular vaginal is very thickened, containing numerous parallel cystic dilatations that protrude into the vaginal cavity

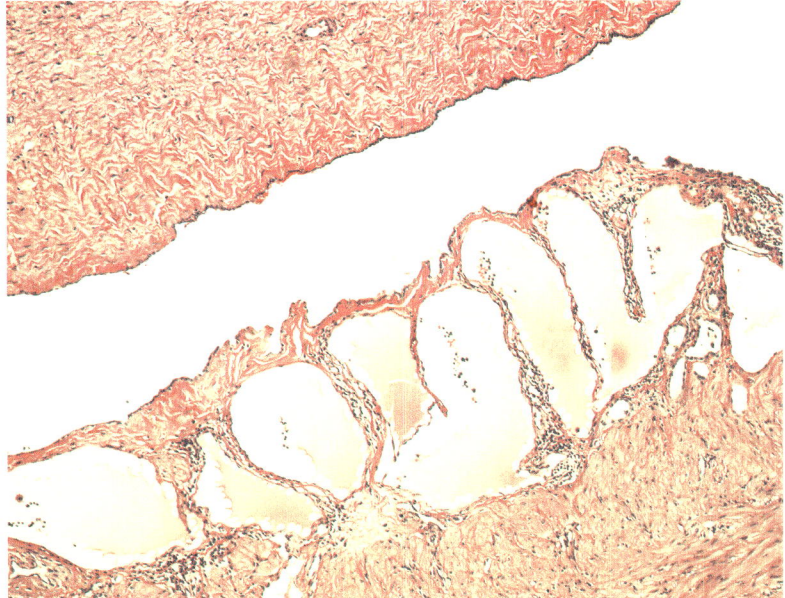

Fig. 17.12 Secondary vaginal lymphangiectasias. Lymphatic dilatations located between the submesothelial layer and the underlying dense connective tissue. The thin-walled cavities contain eosinophilic fluid and lymphoid cells

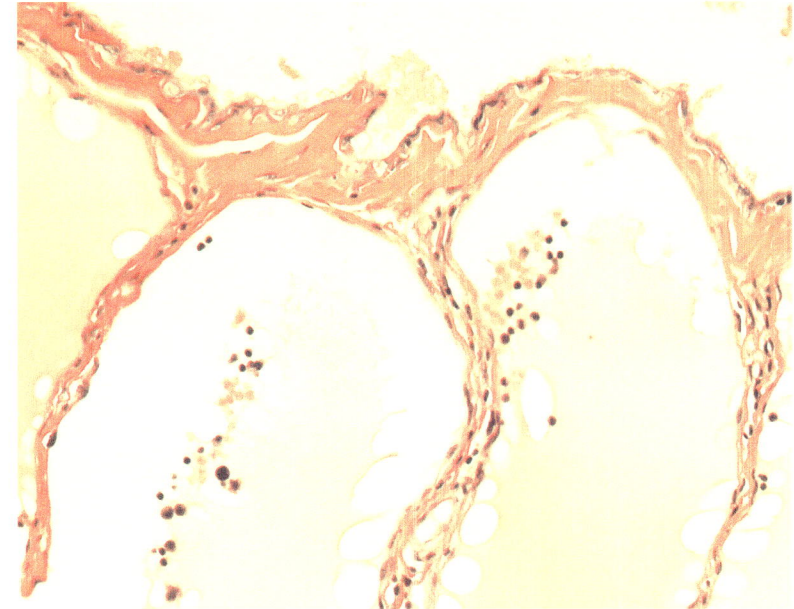

17.2   Testicular Pseudolymphangiectasia. Microcystic Testicular Oedema

This histologic picture is very similar to that of secondary testicular lymphangiectasis. At low magnification, the parenchyma shows a honeycomb appearance due to the microcystic formations separating the testicular lobules or seminiferous tubules. The cavities have irregular contours, with a size exceeding that of the diameter of the seminiferous tubules. At higher magnification, they are lined by cells with flattened nuclei and very thin cytoplasm. Inside the cells there is a slightly eosinophilic fibrillary material in some and amorphous material in others. In the larger cavities, there are fine protrusions of the interstitium consisting of a central vessel surrounded by a minimal amount of connective tissue (Figs. 17.13 and 17.14). Immuno-histochemical study shows that instead of being D2–40 positive (Figs. 17.15 and 17.16), like the cells of the lymphatic vessels, the lining cells are CD34 positive like the telocytes that constitute the testicular architecture (Figs. 17.17 and 17.18). This picture is interpreted as the result of a chronic testicular oedema that has resulted in multiple microcystic formations in the interstitium.

Testicular pseudolymphangiectasias are observed in pubertal patients to older adults. In half of the cases, there is a history of inguinal surgery for hernia or testicular descent and in the remaining cases it is unknown. Testicular pseudolymphangiectasias do not increase testicular size, which is more related to the primary pathology of the testicles in cases of cryptorchidism, or to the frequent testicular atrophy in elderly patients.

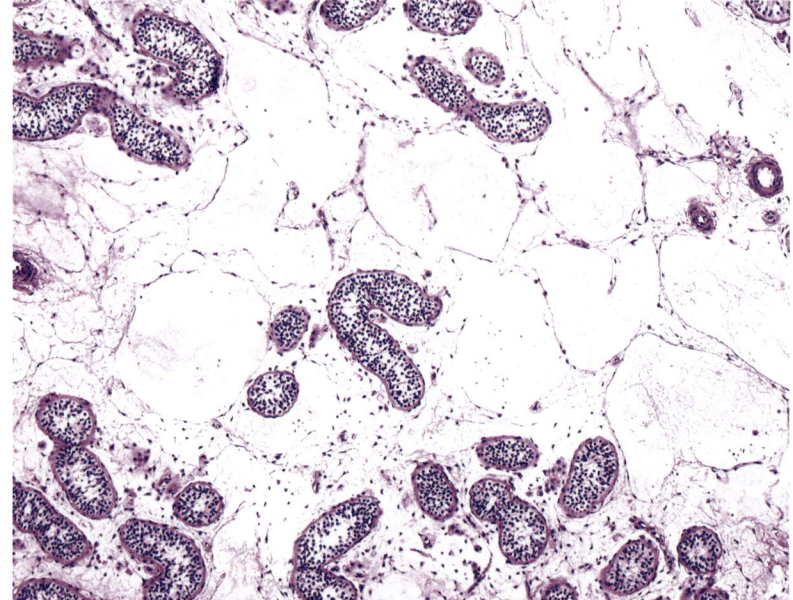

Fig. 17.13 Testicular pseudolymphangiectasias. Microcystic testicular oedema. A 13-year-old patient with a history of inguinal cryptorchidism. Orchiectomy specimen. Seminiferous tubules separated by honeycomb cystic spaces

Fig. 17.14 Testicular pseudolymphangiectasias. Microcystic testicular oedema. Group of cystic spaces with well-defined contours, accompanied by small vessels in their wall, that occupy a large part of the testicular parenchyma

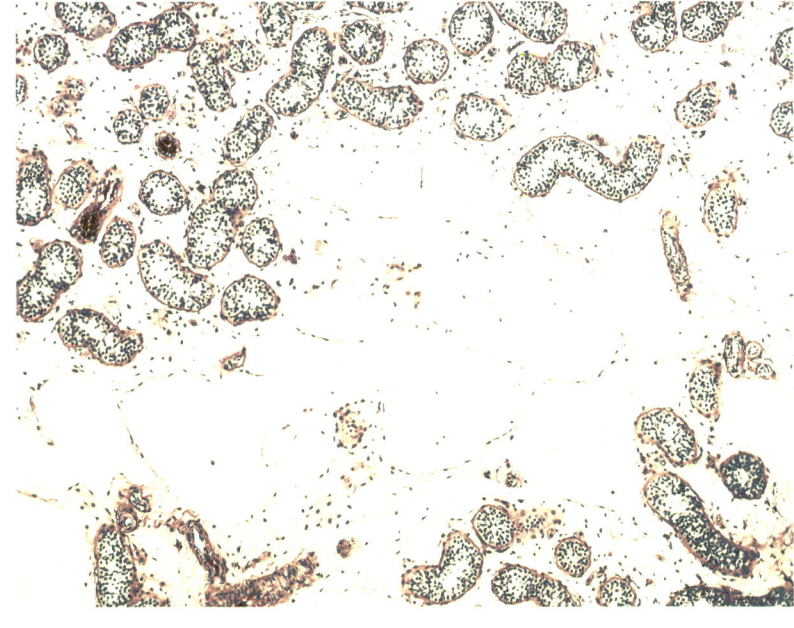

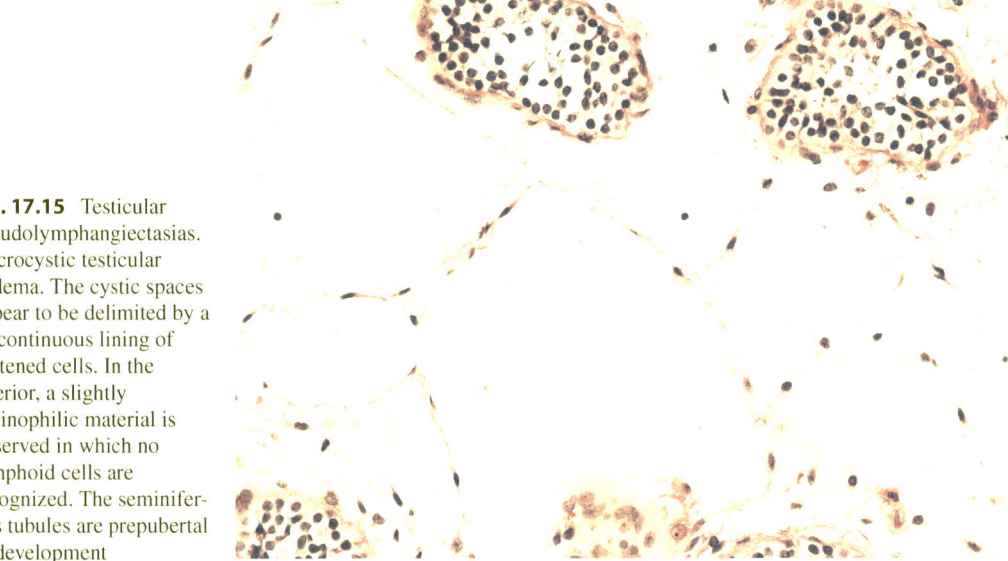

Fig. 17.15 Testicular pseudolymphangiectasias. Microcystic testicular oedema. The cystic spaces appear to be delimited by a discontinuous lining of flattened cells. In the interior, a slightly eosinophilic material is observed in which no lymphoid cells are recognized. The seminiferous tubules are prepubertal in development

Fig. 17.16 Testicular pseudolymphangiectasias. Microcystic testicular oedema. The lining of the cystic spaces is D2–40 negative. As a control, the longitudinal and transverse sections of two lymphatic vessels stand out for their positivity

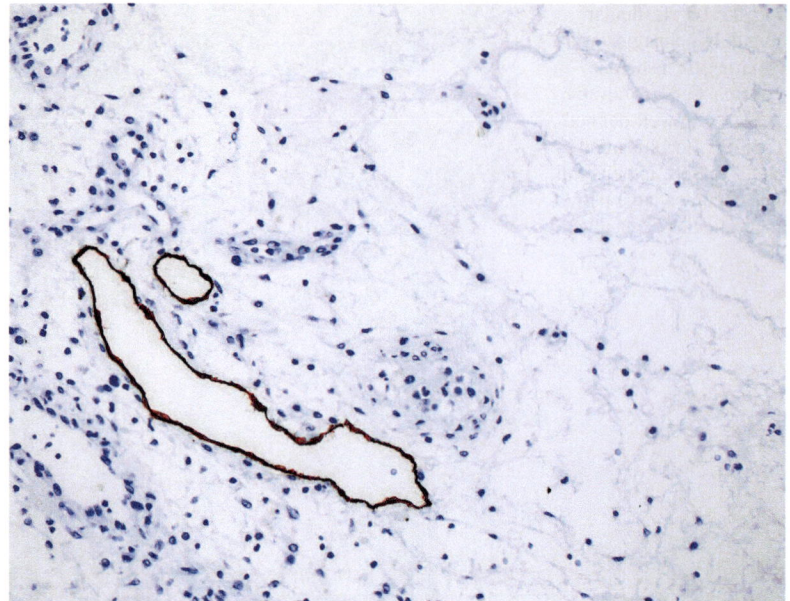

Fig. 17.18 Testicular pseudolymphangiectasias. Microcystic testicular oedema. The lining of the cavities shows immunostaining similar to that of the outer layer of the seminiferous tubule wall (CD34)

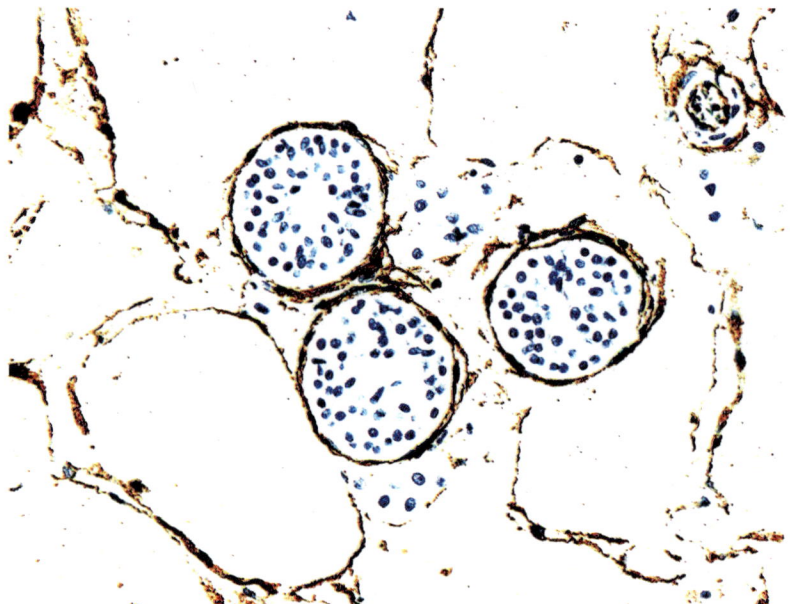

Fig. 17.17 Testicular pseudolymphangiectasias. Microcystic testicular oedema. Cells lining the cavities express CD34 as do cells of the testicular interstitium (telocytes) and the endothelial cells of veins and capillaries

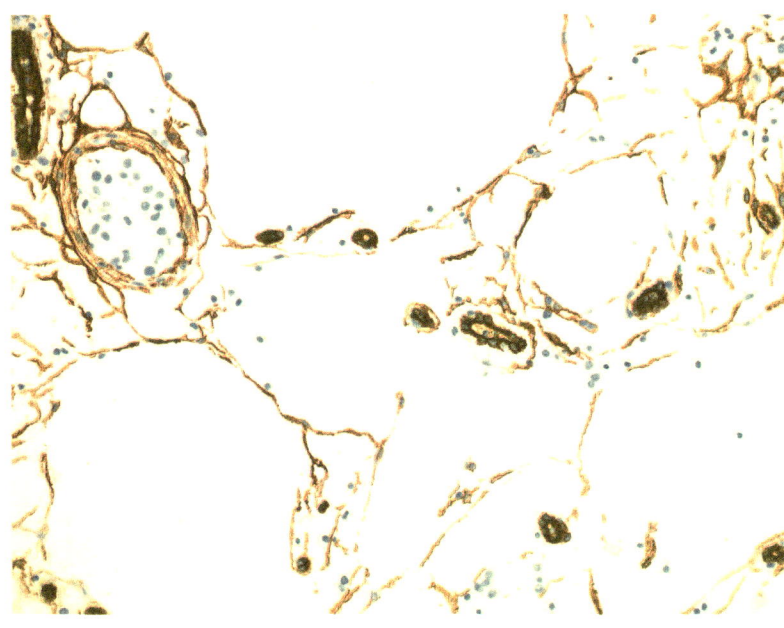

References

1. Nistal M, Paniagua R. Congenital testicular lymphangiectasis. Virchows Arch A Pathol Anat Histol. 1977;377:79–84.
2. Nistal M, Paniagua R, Bravo MP. Testicular lymphangiectasis in Noonan's syndrome. J Urol. 1984;131:759–61.
3. Nistal M, González-Peramato P, Serrano A. Usefulness of histological studies in patients with the androgen insensitivity syndrome. In: Clues in the diagnosis of non-tumoral testicular pathology. Cham: Springer; 2017b. p. 41–8.
4. Nistal M, Garcia-Rojo M, Paniagua R. Congenital testicular lymphangiectasis in children with otherwise normal testes. Histopathology. 1990;17:335–8.
5. Honoré LH. Nonspecific peritesticular fibrosis manifested as testicular enlargement. Arch Surg. 1978;113:814–6.
6. Figueredo-Silva J, Norões J, Dreyer G. Lymphatic endothelial cell in endemic Bancroftian Filariasis: a focus on the lymphatics of the tunica vaginalis testis. J Trop Med. 2018;2018:5134670.
7. Fontaine C, Morfoisse F, Tatin F, Zamora A, Zahreddine R, Henrion D, Arnal JF, Lenfant F, Garmy-Susini B. The impact of estrogen receptor in arterial and lymphatic vascular diseases. Int J Mol Sci. 2020;21:3244.

18.1 Lymphangioma of Paratesticular Structures

Lymphangiomas are congenital lymphatic malformations that accumulate fluid in their cavities, most of which consequently have a cystic appearance. Most lymphatic malformations are primary and develop in the head and neck (75%), axilla (20%), mediastinum, retroperitoneum, mesentery, and, exceptionally in liver, pancreas, kidneys, spleen, intestine, bones, urinary bladder, scrotum or inguinal region, (5%). Most lymphatic malformations are diagnosed in the first 2 years of life and it is estimated that more than 50% are already present at birth [1].

Primary lymphatic malformations in adults are very rare, and even rarer are those located in the paratesticular structures. Half a dozen cases have been described affecting the epididymis [2, 3] and a similar number in the spermatic cord or inguinal region [4, 5]. Both clinically and ultrasonographically, epididymal lymphangiomas manifest as cystic formations. Lymphangiomas of the spermatic cord are described as soft, painless masses that remain stable for years until, due to fluid accumulation in the cysts or trauma, they rapidly increase in size.

Macroscopically, they are lobulated, elastic formations that partially collapse when cut. Histologically, they consist of multiple cavities lined by an endothelium. The wall of the cavities is thin and may contain clusters of lymphocytes. Inside there is a fluid with small amounts of flocculated material and occasional lymphocytes. In some cases, the cavities have isolated red blood cells (Figs. 18.1 and 18.2).

The differential diagnosis should include both tumour and nontumour cystic lesions: hydrocele, hernias, spermatocele, varicocele, ectasia of the rete testis, dermoid and epidermoid cysts and teratomas.

The treatment of paratesticular lymphatic malformations should be a complete resection, to avoid recurrence, and sparing of the intrascrotal structures and spermatic cord.

Secondary lymphangiomas of the paratesticular structures are even rarer and have been described after herniorrhaphy or a surgery for rectal carcinoma [6].

© The Author(s), under exclusive license to Springer Nature Switzerland AG 2024
M. Nistal, P. González-Peramato, *Testicular Vascular Lesions*,
https://doi.org/10.1007/978-3-031-57847-2_18

Fig. 18.1 Lymphangioma of the epididymis. In relation to the tail of the epididymis, there is a multicamera cystic formation in the form of a cap surrounding the epididymis

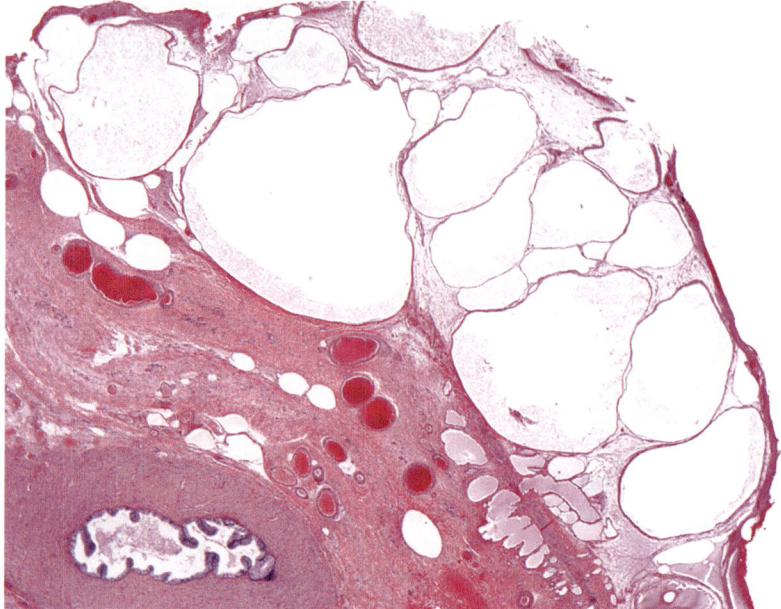

Fig. 18.2 Lymphangioma of the epididymis. The cavities are attached to each other and have a thin wall with hardly any connective tissue between them. They contain a slightly eosinophilic fluid. No cells are observed inside the cavities

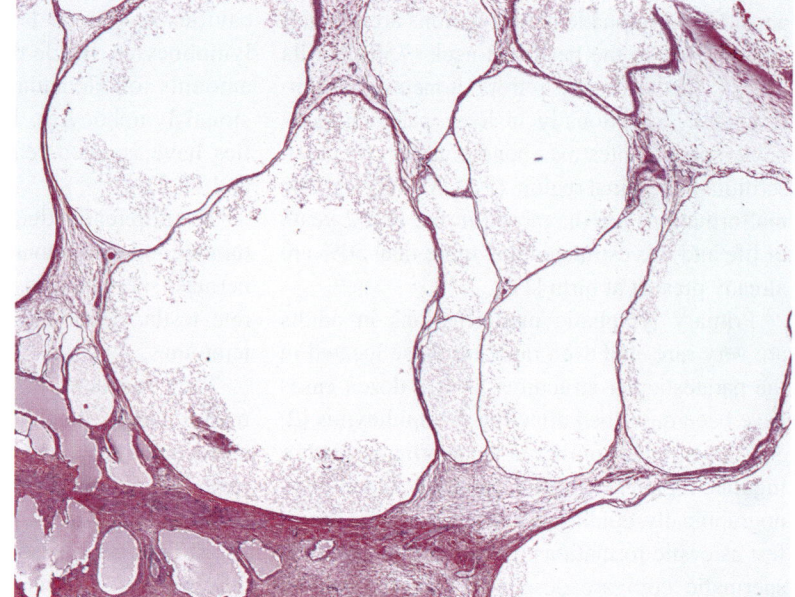

18.2 Benign Lymphangioendothelioma

A term introduced by Jones et al. in 1990 [7] to refer to a slow-growing, nontumourous, malformative process of the dermal lymphatic vessels. It was originally called acquired progressive lymphangioma. It presents as an asymptomatic, well-circumscribed erythematous or hyperpigmented plaque, flat or with small papules. It affects the skin of the thigh (33%), upper limb (20%), head and neck (20%), trunk (18%), and shoulder (8%) [8], and, in isolated cases breast or oral cavity. It has no preferential age or sexual predilection. It can be present already in childhood and undergo a rapid growth in the adult when associated with

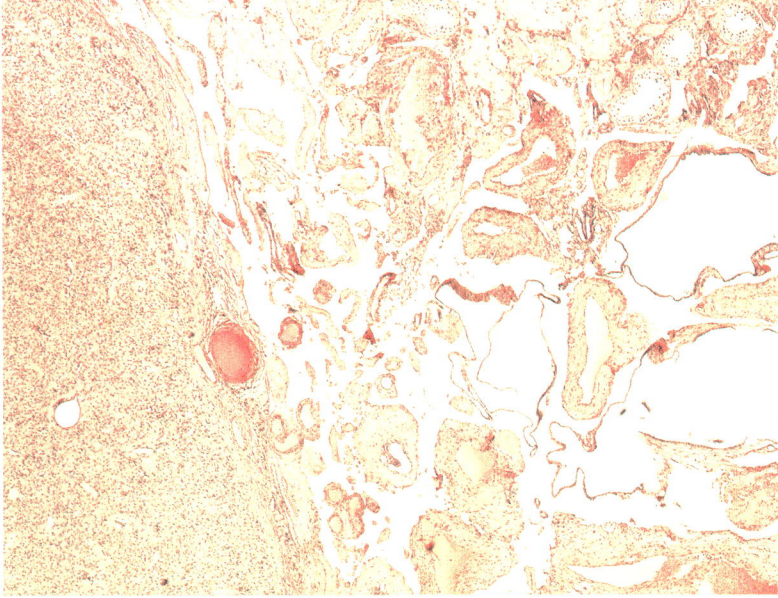

Fig. 18.3 Benign lymphangioendothelioma. A 56-year-old patient with a history of long-standing hydrocele and testicular enlargement. Part of the parenchyma is occupied by a well-demarcated Leydig cell tumour. The rest is constituted by multiple cavities of different sizes and thick-walled vessels dissecting the seminiferous tubules

Fig. 18.4 Intense cytoplasmic positivity for calretinin in most of the Leydig cell tumour cells

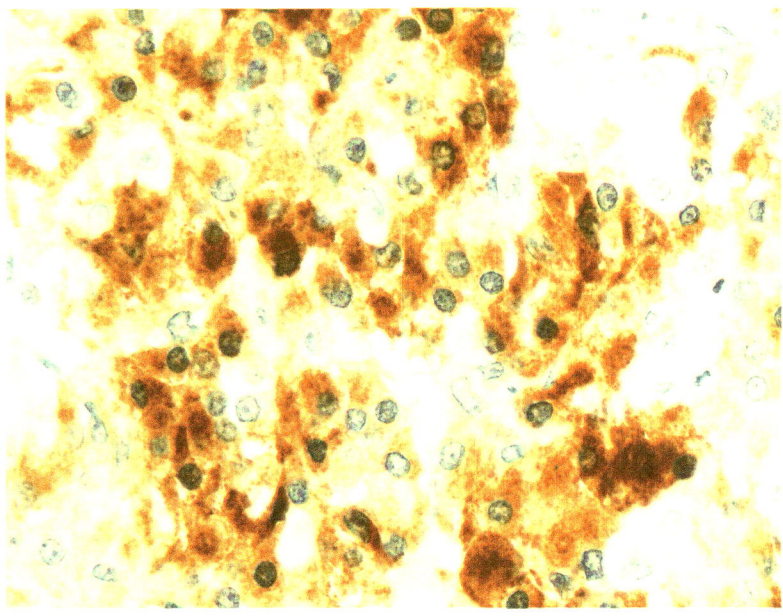

another pathology. Incomplete excisions are followed by relapses [9]. The case we have observed was associated with a histologically benign Leydig cell tumour (Figs. 18.3 and 18.4). In isolated forms significant regression can be achieved with sirolimus [10].

Histologically, it consists of the presence of abundant anastomosed, thin-walled, irregularly contoured vessels lined by endothelial cells, which dissect the pre-existing structures. The endothelial cells do not show atypia, hob nailing, hyperchromasia or mitotic activity. They may show papillary proliferations projecting into the lymphatic cavities. It is not accompanied by haemorrhage, iron deposition or inflammatory phenomena. The endothelial cells express D2-40 and in many cases also CD31. They are negative for human herpervirus-8 and WT-1 (Figs. 18.5, 18.6, 18.7 and 18.8).

Fig. 18.5 Benign lymphangioendothelioma. Testicular parenchyma replaced by a proliferation of lymphatic vessels, that are otherwise optically empty spaces into which digitiform formations of variable size protrude (D2-40)

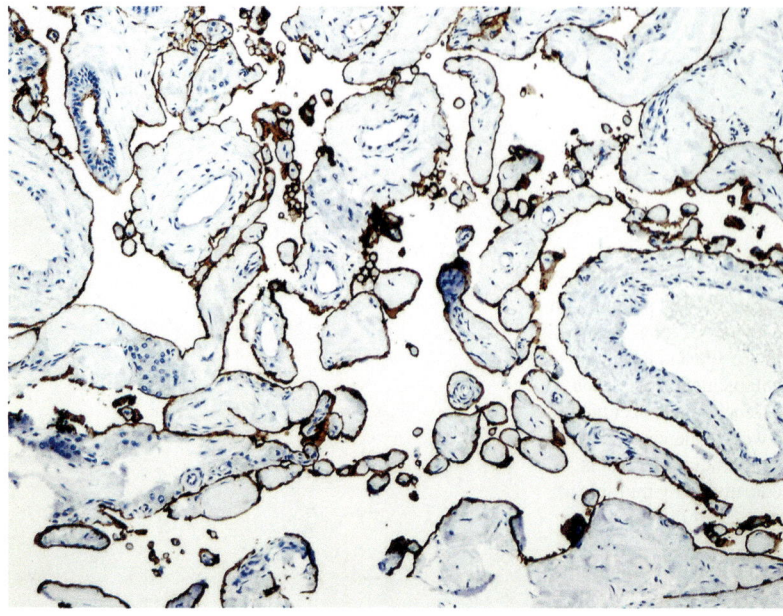

Fig. 18.6 Benign lymphangioendothelioma. Thick intratesticular lymphatic vessel surrounded by numerous interconnected cavities with small papillary formations in its wall

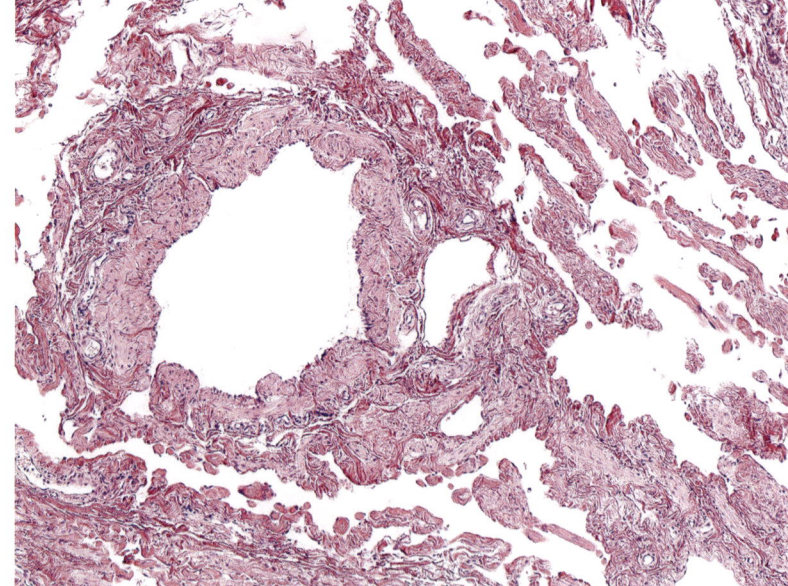

In the testis, the neoformed lymphatic vessels are very numerous in the parenchyma and the vascular tunica of the albuginea, the testicular mediastinum, the parietal layer of the testicular tunica vaginalis and in the initial portion of the spermatic cord. In the parietal layer of the testicular tunica vaginalis, the vessels are very often arranged in cisterns parallel to each other and parallel to the mesothelial surface. The stomata are very extensive and frequent. In the initial portion of the spermatic cord, they are arranged around both arterial and venous vessels or lymphatic collectors (Figs. 18.9, 18.10, 18.11 and 18.12).

The different differential diagnoses posed by cutaneous lesions, Kaposi's sarcoma, and well-differentiated angiosarcoma, are easy to exclude.

Fig. 18.7 Benign lymphangioendothelioma. Cluster of nontumourous Leydig cells with abundant lipofuscin in contact with neoformed lymphatic vascular clefts (D2–40)

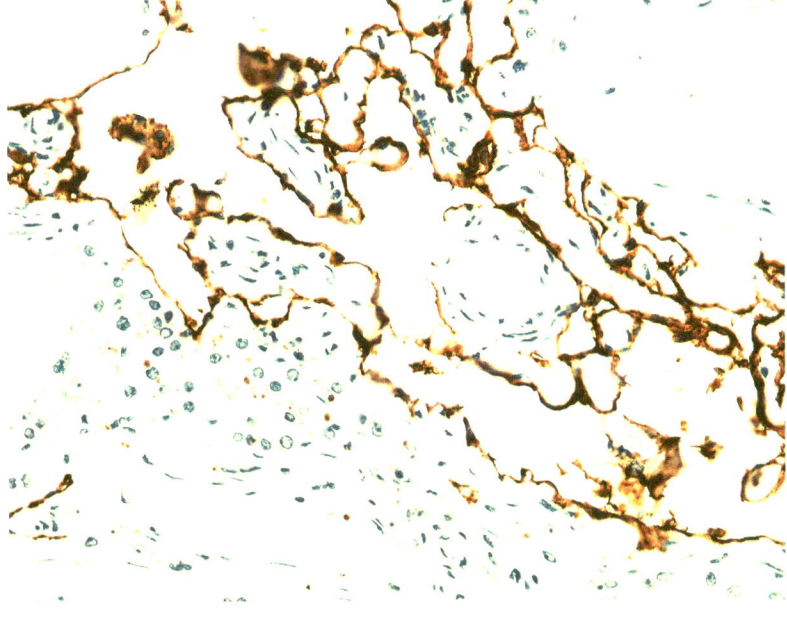

Fig. 18.8 Benign lymphangioendothelioma. Testicular mediastinum occupied by cystic dilatations of lymphatic vessels surrounding arterioles and venules and distorting the architecture of the rete testis (D2–40)

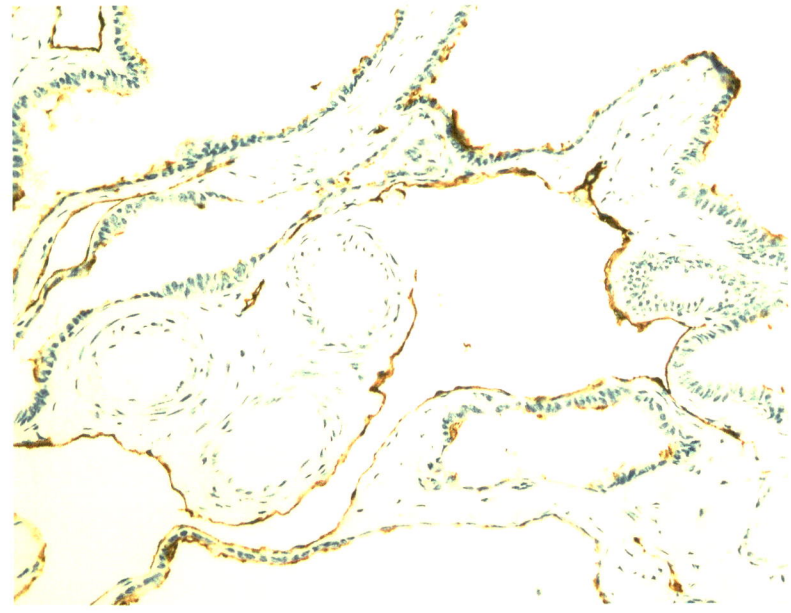

Kaposi's sarcoma is ruled out morphologically by the absence of spindle cell proliferation and lymphoplasmacytic infiltrate and immunohistochemically by the absence of HHV-8 nuclear expression. Morphologically well-differentiated angiosarcoma may also present papillae inside the cavities, but the endothelial cells show large hyperchromatic nuclei, evident proliferation estimated with Ki67 and, in the case of post-irradiation, angiosarcomas c-myc gene amplification [11].

Among the factors involved in the aetiology of benign lymphangioendothelioma is vascular endothelial growth factor (VEGT), which promotes angiogenesis by upregulating the mammalian target of rapamycin.

Fig. 18.9 Benign lymphangioendothelioma. The testicular parenchyma has marked ectasia of the seminiferous tubules and sclerosed tubules at the periphery. A fibrous band separates this parenchyma from the proliferation of lymphatic vessels whose cisterns are arranged perpendicular to it

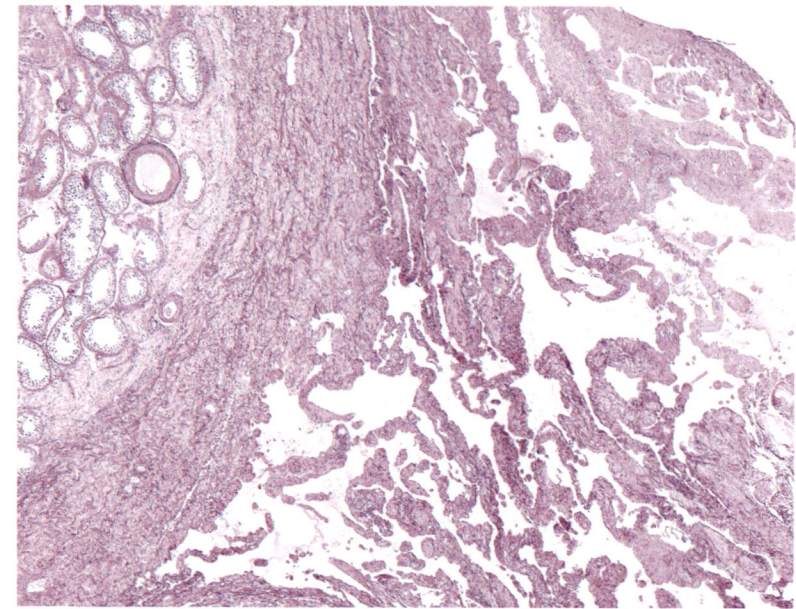

Fig. 18.10 Benign lymphangioendothelioma. The surface of the albuginea at the lower pole of the testis shows neoformation of lymphatic vessels extending to the paratesticular structures (D2–40)

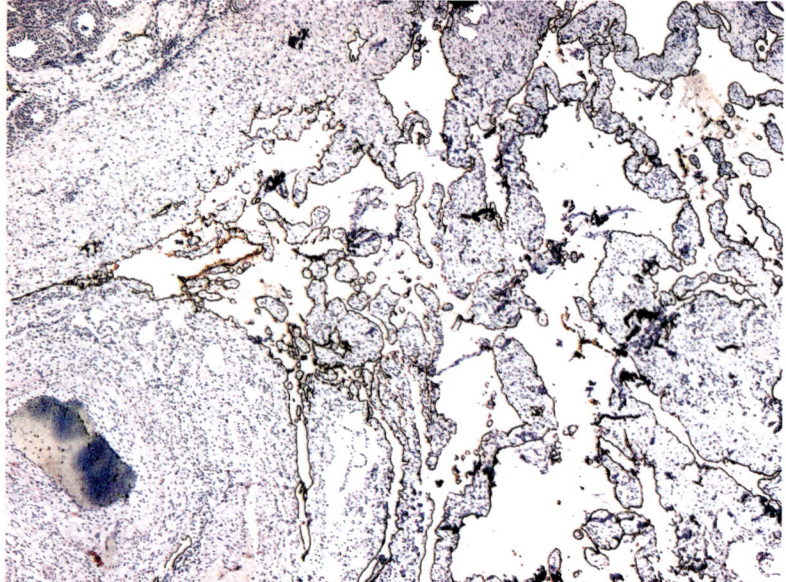

Fig. 18.11 Benign lymphangioendothelioma. Parietal layer of the testicular tunica vaginalis. Intense neoformation and dilatation of the vessels of both the submesothelial and deep plexus located in the dense connective tissue (D2-40)

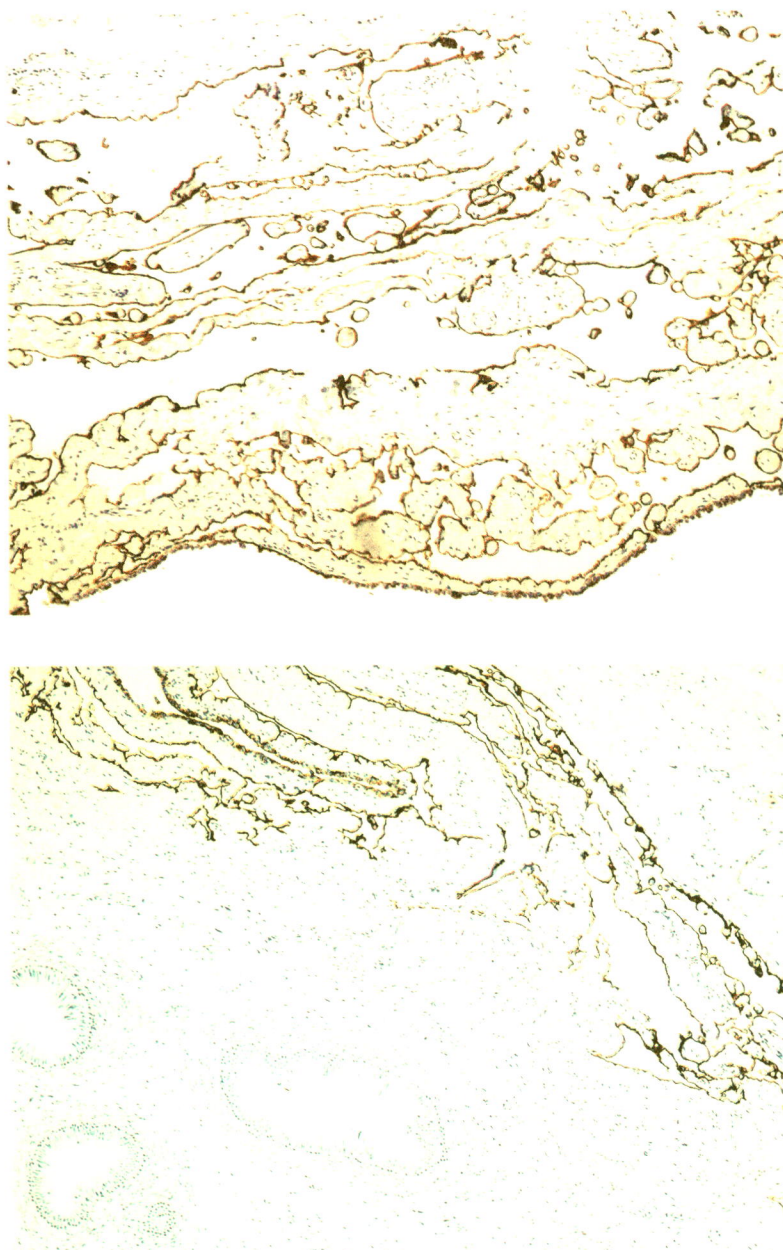

Fig. 18.12 Benign lymphangioendothelioma. The section of the body of the epididymis shows numerous neoformed lymphatic vessels in the retroepididymal tissue (D2–40)

18.3 Haemangiolymphangioma

Haemangiolymphangioma is a mixed vascular malformation of lymphatic vessels and blood vessels that can occur at any age. It is described in locations such as neck, axilla, abdominal cavity, and extremities [12–14]. Exceptionally, it has also been reported in other locations such as the oral cavity [15]. It can be multiple or affect several anatomical regions as in thoraco-abdominal haemolymphangiomas [16].

Isolated cases have been published in the testis and spermatic cord [17–19]. None of the three cases was associated with Klippel-Trenaunay-Weber syndrome. It is a benign process but tends to recur. Histologically, it shows a double haemangiomatous and lymphangiomatous component. The vessels, with walls of variable thickness, appear dilated, some are lined by endothelial cells and contain abundant erythrocytes, and others, also lined by endothelial cells, contain only an eosinophilic and proteinaceous fluid reminiscent of lymphatic vessels. Immunohistochemically, the former are lined by CD31 and CD34 positive endothelial cells while the latter are preferentially lined by D2–40 positive cells).

References

1. Ali AY, Abdi AM, Basar D, Mohamed SS, İbrahim İG. Rare case cystic scrotal lymphangioma presented as a hydrocele. Int J Surg Case Rep. 2022;93:106959.
2. Postius J, Manzano C, Concepción T, Castro D, Gutierrez P, Bañares F. Epididymal lymphangioma. J Urol. 2000;163:550–1.
3. Kok KY, Telesinghe PU. Lymphangioma of the epididymis. Singapore Med J. 2002;43:249–50.
4. Patoulias I, Prodromou K, Feidantsis T, Kallergis I, Koutsoumis G. Cystic lymphangioma of the inguinal and scrotal regions in childhood—report of three cases. Hippokratia. 2014;18:88–91.
5. Oukhouya MA. Cystic lymphangioma of the spermatic cord: about case. Pan Afr Med J. 2018;31:191.
6. Haroon M, Nisha Y, Iqubal K. Epididymal cystic Lymphangioma presenting as scrotal swelling in a post surgery case of carcinoma rectum—a case report. J Clin Diagn Res. 2017;11:TD03–4.
7. Jones EW, Winkelmann RK, Zachary CB, Reda AM. Benign lymphangioendothelioma. J Am Acad Dermatol. 1990;23(2 Pt 1):229–35.
8. Guillou L, Fletcher CD. Benign lymphangioendothelioma (acquired progressive lymphangioma): a lesion not to be confused with well-differentiated angiosarcoma and patch stage Kaposi's sarcoma: clinico-pathologic analysis of a series. Am J Surg Pathol. 2000;24:1047–57.
9. Lu W, Cao Y, Zeng F, Chen C, Yang Z, Qi Z, Yang X. Surgical treatment for benign Lymphangioendothelioma after two incomplete excisions: a case report and literature review. Clin Cosmet Investig Dermatol. 2023;16:2697–719.
10. Hunt KM, Herrmann JL, Andea AA, Groysman V, Beckum K. Sirolimus-associated regression of benign lymphangioendothelioma. J Am Acad Dermatol. 2014;71(5):e221–2.
11. Schnebelen AM, Page J, Gardner JM, Shalin SC. Benign lymphangioendothelioma presenting as a giant flank mass. J Cutan Pathol. 2015;42:217–21.
12. Demiri CD, Kaselas C, Godosis D, Neofytou A, Spyridakis I. Abdominal Lymphangioma and hemangioma in a newborn. Case Rep Pediatr. 2019;2019:6879168.
13. Pupić-Bakrač J, Pupić-Bakrač A, Novaković J, Skitarelić N. Congenital neck masses. J Craniofac Surg. 2021;32:1417–20.
14. Lim HJ, Shin KS, Lee JE, You SK, Kim KH. Rare case of large Hemolymphangioma in the small bowel mesentery: a case report. J Korean Soc Radiol. 2023;84:504–11.
15. Ferreira-Santos RI, Santos KA, Scherma AP, León JE, Kaminagakura E. Unveiling an oral hemangiolymphangioma. Autops Case Rep. 2023;13:e2023435.
16. García Roa MD, Ruiz Carazo E, Moya Sánchez E, López MG. Multiple lymphangiohemangiomas with thoracic and abdominal involvement: a case report. Radiologia (Engl Ed). 2019;61:85–9.
17. Shin YS, Doo AR, Kim MK, Jeong YB, Kim HJ. Cavernous Hemangiolymphangioma of the testis without cutaneous Hemangiomatosis in an elderly patient. Korean J Urol. 2012;53:810–2.
18. Xu R, Shi TM, Liu SJ, Wang XL. Neonatal testicular hemangiolymphangioma: a case report. Arch Iran Med. 2015;18:386–8.
19. Rogel-Rodríguez JF, Gil-García JF, Velasco-García P, Romero-Espinoza F, Zaragoza-Salas T, Muñoz-Lumbreras G. Hemangiolymphangioma of the spermatic cord in a 17 year-old: a case report. Cir Cir. 2016;84:164–8.

Pathology Secondary
to Metastatic Tumours
in the Lymphatic Vessels
of the Spermatic Cord

19

19.1 Anterograde and Retrograde Carcinomatous Lymphangitis

The lymphatic vessels emerging from the testicle are grouped into two plexuses, superficial and deep. Four or five collectors arise from them and join the spermatic cord. They ascend into the spermatic cord along with the blood vessels, pass through the anterior aspect of the psoas muscle, and drain into the para-aortic and para-cava lymph nodes at the level of the renal hilum [1]. The efferent lymphatic vessels from these nodes as well as the intestinal lymphatic duct formed by collectors from the pre-aortic and intestinal trunks, converge in the cisterna chyli, which drains into the thoracic duct [2].

Most testicular tumours, apart from their ability to directly infiltrate the paratesticular structures, often spread via this lymphatic pathway (anterograde carcinomatous lymphangitis), thus reaching the para-aortic lymphatic vessels at the level of the L2 vertebra [3–6]. Metastases can be observed in the inguinal lymph nodes when the lymphatic pathway is altered, but only in less than 2% of tumours and when there is a history of previous inguinal surgery (testicular descent, herniorrhaphy, and lymphadenectomy), [7, 8]. Exceptions to these behaviours are two tumours, choriocarcinoma and yolk sac tumour, which usually spread via a haematogenous route [9, 10].

Histologically, the lesions of the lymphatic vessel wall range from minimal, such as reactive changes in the endothelial cells with prominent hyperchromatic nuclei and isolated lymphocytes in the wall, to rings of fibrous tissue with abundant inflammatory cells in cases where the tumour cells occupy the entire lumen. The first situation is more frequent in seminoma, the second in embryonal carcinoma (Figs. 19.1 and 19.2).

Retrograde lymphangitis is seen in advanced retroperitoneal tumours that have colonised or destroyed retroperitoneal lymph nodes [11] or in tumours of the colon and rectum [12, 13].

Fig. 19.1 Carcinomatous lymphangitis. Lymphatic vessel of the spermatic cord occupied by a mixture of lymphoid cells and large cells. The presence in these cells of vesicular nuclei with prominent nucleoli and a large, clear cytoplasm suggest seminoma cells. In the vessel wall, only the focal presence of some lymphoid cells stands out. The testicular tumour presented two patterns, one predominant, seminoma, and the other formed by a postpubertal teratoma

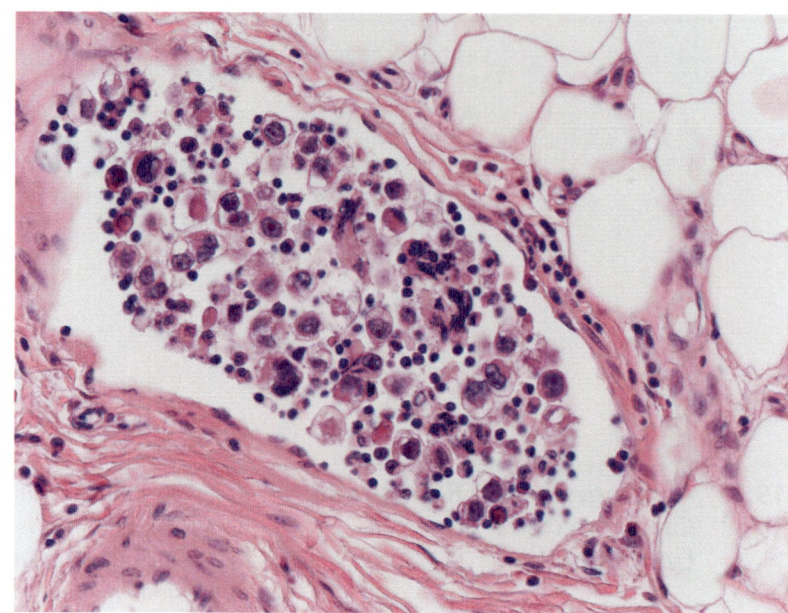

Fig. 19.2 Carcinomatous lymphangitis. Lymphatic vessel of the spermatic cord occupied by cells arranged in a solid and pseudoglandular pattern, typical characteristics of an embryonal carcinoma. The lymphatic vessel has circumferential fibrosis and lymphoid infiltrates. A second seminoma component was observed in the original tumour

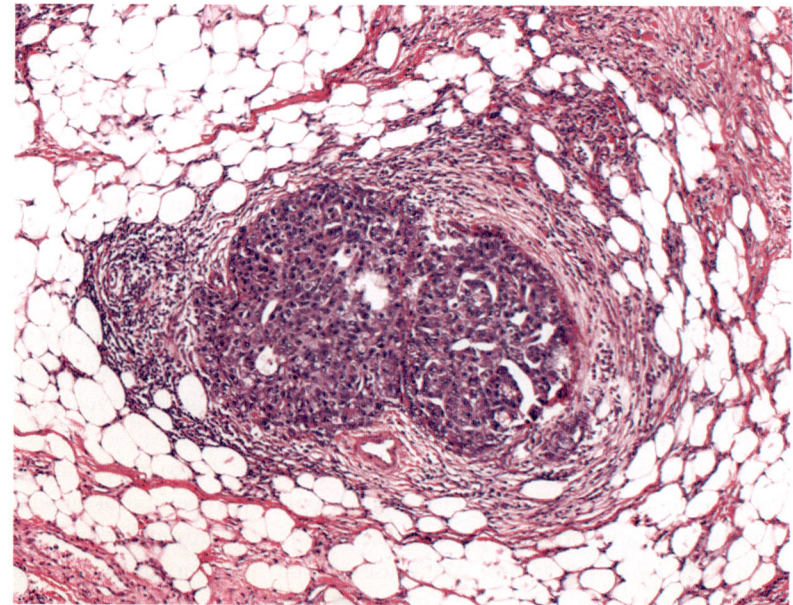

19.2 Sarcoid-like Granulomatous Lymphangitis of the Spermatic Cord Associated with Testicular Germ Cell Tumours (Intravascular Granulomas)

Sarcoid-like reactions have been described in response to both haematological and solid tumours. Lesions may be seen within a tumour, in local lymph nodes or in other nodes unrelated to the tumour. In the genitourinary tract, the sarcoid-like reactions are frequently seen within testicular tumours such as seminoma [14] and exceptionally in renal carcinoma [15]. The most frequently observed distant granulomatous lymph node involvement (in the retroperitonea and/or mediastinal region) generally occurs in seminoma. On the other hand, the association of seminoma and sarcoidosis is still under discussion [16–18].

Sarcoid-like granulomatous lymphangitis of the spermatic cord refers not only to the presence of granulomas inside the lymphatic vessels of the spermatic cord, but also in the wall of the lymphatic vessels of the spermatic cord, in patients with testicular cancer. In the cases in our series, most of the lymphatic vessels showed dilatation of the lumen. When the lymphatic vessel involvement was mural,

the infiltrate was rich in lymphocytes. In granulomas located in the lumen of the lymphatic vessel, there were clusters of epithelioid cells and some lymphocytes that were or were not associated with Langerhans-type giant cells (Figs. 19.3, 19.4, 19.5, 19.6, 19.7 and 19.8). Immunohistochemistry showed positivity for D2–40 in the endothelium of the lymphatic vessels, abundant T lymphocytes in

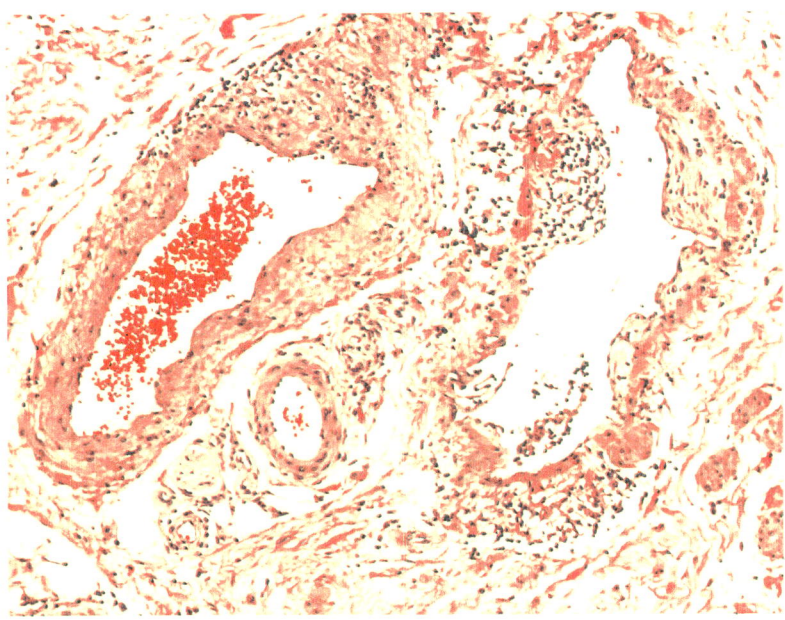

Fig. 19.3 Granulomatous lymphangitis. Cross sections of a vein and a lymphatic collector. The wall of the latter shows focal infiltrates of lymphoid cells in both the intima and the adventitia. The testicular tumour in this and the next two figures was a seminoma in a 26-year-old patient

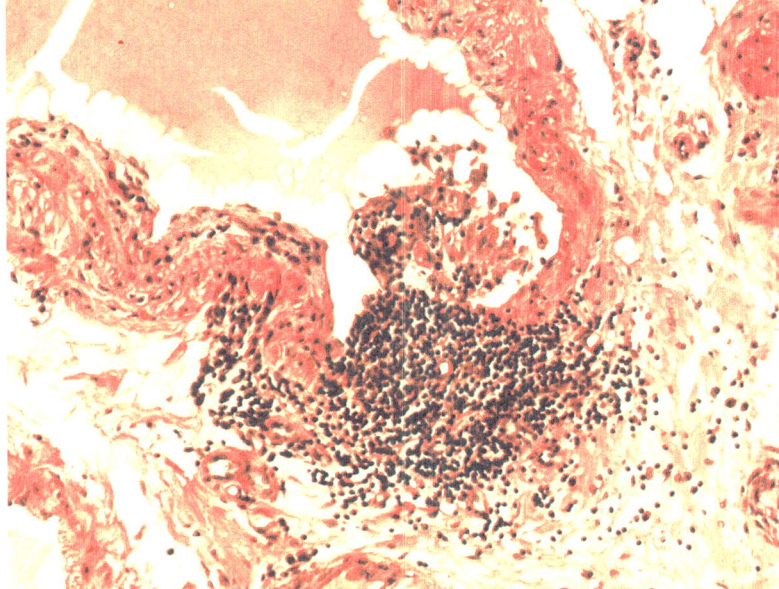

Fig. 19.4 Granulomatous lymphangitis. Wall of a lymphatic vessel focally showing a transmural infiltrate of lymphoid cells extending into the perivascular connective tissue

Fig. 19.5 Granuloma-
tous lymphangitis. In
this detail of the
previous figure the
transmural infiltrate is
rich in lymphocytes
while the inflitrate
protruding into the
vessel is preferentially
formed by epithelioid
cells

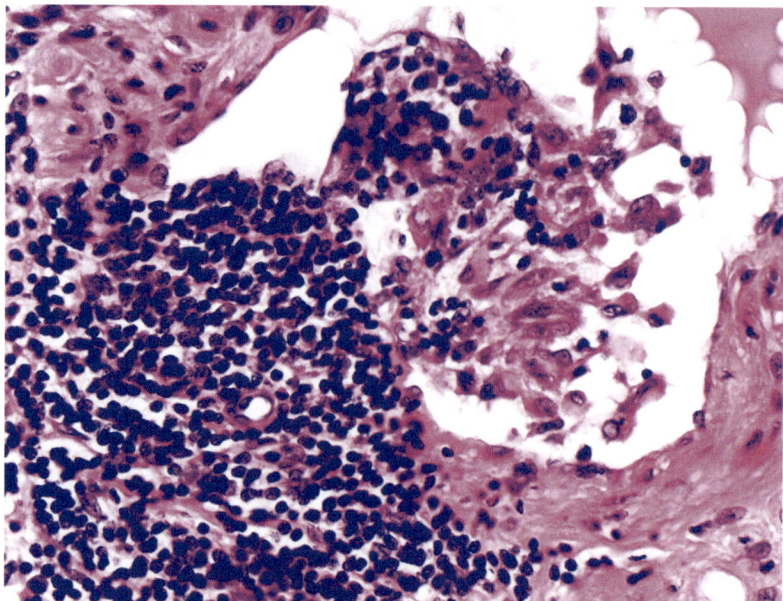

Fig. 19.6 Granuloma-
tous lymphangitis.
Longitudinal section of
a moderately-dilated
lymphatic vessel of the
spermatic cord
containing several
clusters of free lymphoid
cells in the lumen. This
figure and the next two
belong to a 27-year-old
patient with a pure
testicular seminoma

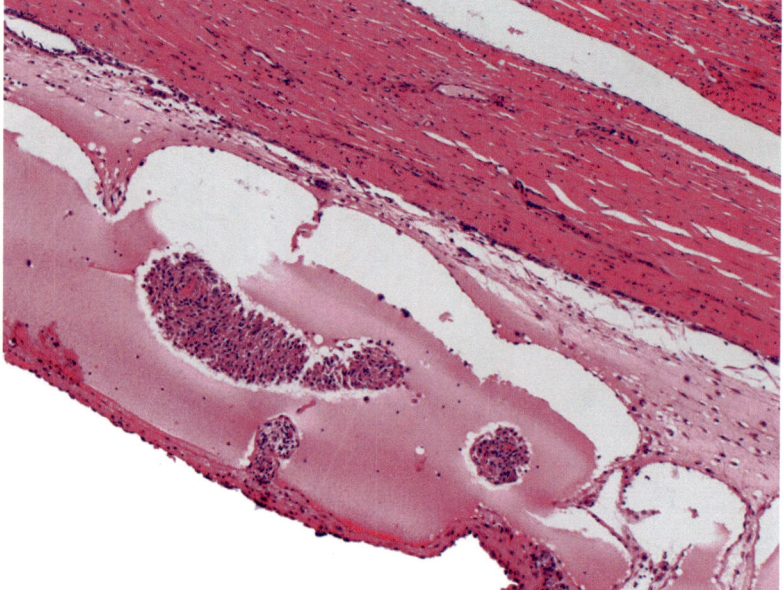

the mural lesions and numerous CD68-positive
macrophages in both mural and intravascular granulomas. No OCT3/4 positive cells were observed in
any case, ruling out the presence of tumour cells.

In all cases where this granulomatous reaction
was observed in our material, the testicular tumour
was either a pure seminoma or had a seminoma
component. It was not necessarily associated with
sarcoid-like granulomas in the tumour parenchyma.
In all cases, the disease was confined to the testis.

The presence of granulomas does not appear to be
associated with tumour progression or recurrence.

The pathogenesis of this granulomatous reaction is probably similar to the accepted explanation for granulomatous lymph node lesions,
which, in summary, consists of an antineoplastic
immune response triggered by tumour-derived
antigens causing CD4+ T lymphocyte activation
and formation of a non-caseating granuloma similar to the granuloma of sarcoidosis.

Fig. 19.7 Granuloma-
tous lymphangitis.
Detail of a conglomerate
of lymphoid cells in the
previous figure. There is
a great cellular
pleomorphism. Next to
the lymphocytes, the
epithelioid cells stand
out due to the larger size
of their nucleus and the
ample eosinophilic
cytoplasm. At one end of
the conglomerate, the
epithelioid cells are
grouped together
forming a small
granuloma. Immunos-
taining with OCT3/4
was negative

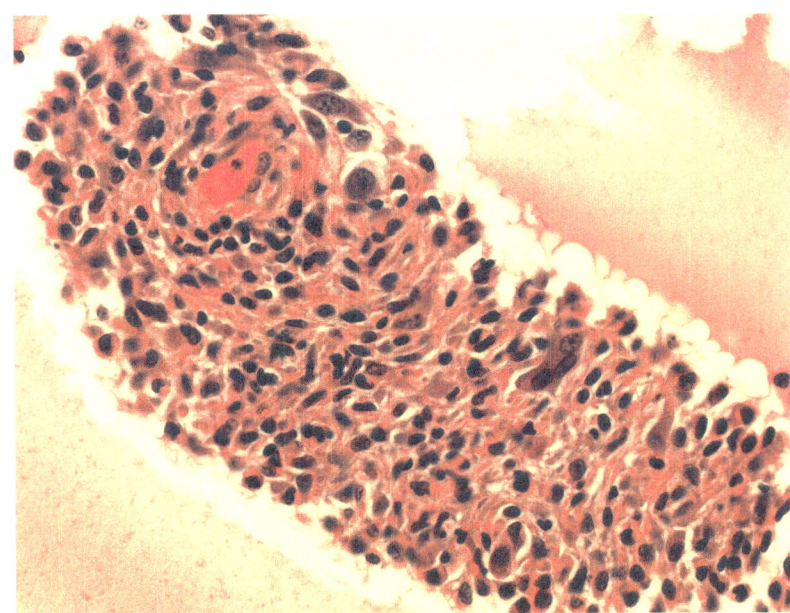

Fig. 19.8 Granuloma-
tous lymphangitis. Cross
section of several
lymphatic vessels. Inside
one of them there is a
group of epithelioid
cells accompanied by
some lymphocytes and a
giant multinucleated
Langhans-type cell

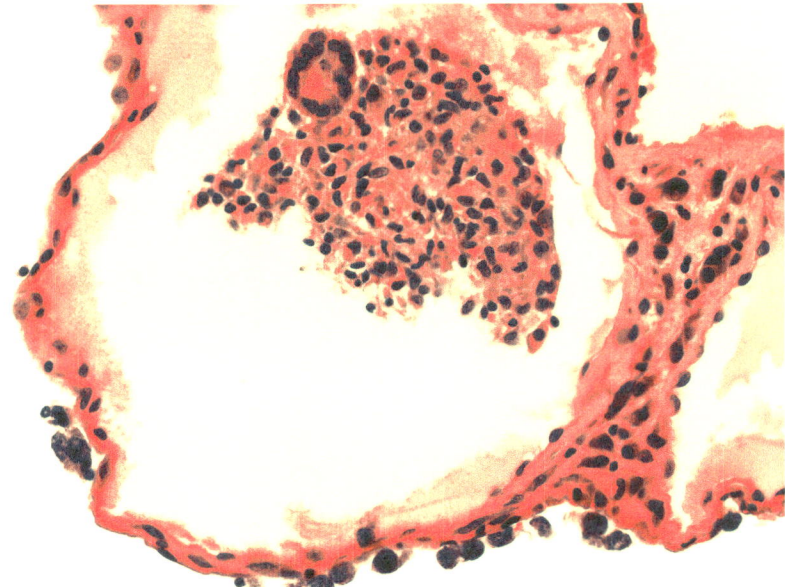

References

1. Paño B, Sebastià C, Buñesch L, Mestres J, Salvador R, Macías NG, Nicolau C. Pathways of lymphatic spread in male urogenital pelvic malignancies. Radiographics. 2011;31:135–60.
2. Jamieson JK, Dobson JF. The lymphatics of the testicle. Lancet. 1910;1:493–e495.
3. Hale GR, Teplitsky S, Truong H, Gold SA, Bloom JB, Agarwal PK. Lymph node imaging in testicular cancer. Transl Androl Urol. 2018;7:864–74.
4. O'Shea A, Kilcoyne A, Hedgire SS, Harisinghani MG. Pelvic lymph nodes and pathways of disease spread in male pelvic malignancies. Abdom Radiol (NY). 2020;45:2198–212.
5. Al-Obaidy KI, Magers MJ, Idrees MT. Testicular cancer: contemporary updates in staging. Surg Pathol Clin. 2022;15:745–57.
6. Kılınç F, Tas Ayçiçek S, Esen HH. Histopathological analysis in testicular tumors: 10 years of experience. Int J Surg Pathol. 2023;32:331.
7. Barreiro D, Blanco F, Parise ML, Caradonti M, Castro F, Lafos N. Abscessed inguinal metastasis of testicular tumor. Case report. Urol Case Rep. 2017;12:9–10.

8. Li M, Stallwood-Hall C, Cundy TP, Jay A. Inguinal node metastases in testicular cancer following previous childhood orchidopexy. ANZ J Surg. 2019;89:1674–6.

9. Shabani S, Pritchard N, Padhya TA, Mifsud M. Head and neck cutaneous metastasis of testicular choriocarcinoma. BMJ Case Rep. 2020;13(2):e233337.

10. Behera P, Ahuja A, Bhardwaj M. Pure yolk sac tumor of testis with lung metastasis in an adult patient—case report. Med Pharm Rep. 2021;94:252–5.

11. Park S, Moon SK, Lim JW. Mechanism of metastasis to the spermatic cord and testis from advanced gastric cancer: a case report. BMC Gastroenterol. 2020;20:119.

12. Hatoum HA, Abi Saad GS, Otrock ZK, Barada KA, Shamseddine AI. Metastasis of colorectal carcinoma to the testes: clinical presentation and possible pathways. Int J Clin Oncol. 2011;16:203–9.

13. Wu JM, Zhang A, Dong Y, Lin SH, Meng JC, Fang CT. Colorectal cancer with testicular metastasis: a case report and literature review. Medicine (Baltimore). 2023;102:e33214.

14. Downes MR, Cheung CC, Pintilie M, Chung P, van der Kwast TH. Assessment of intravascular granulomas in testicular seminomas and their association with tumour relapse and dissemination. J Clin Pathol. 2016;69:47–52.

15. Russell DH. Granulomata in clear cell renal cell carcinoma: an uncommon presentation of a common cancer, not two separate entities. Clin Pathol. 2020;13:2632010X20954215.

16. Kita-Milczarska K, Górska L, Kuziemski K, Sejda A, Jassem E, Biernat W. Współistnienie sarkoidozy i nasieniaka jądra—opis przypadku [Coexistence of sarcoidosis with seminoma—a case report]. Pneumonol Alergol Pol. 2013;81:145–8.

17. Liepe K. False-positive finding in FDG-PET in a patient with seminoma and sarcoidosis. Acta Clin Belg. 2015;70:138–40.

18. Bhatti P, Waight M, Bromage D, Sado D. Cardiac sarcoidosis in a patient with testicular seminoma. BMJ Case Rep. 2019;12:e229912.

GPSR Compliance

The European Union's (EU) General Product Safety Regulation (GPSR) is a set of rules that requires consumer products to be safe and our obligations to ensure this.

If you have any concerns about our products, you can contact us on ProductSafety@springernature.com

In case Publisher is established outside the EU, the EU authorized representative is:

Springer Nature Customer Service Center GmbH
Europaplatz 3
69115 Heidelberg, Germany

Batch number: 10091943

Printed by Printforce, the Netherlands